THE OPHTHALMIC LASER
HANDBOOK

The Ophthalmic Laser Handbook

Lars Freisberg, M.D.
Private Practice
Co-Founder Tulsa Retina Consultants
Co-Founder Tulsa Retina Research
Ophthalmology Board Certified in USA,
    Germany, Norway
Tulsa, Oklahoma

Nate Lighthizer, O.D., F.A.A.O.
Associate Professor of Optometry
Associate Dean
Director of Continuing Education
Chief of Specialty Care Clinics
Northeastern State University
    Oklahoma College of Optometry
Tahlequah, Oklahoma

**Leonid Skorin, Jr., D.O., O.D.,
M.S., F.A.A.O., F.A.O.C.O.**
Consultant, Department of Surgery
Community Division of Ophthalmology
Mayo Clinic Health System in Albert Lea
    and Austin
Albert Lea, Minnesota
Assistant Professor of Ophthalmology
Mayo Clinic College of Medicine
    and Science
Rochester, Minnesota

**Karl Stonecipher, M.D.,
F.A.A.O.**
Clinical Associate Professor
    of Ophthalmology
University of North Carolina
Medical Director
Laser Defined Vision
Physicians Protocol Cosmetic
Physicians Protocol Research
Greensboro, North Carolina

**Aaron B. Zimmerman, O.D.,
M.S., F.A.A.O.**
Professor of Clinical Optometry
The Ohio State University College
    of Optometry
Columbus, Ohio

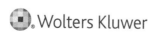. Wolters Kluwer

Philadelphia · Baltimore · New York · London
Buenos Aires · Hong Kong · Sydney · Tokyo

Acquisitions Editor: Chris Teja
Development Editor: Eric McDermott
Editorial Coordinator: Nancy Antony
Marketing Manager: Phyllis Hitner
Production Project Manager: Kirstin Johnson
Design Coordinator: Stephen Druding
Manufacturing Coordinator: Beth Welsh
Prepress Vendor: Lumina Datamatics

9 8 7 6 5 4 3

Printed in the United States of America

Library of Congress Cataloging-in-Publication Data

Names: Lighthizer, Nate, editor.
Title: The ophthalmic laser handbook / [edited by] Lars Freisberg, MD,
  Private Practice, Co-Founder Tulsa Retina Consultants, Co-Founder Tulsa
  Retina Research, Ophthalmology Board Certified in USA, Germany, Norway,
  Tulsa, Oklahoma and [four others].
Description: Philadelphia : Wolters Kluwer, [2022] | Includes
  bibliographical references and index.
Identifiers: LCCN 2021027597 | ISBN 9781975170172 (hardback) | ISBN
  9781975170202 (ebook)
Subjects: LCSH: Lasers in ophthalmology. | Eye--Laser surgery. | BISAC:
  MEDICAL / Optometry | MEDICAL / Ophthalmology
Classification: LCC RE86 .L73 2022 | DDC 617.7/190598--dc23
LC record available at https://lccn.loc.gov/2021027597

shop.lww.com

MPP1023

This book is dedicated to our trainers and trainees. Without both of you, this book would not exist.

It is also dedicated to our families. Thank you so much for your support throughout the years.

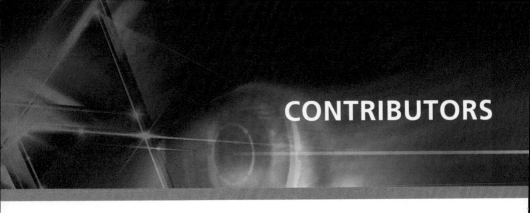

CONTRIBUTORS

John P. Berdahl, M.D.
Associate Professor
University of South Dakota
Adjunct Clinical Professor
University of Utah
Fellowship Director
Vance Thompson Vision
Sioux Falls, South Dakota

Adam R. Bleeker, M.D.
University of South Dakota Sanford School
  of Medicine
Sioux Falls, South Dakota

Stephen Brint, M.D., F.A.C.S.
Associate Clinical Professor
  of Ophthalmology
Tulane University
New Orleans, Louisiana

Richard E. Castillo, O.D., D.O., F.A.S.O.S.
Ophthalmology & Procedural Optometry
Professor
Assistant Dean for Surgical Training &
  Education
Northeastern State University Oklahoma
  College of Optometry
Tahlequah, Oklahoma

Y. Ralph Chu, M.D.
Chief Executive Officer
Chief Medical Director
Chu Vision Institute
Bloomington, Minnesota

Jason Ellen, O.D.
President – Oklahoma Medical Eye Group
Director of Residency Program –
  OMEG/NSUOCO
Adjunct Faculty
Northeastern State University Oklahoma
  College of Optometry
Tulsa, Oklahoma

Michael D. Greenwood, M.D.
Cataract, Refractive, Cornea,
  Glaucoma Surgeon
Vance Thompson Vision
West Fargo, North Dakota

D. Rex Hamilton, M.D., M.S., F.A.C.S.
Founder and Medical Director
Hamilton Eye Institute
Los Angeles, California

Jessica Heckman, O.D.
Vice President of Clinical Affairs
Optometric Residency Director
Chu Vision Institute
Bloomington, Minnesota

Alan R. Hromas, M.D.
Vitreoretinal Disease & Surgery
Tulsa Retina Consultants
Tulsa, Oklahoma

Sophia Leung, O.D., F.A.A.O.
Diplomate, American Board of Optometry
Advanced Glaucoma and Cornea Fellow
Oklahoma Medical Eye Group
Tulsa, Oklahoma
Chair, Continuing Education
Chair, Emerging Trends Committee
Council Member
Alberta Association of Optometrists
Edmonton, Alberta

Nate Lighthizer, O.D., F.A.A.O.
Associate Professor of Optometry
Associate Dean
Director of Continuing Education
Chief of Specialty Care Clinics
Northeastern State University Oklahoma
   College of Optometry
Tahlequah, Oklahoma

Jessica Mathew, O.D., Ph.D., F.A.A.O.
Medical Director—Contact Lenses and
   Refractive Surgery
Medical Affairs, North America
Alcon Vision LLC
Fort Worth, Texas

Marguerite B. McDonald, M.D., F.A.C.S.
Clinical Professor of Ophthalmology
NYU Langone Medical Center, New York
Clinical Professor of Ophthalmology
Tulane University Health Sciences Center
New Orleans, Louisiana
Private Practice
Ophthalmic Consultants of Long Island
Oceanside, New York

Selina R. McGee, O.D., F.A.A.O.
Diplomate, American Board of Optometry
Founder Bespoke Vision
Founder Precision Vision of Edmond
Adjunct Faculty
Northeastern State University Oklahoma
   College of Optometry
Edmond, Oklahoma

Jeff M. Miller, O.D., F.A.A.O.
Professor of Optometry
Glaucoma Service Chief
Assistant Dean for Academic Affairs
Northeastern State University Oklahoma
   College of Optometry
Tahlequah, Oklahoma

Myranda R. Partin, O.D.
Oklahoma Eye Surgeons, PLLC
Oklahoma City, Oklahoma

Nicholas C. Risbrudt, O.D.
Cataract, Refractive, Cornea & Glaucoma
   Surgery
Vance Thompson Vision
West Fargo, North Dakota

Steven R. Sarkisian, Jr., M.D.
Founder and CEO
Oklahoma Eye Surgeons, PLLC
Oklahoma City, Oklahoma

Justin A. Schweitzer, O.D., F.A.A.O.
Director of Optometric Externs
Adjunct Clinical Professor
Illinois College of Optometry
Vance Thompson Vision
Sioux Falls, South Dakota

James R. Singer, D.O.
Vitreoretinal Surgeon
Director of Clinical Research
Iowa Retina Consultants
West Des Moines, Iowa

I. Paul Singh, M.D., F.A.C.S.
President
The Eye Centers of Racine and Kenosha
Surgical Instructor
The Chicago Medical School
Racine, Wisconsin

Leonid Skorin, Jr., D.O., O.D., M.S., F.A.A.O., F.A.O.C.O.
Consultant, Department of Surgery
Community Division of Ophthalmology
Mayo Clinic Health System in Albert Lea
    and Austin
Albert Lea, Minnesota
Assistant Professor of Ophthalmology
Mayo Clinic College of Medicine and
    Science
Rochester, Minnesota

Karl Stonecipher, M.D., F.A.A.O.
Clinical Associate Professor of
    Ophthalmology
University of North Carolina
Medical Director
Laser Defined Vision
Physicians Protocol Cosmetic
Physicians Protocol Research
Greensboro, North Carolina

Andrew S. Whitley, O.D.
Adjunct Faculty
Northeastern State University Oklahoma
    College of Optometry
Clay-Rhynes Eye Clinic
Alliance Hospital
Durant, Oklahoma

Neal Whittle, O.D.
Associate Professor
Chief of Electrodiagnostics Clinic
Northeastern State University Oklahoma
    College of Optometry
Tahlequah, Oklahoma

Aaron B. Zimmerman, O.D., M.S., F.A.A.O.
Professor of Clinical Optometry
The Ohio State University College of
    Optometry
Columbus, Ohio

SECTION & CHAPTER EDITORS

Audrey E. Ahuero, M.D., F.A.C.S.
Ophthalmic Plastic and Reconstructive
  Surgeon
Ophthalmic Plastic Surgeons of Texas
Houston, Texas

John P. Berdahl, M.D.
Associate Professor
University of South Dakota
Adjunct Clinical Professor
University of Utah
Fellowship Director
Vance Thompson Vision
Sioux Falls, South Dakota

Richard E. Castillo, O.D., D.O., F.A.S.O.S.
Ophthalmology & Procedural Optometry
Professor
Assistant Dean for Surgical Training &
  Education
Northeastern State University Oklahoma
  College of Optometry
Tahlequah, Oklahoma

Y. Ralph Chu, M.D.
Chief Executive Officer
Chief Medical Director
Chu Vision Institute
Bloomington, Minnesota

Ralph P. Crew, D.O., F.A.O.C.O.
Clinical Professor
Department of Ophthalmology and
  Neurology
Michigan State University College
  of Osteopathic Medicine
East Lansing, Michigan
Crew Boss Eye Associates
Big Rapids, Michigan

Lars Freisberg, M.D.
Private Practice
Co-Founder Tulsa Retina Consultants
Co-Founder Tulsa Retina Research
Ophthalmology Board Certified in USA
Germany, Norway
Tulsa, Oklahoma

Michael D. Greenwood, M.D.
Cataract, Refractive, Cornea, Glaucoma
  Surgeon
Vance Thompson Vision
West Fargo, North Dakota

Alan R. Hromas, M.D.
Vitreoretinal Disease & Surgery
Tulsa Retina Consultants
Tulsa, Oklahoma

Richard F. Multack, O.D., D.O., F.O.C.O.O.,
M.B.A.
Chief Medical Officer
Advocate Southland Healthcare Network
Hazel Crest, Illinois
Professor Department of Surgery,
   Chair of Ophthalmology (retired) -
   MWU/CCOM
Downers Grove, Illinois
Founder Multack Eye Care and Associates
Olympia Fields and Frankfort, Illinois

Leonid Skorin, Jr., D.O., O.D., M.S.,
F.A.A.O., F.A.O.C.O.
Consultant, Department of Surgery
Community Division of Ophthalmology
Mayo Clinic Health System in Albert Lea
   and Austin
Albert Lea, Minnesota
Assistant Professor of Ophthalmology
Mayo Clinic College of Medicine and
   Science
Rochester, Minnesota

Karl Stonecipher, M.D., F.A.A.O.
Clinical Associate Professor of
   Ophthalmology
University of North Carolina
Medical Director
Laser Defined Vision
Physicians Protocol Cosmetic
Physicians Protocol Research
Greensboro, North Carolina

PREFACE

As clinicians, we are healers and scientists. As scientists in this modern era, we are wedded to technology. One of these ophthalmic technologies that encompasses our practices is lasers. Ophthalmic lasers have an expansive and multifunctional role in ophthalmology and optometry. They can now be applied to almost every crucial ocular structure in an elegant and efficacious manner. At the same time, this diversification of ophthalmic lasers may make it difficult for practitioners, and especially those in training, to have ready access to all the technical knowledge regarding their practical clinical applications. This is why the idea of gathering such essential laser information for the practicing clinician was conceived. Although there have been previous references published regarding one or another specific laser technique, a more comprehensive source that covers all the fundamental ocular lasers with current clinical relevance has been lacking. We hope *The Ophthalmic Laser Handbook* will fill this void.

The Ophthalmic Laser Handbook has been designed to provide concise, relevant clinical laser information arranged in a consistent easy-to-use format. Most of the chapters contain specific key indications, contraindications, preoperative considerations and procedural points. Postoperative considerations are also thoroughly addressed. This part of the chapter should be of considerable value to those who are comanaging these laser patients. One of the most distinctive assets of this laser handbook are its contributors and section editors. All have significant clinical experience in either performing the laser procedures or comanaging laser patients. Laser treatment involves a dynamic process. This is why *The Ophthalmic Laser Handbook* is both a soft cover text and companion eBook. The eBook contains all of the material found in the soft cover text with an extensive collection of laser surgical videos. As a bonus, we have included several non-laser chapters including corneal cross-linking and intense pulsed light therapy. Although these techniques rely on devices that are not lasers by definition, electromagnetic radiation is used to therapeutically manipulate tissue and these topics seamlessly fit with the overall scheme of our book.

Lars Freisberg
Nate Lighthizer
Leonid Skorin, Jr.
Karl Stonecipher
Aaron B. Zimmerman

ACKNOWLEDGEMENTS

A special acknowledgement and thank you to all of the contributors for this book. Your knowledge, expertise, and experience are truly appreciated.

A special acknowledgement and thank you to Nidek and Telscreen for providing a laser and video capability, respectively, for some of the laser procedures seen in this book.

Finally, we would like to thank the staff at Wolters Kluwer, especially Eric McDermott and Chris Teja, for their support and work on this project.

CONTENTS

Cover Editors/Authors:

Lars Freisberg, M.D.
Nate Lighthizer, O.D.
Leonid Skorin, Jr., D.O., O.D., M.S.
Karl Stonecipher, M.D.
Aaron B. Zimmerman, O.D., M.S.

Section 1 Laser History and Fundamentals 1

Section Editors: Richard E. Castillo, O.D., D.O., Richard F. Multack, O.D., D.O., M.B.A.

Section 4 Cataract and IOL   257

Section 5 Retina and Vitreous   291

Section 6 Oculoplastics   369

SECTION 1

Laser History and Fundamentals

History of Lasers

1

Aaron B. Zimmerman   •   Neal Whittle

The story of the ophthalmic laser and how light interacts with the eye begins with the ancient Greeks. Socrates postulated that looking at a solar eclipse was probably harmful to the eyes and recommended indirect viewing.[1] Unaware of the retinal anatomy and function, he observed what is now known as photoretinitis and photoretinopathy, both of which result from photochemical damage.

The narrative rejoins in the late 1800s, where Max Planck struggled to understand black body radiation and how energy was released in distinct patterns (quanta) relative to temperature. Planck determined that the light energy released from the black body was related to its frequency multiplied by an unknown constant, which he calculated. This theorem was later validated by Einstein in 1905[2] and the constant would become universally known as Planck's constant. Then in 1917, based on the quantum theory of energy, Einstein published an article predicting stimulated emission, the lasing mechanism's fundamental property.

Thirty years later, the German ophthalmologist Meyer-Schwickerath began experimenting with a carbon arc to create thermal lesions on rabbit retinas.[3] The carbon arc did not perform as effectively on human eyes, so he created an instrument that condensed sunlight from his clinic's roof. It was effective but frequently changing weather conditions made the instrument unreliable. In 1951, he presented on using the Beck arc successfully to create thermal retinal lesions on hundreds of patients. Through the use of various light sources, Meyer-Schwickerath was the first to implement photocoagulation on human retinas.[4]

Prior to the laser's development, in 1953, a microwave amplification by stimulated emission of radiation device, the microwave amplification by stimulated emission of radiation (MASER), was invented. This validated the concept of stimulated emission as predicted by Albert Einstein back in 1917. The proof that stimulated emission could work for microwaves emboldened researchers to develop a device that would emit visible light. In 1957, Gordon Gould conceptualized and named the light amplification by stimulated emission of radiation (LASER) device and further described the major components, basic construction, and how it would work.[5] However, Theodore Maiman, who was working in the laboratories of the Hughes Aircraft Company, is often credited with developing the first working LASER device in May of 1960.[6] This particular device was named the ruby laser (Fig. 1.1) and emitted a wavelength of 694.3 nm. Though he did not

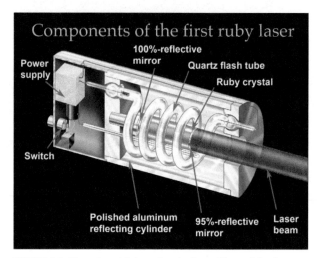

FIGURE 1-1 Theodore Maiman's ruby laser. The solid ruby crystal is stimulated by the flashbulb that is coiled around it. Source: United States Department of Energy. Campbell EM. Laser programs, the first 25 years, 1972–1997. United States: n.p., 1998. Web. doi:10.2172/16710. Available at: https://www.osti.gov/servlets/purl/16710

develop the first functioning laser, Gould had attempted to patent the laser concept and was eventually awarded multiple patents after decades of legal challenges.

Later in 1960, the helium–neon laser was invented by Ali Javan,[7] and in 1962, quotient switching (Q-switching) technology was available, which allowed lasers to produce extremely large pulses of energy.[8] Lasers were quickly being adopted for uses such as range finders, excitation mechanisms for other lasers, and for ophthalmic purposes. The application of using the laser on rabbit retinal tissue was reported by Zaret et al.[9] in 1961 and Kapany in 1963.[10] Documented use of the ruby laser on human retinal tissue was reported by Flocks and Zweng in 1964[11] and by L'esperance in 1966.[12] The rapid expansion of laser applications increased the likelihood of an adverse event, and in 1964 the first documented laser eye injury occurred in a research lab. The first documented laser eye injury occurred in a research lab in 1964.[13]

As use of the ruby laser for retinal procedures was explored, Palanker et al. described that the red wave length was not well absorbed by blood—which limited its efficacy, and the laser was very intense resulting in strong chorioretinal adhesions.[14] Fortunately, in 1964 the argon laser was invented and this would eventually replace the ruby laser as it was much more effective for retinal procedures. The year of 1964 also saw the invention of the carbon dioxide laser and another prominent ophthalmic laser, the neodymium yttrium aluminum garnet (Nd:YAG) laser. The xenon excimer laser was developed in 1970, the Q-switched Nd:YAG in 1977, and the femtosecond in 1990. Each ophthalmic laser, their applications, and major associated milestones will be further discussed in the following section.

ARGON LASER

In 1964, William Bridges developed the argon laser, which, rather than relying on a crystal as the ruby laser did, relied on argon gas as the lasing medium.[15] The argon laser can produce two wavelengths: one is 488 nm and the other a 514-nm band. Due to the emitted beams' blue and green color, this energy could be more effectively absorbed by the retina, which led to its immediate adoption for retinal surgical applications. Numerous publications were produced in the late 1960s and early 1970s, describing the merits of argon laser retinal surgery. Since 1970, the use of continuous wave lasers, such as the argon laser, has been widely accepted for treating retinal vascular conditions.[14]

In the late 1960s and into the 1970s, individuals began exploring how lasers could be applied to anterior segment structures such as the iris and anterior chamber angle. In 1967, Snyder used the ruby laser to study laser peripheral iridotomy on rabbit irises. He determined that the laser parameters available at that time would allow for either successful iridotomy with associated retinal damage, or minimal retinal damage but with a lower successful iridotomy rate. Beckman and Sugar performed further investigation in 1973, by comparing how effective the ruby, Nd:YAG, and argon lasers were for producing a laser iridectomy.[16] While their results suggested that the ruby was superior to the other two, Khuri successfully created laser peripheral iridotomy (LPI) in rabbit irises through the use of the argon laser.[17] Then in 1975 Abraham and Miller further described successful LPI procedures through the use of the argon laser.[18]

Primitive laser-induced procedures to the trabecular meshwork were first attempted in Russia by Krasnov, where he used a Q-switched ruby laser to "puncture" the trabecular meshwork.[19] In the United States, Worthen and Wickham performed trabeculotomy on monkeys using the continuous-wave argon laser.[20] In 1979, using a very similar procedure to modern-day argon laser trabeculoplasty (ALT), Wise and Witter successfully demonstrated on 41 eyes that argon laser modifications to the angle could reduce intraocular pressure (IOP) for at least three months.[21] In 1981, Wise published an article explaining that the argon trabeculoplasty effects lasted for much longer than three months.[22] Further refinements of ALT were proposed by Schwartz & Spaeth, which included reducing the extent of treatment from 360° to 180°.[23] As adoption of the technique increased, the National Eye Institute funded the Glaucoma Laser Trial (GLT). The initial report from the GLT was published in 1989 and discussed the acute effects of ALT.[24] Multiple publications between 1989 to1995 were produced by this group. The overall conclusion was that initial treatment with ALT was as efficacious as topical medication.

Early attempts at separating the iris root from the angle, modern-day argon laser peripheral iridoplasty, was recorded in 1977.[25] The initial technique was performed using a Q-switched laser and with iris-penetrating lesions for 90° of the angle. In 1979, Kimbrough et al. described the argon laser being applied to the peripheral iris to "shrink" the stroma, resulting in less occlusion of the trabecular meshwork.[26] The procedure was further perfected by Ritch in 1982.[27]

Today, the argon laser is becoming increasingly more difficult to find. With the development of the frequency-doubled Nd:YAG and other diode lasers, it is no longer necessary to use the relatively large argon laser. Though the argon laser is slowly going extinct, the names of surgical procedures such as argon laser peripheral iridoplasty, ALT, and argon peripheral iridotomy persist.

NEODYMIUM: YTTRIUM ALUMINUM GARNET

The Nd:YAG laser, invented by Geusic, Marcos, and Van Uitert in 1964 while working at Bell Labs,[28] uses a synthetic crystal as the laser medium. The Nd:YAG laser, when first developed, was a continuous-wave laser emitting a 1064-nm infrared beam. Today, the Q-switched Nd:YAG is an extremely common ophthalmic laser as it is routinely used for posterior capsulotomies and laser peripheral iridotomies. Although Q-switching was discovered in 1962 by McClung and Hellwarth[8] and the Nd:YAG was discovered in 1964, the ophthalmic utility of the Q-switched Nd:YAG was not realized until the late 1970s.

As described by Gloor, Fankhauser and Aron-Rosa were independently experimenting with pulsed lasers in the late 1970s.[29] In 1977, Van der Zypen and Fankhauser evaluated Q-switched Nd:YAG procedures on animals[30] while Aron-Rosa was investigating a mode-locked version.[29] Aron-Rosa published the first manuscript on Q-switched Nd:YAG applications in 1980,[31] followed by Fankhauser, Roussel, and Steffen.[32]

The Nd:YAG laser was available in the American market[33] in 1982 and quickly became the laser of choice for laser iridotomy,[34] but its primary application was for posterior capsule opacification (PCO). The laser allowed for effective disruption of any posterior capsule opacities without entering the eye with instruments, which reduced the risk of endophthalmitis.[35] The instant improvement in visual acuity demonstrated by Aron-Rosa[31] in 1980 and Terry et al.[36] occurred in over 90% of each of their studies with a relatively non-invasive and fast procedure laid the foundation for this laser to become a primary workhorse for PCO and LPI. Today, the Q-switched Nd:YAG is heavily used and is being investigated for vitreolysis, with a recent study demonstrating favorable outcomes.[37]

The frequency-doubled Q-switched Nd:YAG uses an auxiliary crystal of potassium-titanyl-phosphate (KTP) in the resonance cavity to halve the 1064-nm wavelength, or double the frequency, of the Nd:YAG, which results in a 532-nm visible green beam. The frequency-doubled Nd:YAG was first reported by Alex Jalkh et al. out of Boston in 1988.[38] The initial version of the frequency-doubled Nd:YAG was a continuous wave laser with the pulsed Q-switched version being introduced in the 1990s.

In 1995, Mark Latina and Carl Park described a new procedure using a frequency-doubled Q-switched Nd:YAG (532 nm) laser to target the trabecular meshwork's pigmented cells selectively.[39] The term they gave the procedure was *selective laser trabeculoplasty (SLT)*. The Q-switched mechanism allowed for a pulse with a duration of a few nanoseconds, which is less than the thermal relaxation time of melanosomes. This minimizes heat transfer to adjacent tissues, specifically the trabecular meshwork. Their first clinical study was published in 1998, where they demonstrated a 23.5% reduction in IOP for 6 months in patients with open-angle glaucoma.[40] In 2001, the U.S. Food and Drug Administration (FDA) approved SLT; it became the preferred method of laser trabeculoplasty as compared to ALT.[41] Recently, the Laser in Glaucoma and Ocular Hypertension Trial Study Group (LiGHT) was developed to investigate SLT as initial treatment for primary open angle glaucoma or ocular hypertension. At 36 months, 75% of 355 subjects remained free of therapeutic drops, and the mean reduction in IOP was 31.4%.[42] It was estimated that there was a 97% chance that SLT was more cost-effective than eye drops.[43]

EXCIMER

The 1980s saw the rise of the excimer laser in corneal refractive surgery. However, the excimer laser story begins in 1970 in Moscow, Russia, where a xenon dimer was used to create a 172-nm ultraviolet wavelength beam.[44] The argon fluoride (ArF) laser was invented in 1976,[45] but the ophthalmic applications of the excimer were not realized until 1980 by Rangaswamy Srinivasin, James Wynne, and Samuel Blum while working at International Business Machines (IBM). They discovered a high level of precision for organic tissues, specifically on turkey bones and cartilage following a Thanksgiving dinner.[46] It was discovered that the excimer made extremely precise cuts with minimal to no damage to the surrounding tissue.

Dr. Stephen Trokel was becoming aware of IBM's excimer laser work and, in 1983, visited with Srinivasin.[47] By the end of that year, Trokel and Srinivasin, along with Bodil Braren, published a manuscript on the photo-ablative tissue interaction of the excimer on cow eyes.[48] They proved that the laser could remove corneal tissue with minimal adjacent collateral damage and at a very precise depth. They concluded that 1 J/cm^2 fluence ablates 1 μm of tissue. Later research by Krueger and Trokel determined that the 193-nm wavelength was the optimal wavelength for the cornea.[49]

In the mid-1980s, Charles Munnerlyn derived an equation that approximated tissue depth that needed to be removed per diopter of refractive error.[50] Munnerlyn, Trokel, and McDonald began collaborating in 1985 by investigating how the excimer laser affected animal and cadaver corneas. They determined minimal corneal haze or scarring following excimer laser application and that the ablated zone would successfully re-epithelialize. An interesting anecdote was that the excimer was located in a trailer next to a large trash compactor. When the trash compactor would run, it would vibrate the trailer. It had turned out that the surgical outcomes were better when the trash compactor would run as it blended the treatment zone more effectively.[51] Another group, David Muller and John Marshall, collaborated on developing an ophthalmic excimer laser which would become Summit Technologies.[52]

Nidek and Meditec were also developing commercial excimer lasers, but their initial application was designated for radial keratotomy.[47] The VISX laser was the first broad-beamed laser and was used by McDonald in 1988 to perform the first photorefractive keratectomy (PRK) procedure on a to-be-enucleated eye and then later on an eye with optic nerve disease.[53,54] Following several trials on diseased eyes, the phased trials seeking FDA approval for PRK began in 1989. Though separated by a few months in late 1995, Summit Technologies received FDA approval for PRK, and then in early 1996, VISX also received approval.

Laser *in situ* keratomileusis (LASIK) was conceptualized, but not named, by Gholam Peyman in 1985 and filed for a U.S. patent in 1989 (U.S. patent 4,840,175. June 20, 1989).[55] In Peyman's original description, a 200-μm section of epithelium and anterior stroma (cap) would be removed, followed by excimer ablation of the stromal bed, and then suturing of the cap back in place. Peyman was influenced by the work of the Columbian ophthalmologist, Jose Barraquer—who had also created a cap, but had used a cryolathe to alter the stromal shape of the cap, and then had sutured it back in place.[56] Peyman's description with the free cap proved to be rather difficult,[47] and in 1988 in Greece, Pallikaris introduced a technique where an epithelial and anterior stromal flap was created with a microkeratome, followed by excimer laser stromal ablation. Pallikaris named the procedure LASIK.[57] It was first performed in the United States in 1993 by Stephen Slade.[58]

According to the FDA's list of approved lasers, in 1998, the Kremer Excimer Laser System was the first laser approved for LASIK.[59] The SVX Apex Plus (Summit Technologies) laser was approved in 1999. Realizing LASIK's huge potential, Nestle-Alcon purchased Summit Technologies for 893 million dollars in May 2000.[60] Advances in excimer laser systems, and their accompanying software, continued to be developed. The number of LASIK procedures performed annually since 1999 in the United States range between 600,000 and 1.4 million, though over the last decade, it is between 600,000 and 700,000 per year.[61]

FEMTOSECOND

The first ophthalmic femtosecond laser was invented by Tibor Juhasz and Ronald Kurtz in the early 1990s at the University of Michigan.[62] According to Kurtz, he met Juhasz at a conference in 1994, and they began testing the laser on several tissues.[63] They were attempting to create a laser microkeratome that they successfully demonstrated using animal models in 1996 to 1997. Following those successful trials, a venture capitalist firm from Michigan backed further development of the ophthalmic femtosecond laser, and in 1997, the Intralase Corporation was established.[62] The Intralase 600c received FDA clearance in December 1999 and became commercially available in 2001 for LASIK flaps.[64]

The femtosecond laser's wavelength allows it to pass through the corneal tissue, and applying the laser for cataract extraction was first performed by Zoltan Nagy in 2008 using the LenSx system.[65] In the following year, 2009, the LenSx 550 was cleared by the FDA in August to assist with cataract extraction.[66] Another application of the femtosecond laser is small incision lenticule extraction or SMILE. This procedure was first performed in 2011 and later received FDA approval in 2016.[67–69] The femtosecond laser is also used for penetrating keratoplasty, which initially occurred in 2005, to create tunnels for implantable corneal ring segments, anterior lamellar keratoplasty, and Descemet stripping with automated endothelial keratoplasty.[62]

MICROPULSE AND DIODE LASERS

Micropulse lasing was first described in 1997 by Thomas Friberg, who later developed Iridex.[70] The OcuLight SL/SLx, an 810-nm continuous-wave diode laser, received FDA clearance in May 2003.[71] Micropulse lasers operate in a continuous-wave mode, but rather than continuously delivering laser energy for a set period of time (generally 100–500 ms), the energy is delivered in a series of micropulses. The tissue is essentially exposed to laser energy for 100–300 μs, followed by an off time of at least 2 ms. The process repeats itself several times for the duration of the 100–500 ms of exposure. The micropulse laser exposure seems to provide a therapeutic benefit to the target tissue without creating permanent damage to the tissue. Micropulse lasers have retinal and glaucoma applications.

The micropulse lasers are a type of diode laser. The diode laser was invented by Robert N. Hall in 1962 while working at General Electric.[72] Rather than using gas, liquid, or a solid crystal as the medium, the diode laser is technically a semiconductor where an electrical current passes through a p–n junction and stimulated emission can occur. If the junction has mirrors capping each end of the resonance cavity, then amplification can result in a laser beam. Diode lasers are small and relatively inexpensive and therefore are prevalent. Common examples of diode lasers are the typical laser pointer or the laser in a DVD player.

In ophthalmology, diode lasers often serve as the alignment beams for common lasers such as the Nd:YAG or frequency-doubled Nd:YAG. In addition to micropulse applications, diode lasers are used for endoscopic cyclophotocoagulation in refractory glaucoma cases, which was first described by Martin Uram in 1992.[73]

Ophthalmic lasers can therapeutically modify all ocular tissues and often allow for significantly less invasive procedures with better outcomes than manual surgery. Following their invention in 1960, lasers took less than one year to be applied for ophthalmic purposes. Continuous advances in ophthalmic laser applications have been made in the last 60 years, and relentless refinement in techniques and innovations in laser technology will only continue to improve surgical structural and functional outcomes in the future.

REFERENCES

1. Michaelides M, Rajendram R, Marshall J, et al. Eclipse retinopathy. *Eye*. 2001;15:148–151.
2. Einstein A. About a heuristic point of view concerning the generation and transformation of light. *Annalen der Physik*. 1905;322(6):132–148.

3. Meyer-Schwickerath G. Optische Pupillenbildung durch Lichtkoagulation. *Ber dtsch Ophtalm Ges.* 1952;57:144–146.
4. Meyer-Schwickerath GR. The history of photocoagulation. *Aust N Z J Ophthalmol.* 1989;17:427–434.
5. Gould RG. The LASER, light amplification by stimulated emission of radiation. In: Franken PA, Sands RH, eds. *The Ann Arbor Conference on Optical Pumping: The University of Michigan, June 15 through June 18, 1959.* Ann Arbor, MI;1959:128.
6. Maiman TH. Stimulated optical radiation in Ruby. *Nature.* 1960;187:493–494.
7. Javan A, Herriott DR, Bennett WR. Population inversion and continuous optical maser oscillation in a gas discharge containing a He-Ne mixture. *Phys Rev Lett.* 1961;6:106–110.
8. Mcclung FJ, Hellwarth RW. Giant optical pulsations from Ruby. *J Appl Phys.* 1962;33:828–829.
9. Zaret MM, Breinin GM, Siegel IM, et al. Ocular lesions produced by an optical maser (Laser). *Science.* 1961;134:1525–1526.
10. Kapany NS, Peppers NA, Zweng HC, et al. Retinal photocoagulation by lasers. *Nature.* 1963;199:146–149.
11. Flocks M, Zweng HC. Laser coagulation of ocular tissues. *Arch Ophthalmol.* 1964;72:604–611.
12. L'Esperance FA, Jr. Clinical comparison of xenon-arc and laser photocoagulation of retinal lesions. *Arch Ophthalmol.* 1966;75:61–67.
13. Rathkey AS. Accidental laser burn of the Macula. *Arch Ophthalmol.* 1965;74:346–348.
14. Palanker DV, Blumenkranz MS, Marmor MF. Fifty years of ophthalmic laser therapy. *Arch Ophthalmol.* 2011;129:1613–1619.
15. Bridges WB. Laser oscillation in singly ionized argon in visible spectrum (Method – Pulsed D-C discharge transitions – 4p to 4s, 4p to 3d E). *Appl Phys Lett.* 1964;4:128–130.
16. Beckman H, Sugar HS. Laser iridectomy therapy of glaucoma. *Arch Ophthalmol.* 1973;90:453–455.
17. Khuri CH. Argon laser iridectomies. *Am J Ophthalmol.* 1973;76:490–493.
18. Abraham RK, Miller GL. Outpatient argon laser iridectomy for angle closure glaucoma: A two-year study. *Trans Sect Ophthalmol Am Acad Ophthalmol Otolaryngol.* 1975;79:OP529–OP537.
19. Krasnov MM. Laseropuncture of anterior chamber angle in glaucoma. *Am J Ophthalmol.* 1973;75:674–678.
20. Worthen DM, Wickham MG. Laser trabeculotomy in monkeys. *Invest Ophthalmol.* 1973;12:707–711.
21. Wise JB, Witter SL. Argon laser therapy for open-angle glaucoma: A pilot study. *Arch Ophthalmol.* 1979;97:319–322.
22. Wise J. BJB. Long-term control of adult open angle glaucoma by argon laser treatment. *Ophthalmology.* 1981;88:197–202.
23. Schwartz LW, Spaeth GL, Traverso C, et al. Variation of techniques on the results of argon laser trabeculoplasty. *Ophthalmology.* 1983;90:781–784.
24. The Glaucoma Laser Trial. I. Acute effects of argon laser trabeculoplasty on intraocular pressure: Glaucoma laser trial research group. *Arch Ophthalmol.* 1989;107:1135–1142.
25. Krasnov MM. Q-switched laser iridectomy and Q-switched laser goniopuncture. *Adv Ophthalmol.* 1977;34:192.
26. Kimbrough RL, Trempe CS, Brockhurst RJ, et al. Angle-closure glaucoma in nanophthalmos. *Am J Ophthalmol.* 1979;88:572–579.
27. Ritch R. Argon laser treatment for medically unresponsive attacks of angle-closure glaucoma. *Am J Ophthalmol.* 1982;94:197–204.
28. Geusic JE, Marcos HM, Vanuitert LG. Laser oscillations in Nd-doped Yttrium Aluminum Yttrium Gallium + Gadolinium Garnets (Continuous operation of Y3a15o12 pulsed operation of Y3ga5o15 + Gd3ga5o12 Rm Temp E). *Appl Phys Lett.* 1964;4:182–184.
29. Gloor BP. Franz Fankhauser: The father of the automated perimeter. *Surv Ophthalmol.* 2009;54:417–425.
30. Van der Zypen E, Fankhauser F. Wirkung des Neodymium (YAG)-Laser auf die Morphologie der pigmentierten Kanincheniris. *Acta Anat.* 1977;99:327.
31. Aron-Rosa D, Aron JJ, Griesemann M, et al. Use of the neodymium-YAG laser to open the posterior capsule after lens implant surgery: A preliminary report. *J Am Intraocul Implant Soc.* 1980;6:352–354.

32. Fankhauser F, Roussel P, Steffen J, et al. Clinical studies on the efficiency of high power laser radiation upon some structures of the anterior segment of the eye: First experiences of the treatment of some pathological conditions of the anterior segment of the human eye by means of a Q-switched laser system. *Int Ophthalmol.* 1981;3:129–139.

33. Katzen LE, Fleischman JA, Trokel SL. The YAG laser: An American experience. *J Am Intraocul Implant Soc.* 1983;9:151–156.

34. Drake MV. Neodymium:YAG laser iridotomy. *Surv Ophthalmol.* 1987;32:171–177.

35. Shah GR, Gills JP, Durham DG, et al. Three thousand YAG lasers in posterior capsulotomies: An analysis of complications and comparison to polishing and surgical discission. *Ophthalmic Surg.* 1986;17:473–477.

36. Terry AC, Stark WJ, Maumenee AE, et al. Neodymium-YAG laser for posterior capsulotomy. *Am J Ophthalmol.* 1983;96:716–720.

37. Shah CP, Heier JS. YAG laser vitreolysis vs. Sham YAG vitreolysis for symptomatic vitreous floaters: A randomized clinical trial. *JAMA Ophthalmol.* 2017;135:918–923.

38. Jalkh AE, Pflibsen K, Pomerantzeff O, et al. A new solid-state, frequency-doubled neodymium-YAG photocoagulation system. *Arch Ophthalmol.* 1988;106:847–849.

39. Latina MA, Park C. Selective targeting of trabecular meshwork cells: In vitro studies of pulsed and CW laser interactions. *Exp Eye Res.* 1995;60:359–371.

40. Latina MA, Sibayan SA, Shin DH, et al. Q-switched 532-nm Nd:YAG laser trabeculoplasty (selective laser trabeculoplasty): A multicenter, pilot, clinical study. *Ophthalmology.* 1998;105:2082–2088; discussion 9-90.

41. Garg A, Gazzard G. Selective laser trabeculoplasty: Past, present, and future. *Eye.* 2018;32:863–876.

42. Garg A, Vickerstaff V, Nathwani N, et al. Primary selective laser trabeculoplasty for open-angle glaucoma and ocular hypertension: Clinical outcomes, predictors of success, and safety from the laser in glaucoma and ocular hypertension trial. *Ophthalmology.* 2019;126:1238–1248.

43. Gazzard G, Konstantakopoulou E, Garway-Heath D, et al. Selective laser trabeculoplasty versus eye drops for first-line treatment of ocular hypertension and glaucoma (LiGHT): A multicentre randomised controlled trial. *Lancet.* 2019;393:1505–1516.

44. Basov NG, Danilychev VA, Popov Y, Khodkevich DD. Zh. Eksp. Fiz. i Tekh. Pis'ma. Red 1970;12:473.

45. Hoffman. High power UV noble-gas-halide lasers. *Appl Phys Lett.* 1976;28:538.

46. IBM 100 – Icons of Progress. Excimer Laser Surgery. 2011. Available at: https://www.ibm.com/ibm/history/ibm100/us/en/icons/excimer/. Accessed September 1, 2020.

47. Krueger RR, Rabinowitz YS, Binder PS. The 25th anniversary of excimer lasers in refractive surgery: Historical review. *J Refract Surg.* 2010;26:749–760.

48. Trokel SL, Srinivasan R, Braren B. Excimer laser surgery of the cornea. *Am J Ophthalmol.* 1983;96:710–715.

49. Krueger RR, Trokel SL, Schubert HD. Interaction of ultraviolet laser light with the cornea. *Invest Ophthalmol Vis Sci.* 1985;26:1455–1464.

50. Munnerlyn CR, Koons SJ, Marshall J. Photorefractive keratectomy: A technique for laser refractive surgery. *J Cataract Refract Surg.* 1988;14:46–52.

51. McDonald M. From a trash compactor to SMILE: 30 years of laser vision correction. 2018. Available at: https://www.healio.com/news/ophthalmology/20181027/from-a-trash-compactor-to-smile-30-years-of-laser-vision-correction.

52. U.S. Food and Drug Administration, Center for Devices and Radiologic Health. ExciMed UV200LA PMA P910067 approval letter March 10, 1995. Retrieved September 1, 2020, from https://www.accessdata.fda.gov/cdrh_docs/pdf/P910067.pdf.

53. McDonald MB, Frantz JM, Klyce SD, et al. Central photorefractive keratectomy for myopia: The blind eye study. *Arch Ophthalmol.* 1990;108:799–808.

54. McDonald MB, Frantz JM, Klyce SD, et al. One-year refractive results of central photorefractive keratectomy for myopia in the nonhuman primate cornea. *Arch Ophthalmol.* 1990;108:40–47.

55. Peyman GA, inventor. Method for modifying corneal curvature. US patent 4,840,175. June 20, 1989. Available at: http://patft.uspto.gov/netacgi/nph-Parser?Sect1=PTO1&Sect2=HITOFF&d=PALL&p=

1&u=%2Fnetahtml%2FPTO%2Fsrchnum.htm&r=1&f=G&l=50&s1=4,840,175.PN.&OS=PN/4, 840,175&RS=PN/4,840,175. Last accessed September 1, 2020.

56. Barraquer JI. Keratomileusis. *Int Surg.* 1967;48:103–117.

57. Pallikaris IG, Papatzanaki ME, Siganos DS, et al. A corneal flap technique for laser in situ keratomileusis: Human studies. *Arch Ophthalmol.* 1991;109:1699–1702.

58. Brint SF, Ostrick DM, Fisher C, et al. Six-month results of the multicenter phase I study of excimer laser myopic keratomileusis. *J Cataract Refract Surg.* 1994;20:610–615.

59. U.S. Food and Drug Administration, Center for Devices and Radiologic Health. Kremer Excimer Laser System PMA P970005 approval letter July 30, 1998. Retrieved September 1, 2020, from https:// www.accessdata.fda.gov/cdrh_docs/pdf/P970005A.pdf.

60. WSJ.com News Roundup May 26, 2000. Nestle'sNestle's Alcon Laboratories to acquire Summit Technologies for $893 million. *The Wall Street Journal* Retrieved from https://www.wsj.com/articles/ SB959361504770500607. Last Accessed September 1, 2020.

61. Helzner J. Can you revive your refractive surgery practice. *Ophthalmology Management.* September 1, 2010. Retrieved from https://www.ophthalmologymanagement.com/issues/2010/september-2010/ can-you-revive-your-refractive-surgery-practice. Last accessed September 1, 2020.

62. Soong HK, Malta JB. Femtosecond lasers in ophthalmology. *Am J Ophthalmol.* 2009;147:189–197 e2.

63. Kurtz R. How developers of the femtosecond ophthalmic surgical laser took a chance and built a company. *Cataract & Refractive Surgery Today.* May 2002. Retrieved from https://crstoday.com/ articles/2002-may/0502_041-html/. Last accessed September 1, 2020.

64. U.S. Food and Drug Administration, Center for Devices and Radiologic Health. Intralase 600C K993153 approval letter December 17, 1999. Retrieved September 1, 2020, from https://www.access-data.fda.gov/cdrh_docs/pdf/K993153.pdf.

65. Nagy ZZ, McAlinden C. Femtosecond laser cataract surgery. *Eye Vis.* 2015;2:11.

66. U.S. Food and Drug Administration, Center for Devices and Radiologic Health. LenSx 550 Laser System K082974 approval letter August 14, 2009. Retrieved September 1, 2020, from https://www. accessdata.fda.gov/cdrh_docs/pdf8/K082947.pdf.

67. Sekundo W, Kunert KS, Blum M. Small incision corneal refractive surgery using the small incision lenticule extraction (SMILE) procedure for the correction of myopia and myopic astigmatism: results of a 6 month prospective study. *Br J Ophthalmol.* 2011;95:335–339.

68. Shah R, Shah S, Sengupta S. Results of small incision lenticule extraction: All-in-one femtosecond laser refractive surgery. *J Cataract Refract Surg.* 2011;37:127–137.

69. U.S. Food and Drug Administration, Center for Devices and Radiologic Health. VisuMax Femtosecond Laser PMA P150040 approval letter September 13, 2016. Retrieved September 1, 2020, from https://www.accessdata.fda.gov/cdrh_docs/pdf15/P150040B.pdf.

70. Friberg TR, Karatza EC. The treatment of macular disease using a micropulsed and continuous wave 810-nm diode laser. *Ophthalmology.* 1997;104:2030–2038.

71. U.S. Food and Drug Administration, Center for Devices and Radiologic Health. IRIS Medical Ocu-Light SL/SLx K020374 approval letter May 3, 2002. Retrieved September 1, 2020, from https://www. accessdata.fda.gov/cdrh_docs/pdf2/K020374.pdf.

72. Hall R. Coherent light emission from GaAs junctions. *Phys Rev Lett.* 1962;9:366–369.

73. Uram M. Ophthalmic laser microendoscope ciliary process ablation in the management of neovascular glaucoma. *Ophthalmology.* 1992;99:1823–1828.

2 Lasers, Liability, and the Doctrine of Informed Consent

Richard E. Castillo

The issue of liability over patient injury at the hands of the health care practitioner predates the profession's formal establishment. Health care practitioners have been dealing with the risk of litigation over the unintended or unexpected consequences of their actions or lack thereof for centuries. As early as the year 1164, in the case of *Everad v. Hopkins*, a servant and his master collected damages against a physician for the practice of "unwholesome medicine." The 1374 case, *Stratton v. Swanlond*, is frequently cited as the "fourteenth-century ancestor" of modern medical malpractice law. Then Chief Justice John Cavendish presided over the case, in which one Agnes of Stratton sued surgeon John Swanlond for breach of contract after he failed to treat and cure her severely mangled hand.[1,2]

Moving ahead into the 21st century, the number of both medical and optometric malpractice cases have seen a dramatic increase.[2–4] Several arguments have been suggested to account for this:

1. The nature of both medical and optometric practice has changed and continues to evolve. Health care today is more dependent than at any time in the past on continuously evolving technology for complicated drug therapies, surgery, and even diagnostics to address more and more illnesses with a broader range of therapies. As more invasive treatments are devised, more patients are injured as a consequence.
2. Malpractice litigation itself has become simpler to initiate and more accessible to the average citizen.
3. Juries today are less sympathetic toward physicians, and more physicians are willing to testify against other physicians in courtrooms.
4. Malpractice law itself continues to evolve, with new causes of action and new concepts of damages being introduced, such as mental distress and manufacturer or product liability.

THE DOCTRINE OF INFORMED CONSENT

The doctrine of informed consent evolved out of recognition and respect for the individual's inherent right to autonomy with regards to all aspects of their being, establishing that the individual has a right to be free from nonconsensual interference with

13

their person or to be forced to act knowingly or unknowingly in a manner against their will.[5] In the present day, the doctrine of informed consent, therefore, guides medical decision-making by establishing limits to the doctor–patient relationship. Therefore, the patient's informed consent to treatment is essential to the practitioner for reducing liability risk insofar as claims of battery or negligent nondisclosure are concerned. A properly executed informed consent serves to underscore the patient's inherent right to autonomy in medical or optometric decision-making, which is the underlying principle in all consent cases, be they medical negligence (specifically negligent nondisclosure) or battery, the two circumstances upon which the majority of medical liability actions are based.[1,5,6]

MEDICAL BATTERY

Battery, at common law, is defined as an intentional unpermitted act causing harmful or offensive contact with the "person" of another.[3]

The legal doctrine of battery protects a patient's physical integrity and dignity from harmful contacts or unwanted physical contacts. Note that physical injury is not required for a battery to have occurred. The doctrine only requires that the patient show they were not informed of the very nature of the touching or contact, as might occur, for example, during a laser or surgical procedure. If a practitioner operates on a structure other than that which he and the patient discussed, a battery has occurred. If the patient is not made aware that the practitioner will perform a specific procedure and has not consented, a claim for battery may be brought forth.

Health care practitioners have legal liability exposure to claims for battery, negligent nondisclosure, and the failure to obtain informed consent. Battery is an intentional tort that does not require proof of negligence or of the intent to harm. Generally, a person commits battery by intentionally touching another individual without consent. The individual may be permitted to recover monetary damages absent bodily injury, although the damages awarded in such circumstances may be nominal. Battery is also a crime punishable by fines and imprisonment, although charges of criminal battery are usually only attached if there has been a significant injury to the recipient of the offense.[4]

CONSENT: EXPRESS OR IMPLIED

In eyecare practice, consent may be expressed (permission that is explicitly given, either verbally or in writing) or implied (an assumption of permission that is inferred from actions) by the patient seeking treatment or their legal guardian. In cases of an emergency, mainly when the patient is unable or incapable of giving express consent, consent may be implied by law. Whether consent is given or implied, some boundaries limit the practitioner's actions. A practitioner exposes themselves to liability for battery if the treatment furnished exceeds the limits of the consent either given or implied.[4]

ELEMENTS OF PROPER DISCLOSURE

While a properly executed, informed consent may be enough for the practitioner to defend a battery claim successfully, several elements must be addressed to deliver a proper and complete disclosure.[1,7,8] These elements include the following:

- Diagnosis
- Nature and purpose of treatment
- Risks and outcomes
- Disclosure of skill or status of risks
- Alternatives to treatment
- Prognosis if treatment is delayed
- Prognosis with treatment
- Disclosure of conflicts of interest

With regards to a discussion of the anticipated benefits and risks of a procedure, if the consent, or the patient's refusal, was not preceded by disclosure of the known material benefits, risks, and alternatives, the practitioner may be open to liability, even if the procedure itself was performed competently without technical error, or if the procedure was declined in the case of patient refusal.[1,9]

PATIENT REFUSAL

In the case of patient refusal, for there to be liability for lack of informed consent, the patient generally must show that the physician was negligent, that there was an injury with sustained damages, and that the negligent nondisclosure was a proximate cause of the injury and damages. A claim brought forth for lack of informed consent is based on professional negligence (medical malpractice). Unlike a claim of battery, which requires proof of an intentional touch without consent, a negligent nondisclosure claim requires proof that the health care practitioner failed to furnish care in conformity with the applicable standard of care, alongside proof of injury, damages, and causation. The determination of whether the standard of care has been met or breached is generally established through the testimony of expert witnesses.[1,2]

Measuring the Standard of Care: the Reasonable Physician versus the Reasonable Person Standard

The standard of care is generally measured and evaluated in either one of two ways when a charge of negligent nondisclosure or lack of informed consent is made. The first way is from the physician's perspective, known as the reasonable physician standard. Under the reasonable physician standard, current information must be disclosed to the patient regarding accepted standards of practice among physicians with similar training and experience in the community, or nationally for care furnished by a subspecialist. This reasonable physician standard is followed by slightly more than one-half of the jurisdictions in the United States. The alternate perspective, followed by slightly less than one-half of the jurisdictions in the United States, is from the patient's perspective, known as the reasonable person standard. Under the reasonable person standard, the patient must be informed of the risks and alternatives that a reasonable person in their position would consider significant and material in deciding whether to undergo the proposed treatment or procedure.[1,10]

Both the reasonable physician standard and the reasonable person standard are evaluated and measured in the objective sense, rather than by the opposing parties' subjective intent to a malpractice suit. Risks that are rare or remote, not deemed severe, or which the average patient would typically know are generally not considered to be material within the context of the charges alleged.[3]

THE INCOMPETENT PATIENT

Patients not competent to make decisions about their health may not give or withhold consent. Cognitive impairment and decision-making capacity should be documented in the medical record. Likewise, minors may not consent to medical treatment, although some states have enacted exceptions by statute. For these individuals, consent must be obtained from a legal guardian or parent. In emergencies, it is usually permissible to perform procedures or furnish treatment necessary to save the patient's life or a vital organ (such as the eye) without express consent when it cannot be obtained in a timely fashion. In this case, like the ubiquitous "Good Samaritan laws," the legal theory of emergency implied consent applies.[7,9]

WITHHOLDING INFORMATION

In atypical cases where the information to be disclosed might have a detrimental effect on the patient's physical or psychological well-being (i.e., a depressed or suicidal patient), some jurisdictions may excuse obtaining informed consent. The scope of this so-called "therapeutic privilege" varies from state to state, and the practitioner should use great caution and consult with their liability carrier's risk management advisor or legal counsel before exercising this option.[2,3,6]

In these exceptional cases, the practitioner needs to consider the ethical issues raised by postponing the disclosure of information to the patient. Ethically, it may be appropriate in these circumstances to postpone or delay disclosure of certain information if early communication could exacerbate the patient's mental status or pose a significant threat to their well-being.[6] However, withholding medical information from patients is generally not an acceptable practice or ethically permissible. Although all information need not be communicated to the at-risk patient immediately or all at once, the practitioner should carefully assess the amount of information a patient can and should receive at any given time.[6]

THE LIMITS OF LICENSURE AND SCOPE OF PRACTICE

Health care practitioners should be aware of the limits of their licensure and scope of practice (statutes and licensing board regulations) as well as the laws in their respective states. Practitioners often have many resources available on consent issues, such as national and state medical and optometric associations. Additionally, professional liability carriers will often guide their insured practitioner on consent issues and may have readily available templates or model consent forms for their client's use.

THE INFORMED CONSENT FORM

In general, an informed consent form identifies the patient, the procedure, the indications, the benefits, and the risks. A generic space on the form can be used to document the physician's disclosures and discussion with the patient and their consent. Some jurisdictions require a witness to sign the consent form. Practitioners in office settings may ask technicians or other office staff to witness. Due to potential conflict-of-interest issues that may be raised in litigation, the practitioner should consider having a family member or friend of the patient also to witness the consent process when possible, in addition to the office staff. Furthermore, there is a requirement of certified translators for patients who do not speak English and a requirement for documents written in the language used by the patient.[3]

In recent years, courts have been criticized for setting standards that do not reflect contemporary medical or optometric practice, interfering with the traditional doctor–patient relationship. Usually, the fault lies with the implementation, not in the actual concept. The concept of informed consent includes the legal concept of consent, but it goes further in that it requires that the patient be a partner in the decision-making process.[3,8,10]

THE DECISION-MAKING PROCESS

Similar to how laws have evolved to clarify and refine informed consent, there has been a transition toward involving the patient more and more in the decision-making process. Conceptually, there are essentially four descriptive models of decision-making:

1. *Conventional medical model*: The health care practitioner decides which procedure(s) to perform; the patient's trust and confidence in the doctor replace the need for consent.
2. *Conventional informed consent model*: The health care practitioner decides which procedure(s) to perform with the patient's express or implied informed consent.
3. *Collaboration*: The health care practitioner and the patient work together to make a joint decision about the procedure.
4. *Patient choice*: The patient decides with the health care practitioner's advice.

In today's health care environment, few patients choose the traditional model, and few choose the fourth model. Most patients and health care practitioners alike are more comfortable with either conventional informed consent or collaboration. Health care practitioners should learn how to use both of these models of decision-making and determine which model to use for a specific patient.[4]

Regardless of the model of decision-making utilized, the practitioner will be held to the standard of informed consent adopted by the state or jurisdiction in which they practice. The health care practitioner must take care to perform all due diligence in assuring that all the necessary disclosures have been made and are adequately documented in the medical record and that a written and signed consent form is utilized at every opportunity.

VERBAL CONSENT

Except in the case of a life- or vital-organ-threatening emergency, there is seldom an exception to the rule that all procedures, whether office or facility based, require a written and signed informed consent. The consent process should include a discussion and disclosure of the material risks and benefits and an opportunity to allow the patient to ask questions and participate in the ultimate decision as to whether they have or reject the procedure or alternative treatment.[7] In some instances (i.e., an illiterate patient), it may be permissible to obtain the patient's verbal consent. Verbal consents should be carefully documented by the health care practitioner in the medical record addressing all the essential points (diagnosis, procedure, material risks, benefits, known complications, and treatment alternatives). Whenever possible, written consent is always advised.[3]

ADDITIONAL ELEMENTS OF THE INFORMED CONSENT PROCESS

The act of discussing the diagnosis and proposed procedure with the patient (parent or guardian), reviewing the possible complications, and the required aftercare is considered part of the consent process.[8] The consent form also serves as a patient education tool, and a copy (with the patient's signature) should be given to the patient or their caregiver as a reference. Patients should be educated during the consent process that results of medical and surgical procedures are not guaranteed. Furthermore, the procedure's consent form should include post-procedure instructions and instructions for contacting the practitioner or an on-call associate if complications occur outside of regular office hours.[11]

Many offices, professional societies, and even liability insurance carriers recommend or even provide patient videos discussing the proposed procedure. Standardized recordings ensure that each patient receives consistent and complete information and can consider all the pertinent information. Standardized video instruction also serves as a record for the defense of a lawsuit. However, a video does not replace and should not be substituted for the patient and the practitioner's discussion.[3,11]

INFORMED CONSENT IS A PROCESS, NOT JUST A FORM

Surgical complications (including those caused by ophthalmic laser procedures) are the foundation of many malpractice suits. The health care practitioner should not rely exclusively on a signed consent form to defend a malpractice suit. Instead, a better strategy would be to strengthen and highlight the entire process that resulted in the patient's consent. This includes all facets of the patient's participation in that process. Understand that during litigation, a practitioner who brings out a convoluted and highly technical consent form, which was signed by the patient at the last minute, with little opportunity for questions or discussion, is not likely to be viewed favorably from the perspective of a jury.[2,8]

The fact is that no printed form, regardless of signature, may necessarily be viewed as prima facie evidence that the patient's consent was informed. A consent form is only one piece in the totality of the evidence accrued, and in current lawsuits, other pieces of evidence, such as the patient's testimony, will be introduced and considered as well. The consent form itself is not a substitute for a candid discussion with the patient about the procedure and the patient's inclusion in the decision-making process, nor is a preprinted consent form a substitute for documentation in the medical record of the discussion and opportunity to ask and have questions answered before the patient signs the form. This aspect of the process should be explicitly stated in the patient's chart.[9,10]

It is counterproductive from the standpoint of defending a lawsuit to utilize a consent form that uses language that is too technical and too long to read and interpret during an office visit. Consent forms are often handed out to patients during registration by nonprofessional office staff, and many are unable to comprehend the procedure even after the written explanation. The consent form should be meaningful to the patient if it is to be of value to the defendant during litigation. Also, as stated earlier, the practitioner should include a narrative of the discussion between doctor and patient during the decision-making process in the medical record.

The health care practitioner should be careful not to overpromise or oversell a procedure. Furthermore, one should never offer a "guarantee" of what a procedure can do. "Never say never and never say always." Medicine, optometry included, is not a science of precision, like Physics, for example, where problems typically have exact solutions and answers are calculated to the nth decimal place. The practice of both medicine and optometry is as much an art as a science, and there are simply too many intangibles when it comes to performing procedures on patients to ever offer a guarantee of results.

CONCLUSION

It is essential to understand that no consent form will protect a health care practitioner from an actual malpractice lawsuit. Competence, experience, and staying current with the ever-evolving science, advances in technology, and the art of clinical care are essential. Recognizing one's professional limits and knowing when to seek advice from a colleague or refer for definitive care are equally essential to avoid litigation.

REFERENCES

1. Beauchamp TL, Childress JF. *Principles of Biomedical Ethics*. 6th ed. New York, NY: Oxford University Press; 2009.
2. Emanuel EJ. Bioethics in the practice of medicine. In: Goldman L, Schafer AI, eds. *Goldman-Cecil Medicine*. 26th ed. Philadelphia, PA: Elsevier; 2020: chap 2.
3. Berg JW, Appelbaum P, Lidz C, et al. The legal requirements for disclosure and consent: History and current status. In: *Informed Consent: Legal Theory and Clinical Practice*. 2nd ed. New York, NY: Oxford University Press; 2001:41–74.
4. United States Department of Health and Human Services website. Informed consent. Available at: www.hhs.gov/ohrp/regulations-and-policy/guidance/informed-consent/index.html. Accessed December 5, 2019.
5. Faden RR, Beauchamp TL. *A History and Theory of Informed Consent*. New York, NY: Oxford University Press; 1986.
6. Grisso T, Appelbaum PS. *Assessing Competence to Consent to Treatment: A Guide for Physicians and Other Health Professionals*. New York, NY: Oxford University Press; 1998.
7. Barry MJ. Involving patients in medical decisions: How can physicians do better? *JAMA*. 1999;282:2356–2357.
8. Robinson G, Merav A. Informed consent: Recall by patients tested postoperatively. *Ann Thorac Surg*. 1976;22:209–212.
9. Solomon J, Schwegman-Melton K. Structured teaching and patient understanding of informed consent. *Crit Care Nurse*. 1987;7:74–79.
10. Lloyd A, Hayes P, Bell P. The role of risk and benefit perception in informed consent for surgery. *Med Decis Making*. 2001;21:141–149.
11. Dawes PJ, O'Keefe L, Adcock S. Informed consent: Using a structured interview changes patients' attitudes towards informed consent. *J Laryngol Otol*. 1993;107:775–779.

SUPPLEMENTAL READING

1. Brennan K. Malpractice: Minimizing your exposure. Review of Ophthalmology. October 14, 2018. Available at: https://www.reviewofophthalmology.com/article/malpractice-minimizing-your-exposure

3 The Basic Science and Mechanism of Laser Components

Neal Whittle • Aaron B. Zimmerman

The word *laser* is an acronym for the words *l*ight *a*mplification by *s*timulated *e*mission of *r*adiation.[1] Each of these terms describes a laser beam's properties and must be fully understood for one to appreciate the nature of laser ophthalmic surgery. The first term to be described is *light*.

Light is a form of electromagnetic radiation (EMR). EMR is energy emitted and absorbed by charged particles; in other words, it is energy emitted and absorbed by matter. EMR exhibits wave-like behavior as it travels through space. As the name suggests, EMR has both electric (E-field) and magnetic (B-field) components. The E-field of EMR is responsible for all observed optical phenomena such as reflection, refraction, diffraction, and interference. In a vacuum, EMR propagates at the speed of light.[2]

Light may be described either as electromagnetic (EM) waves or as the flow of particles (photons). Each of these views is described in this chapter.

LIGHT AS A WAVE

Oscillations cause waves. These oscillations propagate out from the source, inducing further oscillations as the wave moves through space or a medium. There are two types of propagating waves: transverse waves and longitudinal waves.

A *longitudinal wave* is a wave in which the direction of oscillation is in the same plane as the direction of travel. Longitudinal waves are also referred to as compression waves. Sound waves are longitudinal waves.

A *transverse wave* is one in which the oscillation is perpendicular to the direction of travel. A pebble dropped into still water produces transverse waves (ripples) that move outward in two dimensions. EMR propagates as *transverse waves*, meaning that light propagates as a transverse wave as well. Light waves travel very much like ripples on a pond's surface, but light waves propagate in three dimensions. Transverse waves may be *polarized*. The polarization of a light wave is the orientation of the E-field of the EM wave and the direction of oscillation that produced the wave. For example, an EM wave with a vertical oscillation would also have a vertically oriented E-field, and therefore has a vertical polarization.

21

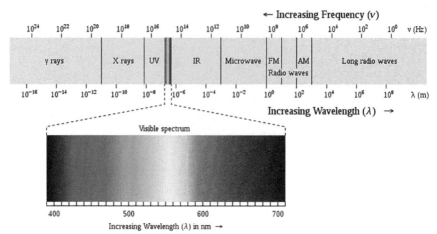

FIGURE 3-1 Electromagnetic spectrum. (Shared by Philip Ronan under the Creative Commons Attribution-Share Alike 3.0 Unported license.) IR, infrared; UV, ultraviolet.

As the source oscillates, new waves continue to form at the frequency (ν, Greek letter *nu*) of the oscillation. The resulting wavelength (λ, Greek letter *lambda*) of the EMR is then fixed by the velocity (c) and the frequency (ν):

$$\lambda = \frac{c}{\nu} \text{ or } \nu = \frac{c}{\lambda} \text{ or } c = \lambda\nu$$

Note that frequency (ν) and wavelength (λ) are inversely proportional, that is, the longer the wavelength, the lower the frequency, and vice versa. EMR waves differ in their wavelength (and their equivalent frequency). The EMR spectrum is a continuum that is arbitrarily broken up into ranges called *bands* (Figure 3.1).

Visible light makes up only a small part of the EM spectrum. The only difference between visible light and the other parts of the EM spectrum is that, as the term suggests, the former may be detected by the human eye. Observe how the visible spectrum is oriented to the rest of the EM spectrum. Blue light has a shorter wavelength and therefore a higher frequency than the other visible wavelengths such as green, yellow, orange, and red. It is also positioned directly next to ultraviolet (UV), whereas red is positioned next to infrared (IR). Therefore, the light wave's wavelength (and frequency) and the particles' energy making up the light wave are related.

LIGHT AS A PARTICLE

As stated earlier, light may be described either as EM waves or as the flow of particles. The particle in question is called the *photon*. The photon is a discrete packet of energy (or quantum) for all forms of EMR, including light. The photon is the force carrier for the EM force, which means that while the EMR wave moves the energy through space, the photon is responsible for the actual transfer of energy or force between particles (i.e., matter).

A photon's energy (and therefore the light wave) is quantified by the equation $E = m(h\nu)$, where h is the Planck's constant, ν is the frequency, and m is an integer, 1, 2, 3 ... . More commonly, the photon equation is displayed like this:

$$E = h\nu$$

This equation provides a relatively complete understanding of how the wave nature of light relates to light's particle nature. As stated earlier, frequency and wavelength are *inversely* proportional, whereas energy is *directly* proportional to frequency. Therefore, when comparing blue light to red light, it may be immediately noticed that blue has a shorter wavelength than red and therefore a higher frequency. The higher frequency of blue light indicates that blue has higher energy. It is well known that UV is harmful to tissue due to its high frequency and high energy[3]; blue light falls on the spectrum adjacent to UV, and red is adjacent to IR.

INTERFERENCE

The oscillation of the E-field of a light wave can be described by a sine wave. As a sine wave, the light wave has amplitude, frequency, wavelength, and phase. The phase of any sine wave is measured in degrees or radians, representing the time or distance elapsed from the source of oscillation in one cycle. The phase that two or more waves have at a point of summation will determine how they interact. When two or more waves come together at a point in space, their energy fields' summation is referred to as *interference*. Interference can occur when light waves from a single source (originally in *phase*) are divided and recombined after traveling through separate paths with different lengths. A phase difference (δ) can result between two waves of the same wavelength (λ) because of either a difference in time of generation (Δt) or a difference in path length (Δx) traveled by waves to reach that point or a combination of both.

When two waves meet at a point in space so that they are in phase ($\delta = 0$ or multiples of 360), they are said to undergo complete *constructive interference*. When two waves undergo constructive interference, their amplitudes add together, thereby amplifying the wave. When two waves are 180° out of phase at a point in space ($\delta = 180$ or multiples of 180), they undergo complete *destructive interference*. Waves that undergo destructive interference cancel out one another's amplitudes. Interference that is neither wholly constructive nor wholly destructive is referred to as *partial interference*.

COHERENCE

When all of the waves in a beam of light have equal wavelength and frequency (i.e., they are the same color) and all have the same phase (crests coincide with crests and troughs with troughs, i.e., $\delta = 0$), then the light is said to be *coherent*. Except for lasers, most light sources do not produce highly coherent light. Most light sources are *incoherent* because they emit polychromatic wavelengths, all of which have different frequencies.

ATOMS AND ENERGY LEVELS

EMR is emitted and absorbed by matter. Atoms are the building blocks of all molecules and are the smallest components of matter representing a chemical element such as hydrogen or helium. An atom is composed of a nucleus of protons (positive charge) and neutrons (neutral), whereas negatively charged electrons "orbit" around the nucleus in regions of space called orbitals. To appreciate the scale, if the nucleus of an atom were the size of a grain of dust on a pitcher's mound, the orbitals making up the remainder of the atom would fill a professional baseball stadium.

There are certain fixed orbits in which electrons orbit an atom. Each of these orbits corresponds to a certain amount of total energy, and an electron can only change from one orbit to another by giving up or receiving an amount of energy, which is the difference in energy between the two orbits. It should be noted that electrons cannot fall anywhere in between orbitals. Thus, photons of a quantal amount of energy are emitted when electrons jump from a higher energy orbit (an outer orbit) to a lower energy orbit (an inner orbit). The amount of energy is $\Delta E = E_{outer} - E_{inner} = h\nu$ (Figure 3.2). Orbitals can also have different shapes. More complex orbital shapes have a higher energy than those that are more simple in shape. These orbitals are also known as energy levels. An energy level is the energy necessary to move an electron from a lower to a higher orbital or to a different orbital shape.

Orbitals farther from the nucleus have a much higher energy level than orbitals closer to the nucleus. The highest energy electrons—the most unstable—are found in the outermost orbitals and are called valence electrons. Valence electrons are responsible for the chemical reactivity of an element and the electrical conductivity of an element.

Once an electron is excited, it cannot maintain the excitation for long. It returns to its previously occupied lower orbital by emitting energy in the form of EMR (*emission*). This energy is emitted as a photon, and this is responsible for the production of light.

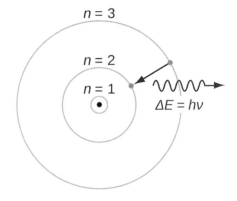

FIGURE 3-2 The Bohr model of the hydrogen atom where the negatively charged electron (green dot) travels in an orbital around the small, positively charged atomic nucleus (black dot). The orbits (gray circles) have an energy level associated with them. The orbits with a larger radius have higher energy, whereas the orbits with a smaller radius have less energy. When an electron jumps between orbits, it is accompanied by an emitted or absorbed amount of electromagnetic energy ($h\nu$). (Shared by JabberWok under the Creative Commons Attribution-Share Alike 3.0 Unported license.)

ABSORPTION

For emission to occur, an atom's electrons must first be elevated to a higher energy level through *absorption* (Figure 3.3). The only frequencies absorbed are those that have just the right amount of energy ($E = h\nu$) to elevate electrons to the particular energy levels available in the atoms. The frequencies a substance strongly absorbs are known as *resonance frequencies*. The type of absorption (and scatter) depends on whether the matter with which the light interacts is rarefied or dense.

Rarefied Gas Made Up of Atoms: Atomic Gas

In a rarefied gas made up of atoms, the resonant frequencies (absorption bands) are extremely narrow. For example, sodium vapor absorbs strongly (and thus scatters strongly) at 589 nm (yellow) but allows most other wavelengths to easily get through. The sodium atom dipoles resonate at $\nu = c/\lambda = (3 \times 10^8 \text{ m/s})/589 \text{ nm} = 5.09 \times 10^{14} \text{ Hz}$ and reemit EMR at the same frequency (and wavelength) but in all directions, a process called *resonant scatter*.

Rarefied Gas Made Up of Molecules

In a rarefied gas made up of molecules, the absorption bands are broader due to interactions between atoms held together in molecules. Scatter is again greatest for wavelengths near the resonant frequencies. For example, air molecules (N_2 and O_2) have a resonant frequency in the UV range. Therefore, most of the scattering of visible light in the atmosphere is for blue light, which is closest to UV, and as a result, the sky appears blue.

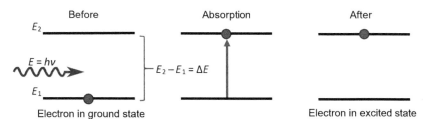

FIGURE 3-3 Absorption. The electron absorbs the energy from the photon. The absorbed photon's energy must have the exact energy required to elevate an electron to a higher energy level.

CONDENSED MATTER: SOLIDS, LIQUIDS, AND DENSE GAS

Opaque Substances

In condensed matter, the absorption bands run together due to the interactions between close neighboring atoms and molecules (*particles*). These particles are so close together that when one particle absorbs EMR, it transfers some of the energy to adjacent particles through *frictional* forces before reradiation can occur, and the energy is converted from EMR energy to the kinetic energy of particle motion (heat). Such matter is opaque to those absorbed wavelengths. The kinetic energy causes lower frequency (ν) oscillations of the particles, so the energy is reradiated as IR light, but the original wavelength is lost.

Transparent Substances

Some solid or liquid materials are, of course, *transparent* to visible light (e.g., glass). These materials have few or no resonant frequencies in the visible spectrum. A material is transparent to wavelengths between the resonant frequencies. Glass is useful optically because it has no resonant frequencies in the visible range of wavelengths. Glass can appear colored if dyes are added, which resonate and absorb specific wavelengths while passing others.

However, transparency depends on the wavelength interacting with the medium. For example, a black plastic trash bag is opaque to all visible wavelengths due to its absorption across the whole visible spectrum but does not absorb IR light. Therefore, you would not see through it with visible light, but it is entirely transparent to IR light. Likewise, glass is transparent to the human eye because it passes visible wavelengths, but it is opaque to specific IR and UV wavelengths (e.g., 193 nm produced by excimer lasers).

Pigments

A pigment is a material that changes the color of reflected or transmitted light as the result of wavelength-selective absorption. These pigmented objects can be transparent or opaque. When illuminated by white light, some visible wavelengths may be absorbed, while others are transmitted or reflected. A shirt that absorbs every visible wavelength except blue wavelengths appears blue to the human eye, as only blue light is reflected from it. A shirt that absorbs *all* visible wavelengths appears black. The same is true for ocular pigments. Melanin, a prominent pigment in the body, absorbs almost all visible wavelengths and appears brown or black. Hemoglobin, the pigment found in blood, absorbs short and medium wavelengths well but reflects longer wavelengths, such as red. Xanthophylls, like lutein and zeaxanthin, strongly absorb shorter wavelengths such as blue but reflect yellows.

Not all observed colors are from pigments. As we can see with the sky, the sky's blue color is produced by scattering by the molecules in the atmosphere rather than by a reflection of a non-absorbed wavelength, like a shirt with blue pigment. There are other ways to produce color by scatter, such as the blue appearance of blue eyes, the blue hue of blood vessels beneath the skin, or even the blue color of some bird feathers. The color is produced by scatter by the iris, skin, and feathers' fine protein structures, respectively. This type of color is called *structural color* and does not rely on absorption or pigmentation to produce a blue color or scatter short wavelengths.

EMISSION

Each element has its own unique set of wavelengths and frequencies it can absorb; it also has a set of wavelengths and frequencies it can emit based on how many electrons it has orbiting the nucleus. As discussed earlier, when an electron jumps from a higher energy level to a lower energy level, the energy difference between the levels is given off in the form of photons, or light. The production of light by an electron changing energy levels is called *emission*. The emission spectra of each element on the periodic table are unique (Figure 3.4). Lasers use both spontaneous and stimulated emission, which is discussed in the following.

If light is produced by heating a solid, the emission is called *incandescence*. In incandescent lamps, a current is run through a high resistance filament so that it heats up, and as a result, it glows in a continuous spectrum containing all visible wavelengths. Its brightness and the spectral distribution of its energy (color) depend on its temperature. Higher temperatures produce shorter wavelengths (or cooler light), whereas lower temperatures produce longer wavelengths (warmer light). This is why 5000K light bulbs look blue, whereas 2800K light bulbs look yellow. Incandescent lights do not have very high efficiency (light output/watt) because a lot of the electrical energy is wasted producing IR light, which is lost as heat.

If light is produced by "cold" emission as opposed to incandescence, the emission is called *luminescence*. In other words, luminescence refers to light emitted by electrons directly excited by energy, such as light or electricity. If the stimulation is by light, the substance sometimes absorbs one wavelength but reemits it at a longer wavelength (i.e., *Stokes' shift*). In this case, electrons raised to a higher energy level return to the

FIGURE 3-4 Emission spectra for hydrogen (top) versus iron (bottom). Each element has its unique spectrum because each element has a unique number of electrons and energy levels. Hydrogen spectrum shared by Adrignola (Creative Commons CC0 1.0 Universal Public Domain Dedication). Iron spectrum shared by Nilda (Public domain via Wikimedia Commons).

original level in *two or more steps*, producing lower energy photons (longer λ). The coating on fluorescent bulbs absorbs UV light and reemits it in the visible spectrum by employing a Stokes' shift. Light emitting diodes (LEDs), fluorescent lamps, and lasers function via luminescence. There are many types of luminescence, but the most common types are listed here:

> *Fluorescence*—If photon emission ceases almost immediately after stimulation is stopped, the process is called fluorescence. An example of fluorescence is the *fluorescein*, which we use to observe the tear film of eyes. When stimulated by blue light, the orange dye fluoresces a bright green.

> *Phosphorescence*—If photon emission following cessation of stimulation takes a significant length of time to stop ($\geq 10^{-7}$ second), then the process is called phosphorescence. In phosphorescence, emission can continue for minutes to hours following the excitation (e.g., a glowstick).

> *Electroluminescence*—This type of luminescence refers to luminescence in response to an electrical current or a strong electrical field. This is how LEDs work.

Spontaneous versus Stimulated Emission

When an electron is elevated to a higher energy level via absorption, the electrons usually stay at the higher energy levels for short times, after which they spontaneously drop to a lower energy level and emit a photon in a process called *spontaneous emission* (Figure 3.5). In other words, the electron falls back to a lower energy level without additional stimulation from an outside source. If the electron falls back to the original orbit from which it was elevated, the released photon has the same energy and, therefore, the same wavelength as the stimulating photon. However, the released photon has a random direction and is not in phase with other spontaneously emitted photons, meaning that they are not coherent.

Although spontaneous emission does not produce coherent light, another process, called *stimulated emission*, can. If an electron at an elevated energy level encounters a photon of the same wavelength as the photon that *would be* emitted if it were to fall to a lower level, then the electron immediately jumps to the lower level and emits a new photon of the same wavelength, direction, phase, and polarization as the stimulating photon. Thus, *one* photon encounters the atom, but *two* coherent photons leave (Figure 3.6).

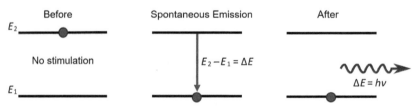

FIGURE 3-5 Spontaneous emission. Note that no external stimulation is required for the electron to return to the lower energy level. The wavelength of the emitted photon (green arrow) is dependent on the energy difference between the two energy levels.

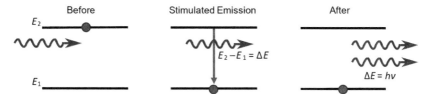

FIGURE 3-6 Stimulated emission. The stimulating photon (green arrows) must be of the same wavelength that the electron would emit on its own if emitted during spontaneous emission.

Since they are coherent with one another, they add together and amplify the beam. Remember that *laser* stands for *l*ight *a*mplification by *s*timulated *e*mission of *r*adiation. We are taking light produced by the medium and then amplifying that light using constructive interference brought about by stimulated emission of radiation.

PROPERTIES OF LASER LIGHT

Laser light is unique because it is highly monochromatic, is highly coherent, is highly directional (minimally divergent), and has a high power density due to those factors. The concentrated nature and high power density of lasers make them very useful for various applications, including ophthalmic surgery.

Monochromatism

As lasers are often used in applications that require monochromatism (including ophthalmic surgery), they are designed in such a way that only allows for a single or very narrow band of wavelengths to be emitted. The wavelength of light emitted by the laser depends on the atoms emitting the light (the medium) and the resonance cavity's length.

Different wavelengths are absorbed in different parts of the eye, depending on the tissue's transparency or resonance frequency.[4] For example, light from the argon–fluoride excimer laser (193 nm) is absorbed strongly by the cornea and does not penetrate deeper into the eye. This, coupled with how it interacts with tissue (discussed later), makes it ideal for corneal surgery. If the excimer laser were polychromatic and emitted light in the visible or IR bands, the laser's visible energy could damage the lens or retina by passing deeper into the eye. On the other hand, retinal surgeon's use visible and IR light for retinal surgeries; therefore, a laser that also emits in the UV range (and therefore would transmit energy to the cornea) would be undesirable. A laser's monochromaticity allows the surgeon to select the appropriate wavelength for the eye's specific target tissue.

Coherence

When a photon is emitted, the wave associated with it has a finite length. When this wave is divided and then recombined after its parts have traveled different distances, its parts will remain coherent only if the difference in distance traveled is shorter than the length of the wave train. This is referred to as the coherence length of the light. If the difference in distance traveled by a split wave is greater than the coherence length, then the two waves no longer share the same original phase relationship and will not interfere. The coherence length of a light wave is also referred to as temporal coherence, and represents the predictability of the phase of the wave a great distance from the source. Light bulbs emit light of short *coherence length* because multiple waves of multiple wavelengths are interacting. Lasers have a *temporal coherence* approaching a plane wave, or infinite coherence length, and a monochromatic nature depending on the lasing substance used. A beam with high temporal coherence can be easily amplified. This leads to a very intense beam, especially compared to that from an incoherent source.

Directionality

Lasers are also highly directional, meaning that they have low divergence or spread over great distances. High directionality is also known as *spatial coherence*. For example, a powerful laser directed at the moon would only spread to a spot size width of 4 miles over a distance of 239,228 miles.[5] Although it seems large, the spread shows a divergence of only 0.001°. A laser beam with high spatial coherence maintains a small beam diameter and focuses on a small spot size.

Most lasers emit far less power (watts) than does a standard light bulb, but they are a more significant vision hazard due to their beams' high collimation (directionality). A standard 100-W incandescent bulb might emit 20 W of visible power, but it is emitted in all directions so that only 0.0016 mW falls on a 1 mm^2 area 1 m away. On the other hand, a 1-mW laser with a 1 mm^2 beam area directs *all* its power onto a 1 mm^2 area 1 m away. All this light could easily enter through the pupil of an eye, and due to the high concentration of the light, it could overwhelm the retinal tissue and cause permanent tissue damage.

Power Density

The highly amplified and highly directional nature of laser light creates a very concentrated beam. *Power density*[6] is the transfer of a specific number of photons per second to a given area (W/cm^2) and can be described by the following equation:

$$\text{Power density} = \frac{W}{cm^2} = \frac{\left(\frac{J}{s}\right)}{cm^2}$$

where
- J (energy) is the number of photons
- s (seconds) is the pulse time
- cm^2 (spot size) is the given area the photons are transferred to

Power density is also referred to as *flux* or *irradiance*. *Fluence* refers to the total number of joules (J) delivered to unit area (cm^2) without consideration of time. Lasers used for ophthalmic purposes can have outputs listed in milliwatts (power) or millijoules (energy). The time component is inherently considered when power is listed. When a laser is programmed to emit a specific energy, that laser will deliver the energy in a specified unit of time; therefore, power output can be calculated.

Consider the following: Two beams of laser light emit 50 photons in a specified unit of time. One laser has a 50-micron spot size diameter, and the other has a 100-micron spot size diameter (Figure 3.7). They both emit the same number of photons in an equal period (equal power), but the smaller spot size (50 microns) has a higher power density (flux) because its photons are confined to a smaller area than the 100-micron spot size. To be exact, a 50-micron spot size has only one quarter of the area of the 100-micron spot size. Therefore, the power density of the 50 μm spot diameter is fourfold higher than that of the 100 μm spot diameter.

The amount of time a laser needs to emit a pulse is also critical to understanding a laser's output. Assume you have two lasers that emit 100 photons (J) with equal spot sizes (cm^2). However, one beam emits its 100 photons over 1 second, whereas the other emits its photons over 1/1,000th of a second. The laser that emits the photons in 1 second has a power of 100 W. The laser that emits the 100 J in 0.001 second has a power of 100,000 W. Ophthalmic lasers do not have energy levels remotely close to those in the previous example. They often use energy levels in micro- or millijoules, but the pulse times can range from femtoseconds (10^{-15} s) to milliseconds (10^{-3} s). Despite the seemingly low energy settings, the resultant power density is high when delivered in very rapid pulse durations.

When considering power density, the energy, spot size, and pulse duration can all be modified independently for effect on the target tissue. Higher energy, a shorter pulse duration, and a smaller spot size all increase power density.

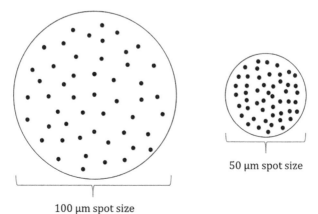

50 μm spot size

100 μm spot size

FIGURE 3-7 Spot size and photon density. Notice that if the number of photons is equal, the smaller spot size has a higher power density.

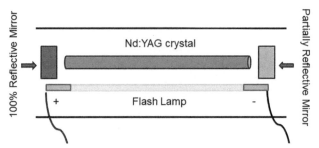

FIGURE 3-8 The three basic components of a laser: (1) the medium, in this example an Nd:YAG crystal; (2) the excitation mechanism, in this case, an optical flash lamp; and (3) the resonance cavity with mirrors on each end.

COMPONENTS OF A LASER

A laser consists of three basic components: a medium, an energy source, and an optical resonator (Figure 3.8).[7] The energy source is what excites the medium to produce the light. The optical resonator (also known as the *resonance cavity*) provides the light amplification to achieve a coherent, powerful beam.

Medium

Recall that photons are emitted by atoms when electrons at higher energy levels drop to vacant lower energy levels (fluorescence). The energy (E) of the photon is equal to the difference in energy between the two levels. For any atom, the possible levels are quantized in set amounts of energy, and thus only specific frequencies and wavelengths are emitted. In other words, the wavelengths of light emitted from a laser depend on what types of atoms produce light in the laser.

Laser mediums can come in many different forms, such as gas, solid state, liquid, and semiconductor lasers. In a gas laser, the lasing substance is a gas suspended in a glass or quartz chamber. The argon and red krypton lasers are ion gas lasers, whereas the excimer laser uses a noble gas (argon) and a halide (fluoride). In a solid state laser, the lasing substance is embedded in a transparent solid such as crystal or glass. In this form, the active lasing substance is referred to as the dopant, whereas the crystal that it is embedded in is called the substrate. A common ophthalmic laser that is solid state is the Nd:YAG laser, which stands for neodymium:yttrium aluminum garnet. The synthetic Nd:YAG crystal serves as the substrate, and the neodymium is the dopant. Another example of a solid state laser is the ruby laser, which was the first visible laser to be invented. The ruby's red color comes from chromium atoms that are embedded in an aluminum oxide crystalline substrate. Lasers that use a liquid medium are commonly known as dye lasers. In a dye laser, an organic dye (the dopant) is dissolved into a solution (the substrate). There are many different dyes that can be used, but most are fluorescent in some way. A unique property of dye lasers is that each laser tends to have a broader range of wavelengths available than most solid or gas lasers, meaning that they are tunable to a specific desired wavelength. One downside to the dye laser is that the dyes used are often highly corrosive or carcinogenic. Dye lasers are not commonly used for ophthalmic purposes.

Another type of laser is the semiconductor laser, a.k.a. the diode laser. The diode laser is an elaboration on the LED. Relatively monochromatic light is produced when electrons cross a junction between n-type and p-type materials. If the two opposite faces of the LED are made to be flat and parallel, a resonance cavity is formed, which produces a laser beam. Unlike the previously mentioned laser types, the beam is as much as 20° divergent and not as coherent. However, it can be collimated optically into a high-power-density beam and used surgically for its thermal effect. In ophthalmology, diode lasers are used as aiming beams, as micropulse lasers, and for endoscopic cyclophotocoagulation.

Excitation Mechanism, or Pump

Lasers require stimulated emission to produce an amplified, coherent beam. Stimulated emission requires electrons to be in their excited states to produce the cascade of photons. However, most electrons are usually in their lowest energy orbit (*ground state*) because lower energy orbitals are more stable, meaning that they absorb rather than emit photons. Then they spontaneously emit noncoherent photons before other photons can trigger stimulated emission. However, certain higher energy levels, called *metastable states*, can hold the elevated electrons for a considerably longer time than normal before the electrons return to a lower energy level. Due to these metastable orbits, energy can be added to elevate more electrons to the higher energy states than are at ground level—a condition referred to as a *population inversion*. Stimulated emission can thus result in a chain reaction of photon emission where most of the energy is converted into a large number of coherent photons.

As the electrons leave the metastable orbits to produce light, additional electrons are elevated to the metastable orbits by adding energy to the system through a *pump mechanism*. The pump energy can be in the form of an electric current (electron collision pumping) or light energy (optical pumping). Optical pumping can be in the form of a flashbulb or another continuous wave (CW) laser.

The type of pump the laser uses varies based on the type of medium the laser uses. For example, gas lasers may be pumped with an electrical pump or optical pump, but the electrical pump is more common. Solid state lasers are only pumped by light, and diode lasers are only pumped electrically.

The Resonance Cavity

The resonance cavity houses the medium and has a 100% reflective mirror on one end and a just-less-than-100% reflective mirror on the opposite end. The photons that are released during stimulated emission can be emitted in any direction. The mirrors allow photons to reflect back and forth as they recruit additional coherent photons in the same direction, creating a cascade effect that significantly amplifies the light energy with the resonance cavity. Because one of the mirrors allows a small percentage of light to pass, with each round trip between mirrors, some of the lasing cavity's energy can be released.

One other requirement is that the length of the cavity must be such that the wavelengths are divisible into the length of a round trip ($2t$) through the laser cavity an integer number of times so that the waves remain in phase with each other with each round trip. This is referred to as a *resonance cavity*. The waves traveling back and forth form a standing wave. A standing wave is a summated, stationary wave formed by interference between two waves traveling in opposite directions. The wavelength of the standing wave depends on the length of the cavity (i.e., the separation of the mirrors). Nearly all other wavelengths in the resonance cavity are suppressed, which means we can make a laser beam monochromatic without using a filter (although there is a notable exception, the Argon Laser which is discussed in "Auxiliary Crystals and Filters".).

LASER OUTPUT

There are four major types of beam duration: continuous, long pulse, Q-switching, and mode locking. Those lasers that lase without interruption are called *CW lasers*. A CW laser requires a continuous pump, such as an electrical current or another CW laser. The effect on the tissue is usually thermal. A long pulse laser emits on the order of milliseconds. That sounds like a short pulse time, but it is long by laser standards. Similar to the CW laser, the long pulse laser has a thermal effect. For both CW and long pulse ophthalmic lasers, the output is usually labeled in power as milliwatts (mW).

However, if one of the resonance cavity mirrors is interrupted by a "shutter" for a period of time while the pump continues to operate, cascades of stimulated emission are delayed, and a greater population inversion is allowed to build up. Then, when the shutter is opened, the energy is released in a burst, usually on the order of pico- or nanoseconds, which results in a pulse of light with extremely high power. This form of pulsing is referred to as *quotient switching* or *Q-switching*.[8] Such lasers can be a greater ocular hazard because they allow high amounts of light energy to be released for exposures too short to be prevented by a lid blink. Q-switching causes plasma formation, even in non-pigmented tissue, resulting in a photodisruptive tissue effect as opposed to a thermal effect. The photodisruptive effect minimizes heat exchange with adjacent tissues, which offers some surgical advantages.

Ophthalmic femtosecond lasers use passive *mode locking* to achieve even shorter pulse times than does a Q-switched laser. Mode-locked lasers make use of an absorber placed in the resonance cavity. The absorber selectively absorbs low-intensity light and transmits high-intensity light. By doing this, the absorber locks the phases of the various random modes inside the cavity, resulting in periodic, intense, regular pulses of constructive interference. Because there are no moving shutters, mode-locked lasers can achieve incredibly low pulse times (femtoseconds), which results in a large power density. For comparison, a mode-locked femtosecond laser pulse is one million times shorter than a Q-switched nanosecond laser pulse.

AUXILIARY CRYSTALS AND FILTERS

Also known as second harmonic generation, *frequency doubling* is a method by which a laser's wavelength can be halved. Frequency doubling is a nonlinear optical process that does not follow the superposition principle and only works at very high light intensities. Two photons are passed through a nonlinear crystal medium. The crystal used in ophthalmic lasers for frequency doubling is potassium-titanyl-phosphate, which creates a second harmonic wave with two photons.[9] The two photons are stacked upon one another in two virtual states, resulting in a single, higher-energy photon at twice the frequency and half the wavelength. This is commonly used in the frequency-doubled Nd:YAG laser, taking it from a 1,064 nm IR laser to a 532 nm visible green laser, which is commonly used in various ophthalmic surgeries.

Sometimes, a filter is required to ensure that the laser being used is monochromatic. Most notably, for ophthalmic surgery, the argon laser is a CW laser with two natural wavelengths, at 488 nm (blue–green) and 513 nm (green). The xanthophyll pigments in the macula strongly absorb blue light; therefore, the 488 nm wavelength is often filtered out of the argon laser beam to protect the macula from stray blue laser light. A green hand-held laser pointer may emit a visible green wavelength and an IR wavelength. The laser pointer may have a filter to inhibit the infrared wavelength from being emitted from the device.

REFERENCES

1. Gound G. The LASER, light amplification by stimulated emission of radiation. *The Ann Arbor Conference on Optical Pumping*. Ann Arbor, MI 1959;15.
2. Michelson AA. Measurement of the velocity of light between Mount Wilson and Mount San Antonio. *Astrophys J*. 1927;65:1–22.
3. Coroneo M. Ultraviolet radiation and the anterior eye. *Eye Contact Lens*. 2011;37:214–224.
4. Boettner EA, Wolter JR. Transmission of the Ocular Media. *Invest Ophth Visual*. 1962;1:776–783.
5. NASA Eclipse Website. Measuring the Moon's distance. 1994. Available at: https://eclipse.gsfc.nasa.gov/SEhelp/ApolloLaser.html. Accessed September 2, 2020.
6. Matys J, Dominiak M, Flieger R. Energy and power density: A key factor in lasers studies. *J Clin Diagn Res*. 2015;9:ZL01–ZL02.
7. Siegman A. *Lasers*. Sausalito, CA: University Science Books; 1986.
8. Mcclung FJ, Hellwarth RW. Giant optical pulsations from ruby. *J Appl Phys*. 1962;33:828.
9. Jalkh AE, Pflibsen K, Pomerantzeff O, et al. A new solid-state, frequency-doubled neodymium-YAG photocoagulation system. *Arch Ophthalmol*. 1988;106:847–849.

4 Laser–Tissue Interactions

Neal Whittle • Aaron B. Zimmerman

Depending on the type of ophthalmic surgery being performed, different tissue responses to laser light may be desired. These laser–tissue interactions can change depending on variables in the laser as well as variables in the tissue. Laser variables include wavelength, spot size, pulse duration, and energy or power level setting. Tissue variables include the type and amount of pigmentation of the tissue as well as the transparency of the tissue to the wavelength of the laser. The combination of the laser parameters and the target tissue results in three basic laser–tissue interactions: (1) photochemical, (2) photothermal, or (3) photodisruptive (sometimes referred to as photomechanical).[1] The laser variables, tissue variables, and laser–tissue interactions will be discussed in the following section.

LASER FACTORS

The first laser variable to consider is the wavelength. Since ophthalmic lasers range from ultraviolet (UV) to infrared (IR) wavelengths, an appropriate wavelength must be selected to interact with a specific tissue. For example, the cornea strongly absorbs UV-B, UV-C, and some IR wavelengths while allowing transmission of visible and near IR.[2] An UV emitting laser, such as the argon-fluoride excimer (193 nm), would be excellent for the cornea, but that wavelength could not reach the iris or the retina. A visible or near-IR wavelength can easily reach the retina, and therefore those wavelengths would be most appropriate for retinal- or iris-related laser procedures (Fig. 4.1).

As described in Chapter 3, spot size, pulse duration, and the energy level all factor into the power density that a laser can deliver. Of the three factors listed, the pulse duration is critical. Ophthalmic lasers are generally classified as either continuous wave (CW) or pulsed. Lasers that are considered CW generally will have pulse durations in the hundreds of milliseconds to second range, and the output is generally listed in milli-Watts (mW). Increasing or lengthening the pulse duration for the CW lasers will result in more tissue response in the form of a deeper or bigger laser burn. Pulsed ophthalmic lasers range from femtoseconds to nanoseconds, and they are programmed to emit pulses in the micro- or milli-joule range.

36

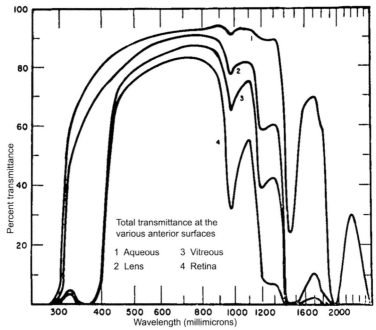

FIGURE 4-1 Ocular transmission of ultraviolet, visible, and infrared radiation.[2] (Reprinted with permission from Boettner EA, Wolter JR. Transmission of the ocular media. *Invest Ophth Visual.* 1962;1:776–783.)

These pulse durations allow for massive differences in power density. The pulsed lasers generally interact with ophthalmic tissues with a photodisruptive or photomechanical mechanism. CW lasers will generally result in photothermal or photochemical outcomes (Fig. 4.2).

If pulse duration and spot size are held constant, increasing the energy setting will result in a higher-power density. However, changing the pulse duration or spot size will have a much more profound effect on power density. Most ophthalmic lasers will have a fixed spot size. Some examples include the neodymium yttrium aluminum garnet (Nd:YAG) (several microns spot size), selective laser trabeculoplasty (SLT) (400 mcm spot size), excimer, and femtosecond lasers. Adjustable spot sizes can be used with argon/green lasers for retinal applications as well as for treating other areas of the eye. In these circumstances, if the laser spot diameter is increased, then the power density will be decreased provided all other variables remained constant. If desiring to keep the power density constant after the spot size was increased, then the power must also be increased. If the laser spot diameter is decreased, then the power must also be decreased if desiring to maintain a constant power density. Spot size can also be affected by a magnifying laser lens. Assuming all laser parameters are held constant, a magnifying lens will decrease the spot size and increase power density.

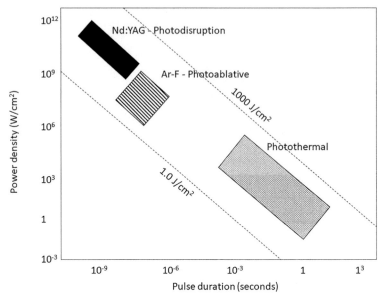

FIGURE 4-2 Power density versus pulse duration. Adapted from Boulnois 1986.[3] Ar-F, argon fluoride laser; Nd:YAG, neodymium yttrium aluminum garnet.

The number of laser applications must be recorded to report the *total cumulative energy dose during a procedure*. The risk of complications from the laser procedure increases in proportion to the total cumulative dose of energy delivered into the eye. Therefore, the best rule-of-thumb is **Use the lowest energy setting, the least number of shots, and the lowest duration possible to accomplish the desired effect.** This does not mean to always use the lowest energy possible. Consider a Nd:YAG capsulotomy: if the tissue is not responding well to 1.5 mJ of energy and it takes 100 shots to clear the posterior capsule, the total cumulative energy is 150 mJ. If instead the energy were increased until the tissue responded better, perhaps 2.5 mJ, and it only took 35 shots to clear the capsule, the total energy would then be 87.5 mJ. By increasing the energy of the individual shot slightly to achieve a better tissue response, the total cumulative energy is less, and the patient has a smaller chance of complications than if the physician had used many more shots with a lower energy.

TISSUE FACTORS

There are some lasers that are considered *pigment independent* and some that are considered *pigment dependent*. A pigment-independent laser does not need pigment to affect the targeted tissue. Examples of nonpigmented tissue would be the cornea, lens, and vitreous. Lasers that are effective on nonpigmented tissues need to be focused at the plane of the target tissue. A femtosecond laser focuses its energy at specific preprogrammed corneal depths. An Nd:YAG uses an alignment system to ensure that the laser is focused at a specific plane. A pigment-independent laser can be used on pigmented tissues, but whether the tissue is transparent or pigmented does not dramatically change how the laser interacts with the tissue[4,5].

With pigment-dependent lasers, a pigment is required to transfer the energy from the laser to the tissue. Absorption of laser light by a pigment is converted to heat, meaning pigment-dependent lasers have a thermal effect on the tissue. The primary ocular pigments are melanin, hemoglobin, and the macula's xanthophylls (Fig. 4.3). Melanin is heavily present in the iris and retinal pigment epithelium (RPE). Melanin absorbs across the entire visible spectrum, which gives it a brown to black color. It absorbs IR less effectively.[4,5] The less efficient the absorption of a wavelength, the more that wavelength is transmitted through, and therefore the deeper its penetration into the tissue. Therefore, a red or IR laser would be ideal for coagulating structures deep to the RPE, while the RPE would almost fully absorb a green laser.

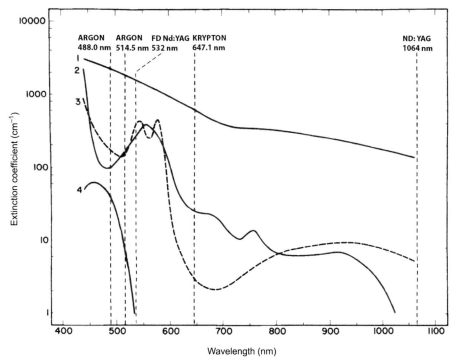

FIGURE 4-3 Visible absorption spectrum for melanin (curve 1), reduced hemoglobin (curve 2), oxyhemoglobin (curve 3), and macular xanthophyll (curve 4). Also shown are some common visible and infrared wavelength ocular lasers, showing the degree to which they are absorbed by each ocular pigment. For example, the FD Nd:YAG 532-nm laser is absorbed much more strongly by melanin compared to xanthophyll.[6] (Reprinted with permission from Mainster MA. Wavelength selection in macular photocoagulation. *Opthalmology.* 1986;93(7):952–958.) FD, frequency-doubled; Nd:YAG, neodymium yttrium aluminum garnet.

Hemoglobin is the iron-containing pigment that is present in the blood. It absorbs blue and green wavelengths very effectively. Yellows and oranges are less efficiently absorbed by hemoglobin while red wavelengths are the least absorbed.[7] A red krypton laser or an IR laser is often used to photocoagulate targets deep to regions of hemorrhage, allowing for coagulation of the bleeding structures without denaturing the blood just above it.

The xanthophylls in the macula (lutein and zeaxanthin) are pigments in the carotenoid group. Lutein is mostly present in the peripheral retina, while zeaxanthin is concentrated in the central retina. Xanthophylls are a brownish-yellow pigment, which are mostly present in the plexiform layers of the retina. They absorb UV and blue wavelengths very effectively, while absorption of longer wavelengths is less effective (green to red).[8] The blue 488-nm wavelength of an argon laser would be strongly absorbed by xanthophylls and would cause undesired damage to the macular region. Therefore, this wavelength is often filtered, allowing for only the green wavelength to exit the laser.

For pigment-dependent tissue interactions such as photocoagulation and photothermolysis, the level of pigment in the tissue can change what energy or power setting you might need to get the desired tissue response. For example, SLT is a pigment-dependent procedure in which a green SLT laser targets the melanosomes in the trabecular meshwork (TM).[9] The greater the level of pigment, the greater the absorption of the green laser light. Therefore, TMs with lighter pigment will need a higher energy setting than TMs with heavier pigment to have an equivalent tissue response.

If there is a loss in lens, aqueous, corneal, or vitreal transparency for any reason, the transmission of laser light directed towards the retina is reduced. If there is sclerosis or brunescence in the lens, the lens will begin absorbing more visible light intended to reach the retina, causing thermal effects in the lens and potentially speeding up cataract progression. Occasionally, a cataract extraction must be performed before a retinal laser procedure due to poor lens transparency. If there is significant corneal scarring, infiltration, or edema, the cornea will also absorb more laser light rather than transmitting it. This increases the chance of corneal burn. Inflammatory cells, flare, hyphema, and hemorrhages can reduce the transparency of the aqueous and vitreous. In this case, heating these protein-rich fluids can cause them to denature or coagulate, leading to inflammation.

LASER–TISSUE INTERACTIONS

Photothermal—Photocoagulation

Photocoagulation is a pigment-dependent interaction in which laser light is absorbed by one of the ocular pigments (usually melanin) and converted to heat. This heat causes a localized increase in temperature of about 50°F to 86°F (10°C–20°C increase). The tissue proteins are denatured, blood is coagulated, and moderate inflammation is induced. The inflammatory response, if controlled, can be very beneficial. For example, using a thermal laser to create scarring and adhesions can help control retinal holes, control tears, and repair detachments. There is also target and collateral tissue atrophy due to heat exchange with adjacent tissue for each laser spot.[10] When controlled, this can help reduce the relative oxygen demand of poorly perfused ischemic tissue, such as with pan-retinal photocoagulation for diabetic retinopathy.[11]

Photocoagulation not only denatures cellular proteins but can also affects collagen. The heat absorbed from the photothermal interaction causes collagen to contract, thus altering structural anatomy. Argon laser trabeculoplasty uses this effect.[12] A series of laser spots are spaced out over the patient's TM. The laser spots cause a local contraction of the collagen fibers in the TM, stretching them out and allowing better aqueous outflow from the anterior chamber into Schlemm's canal. Another example is a laser iridoplasty used to treat plateau iris.[13] In an iridoplasty, a thermal laser with a large spot size (and therefore low power density) is used to warm the collagen on the peripheral iris without denaturing the iris proteins. This causes a local contraction and draws the peripheral iris out and away from the angle. Focal photocoagulation is occasionally used to shrink the collagen in a blood vessel wall to lead to occlusion and stop bleeding or as a pretreatment prior to an iridotomy.

Photothermal—Photovaporization

Photovaporization is a form of photothermal tissue interaction and is very similar to photocoagulation in that it is a pigment-dependent tissue interaction. However, instead of warming the tissues to 50°F to 60°F, the tissues are instead warmed to 140°F to 212°F (60°C–100°C increase). Thus, instead of just denaturing proteins, the cellular water content boils and results in vaporization of the cellular contents. Photovaporization is desired when trying to burn a hole or channel through pigmented tissue like during a thermal iridotomy. It is rare in other ophthalmic surgeries due to the large amounts of inflammation and collateral damage introduced.

Photodisruption

Photodisruption is pigment independent, which means that the laser can affect pigmented as well as nonpigmented tissue. Photodisruption involves delivering large amounts of energy to very small focal spots in a very brief duration of time, resulting in a large power density. There is an instantaneous, localized temperature rise that occurs. The tissue is warmed by over 15,000°C, and the involved molecules are stripped of their electrons. In doing so, the involved tissue is explosively reduced to plasma. The plasma rapidly expands, causing an acoustic shockwave where most energy is directed anteriorly towards the front of the eye and physician.[14] This shockwave physically cleaves the tissue in its path.[15] The explosive laser–tissue interaction has a mechanical component, so it is sometimes described as a photomechanical disruption.

Even though the ionized tissue has a large increase in temperature, the temperature rise is so short that very little heat is transmitted to the adjacent tissue. This is because the laser energy is delivered in less time than the tissue's thermal relaxation time. If the laser energy is applied to a tissue for longer than the thermal relaxation time, heat is exchanged with the adjacent tissue, resulting in collateral damage. Since a photodisruptive laser has a mechanical tissue effect, a hemorrhage can result if a blood vessel is damaged. The localized, high heat during the interaction cannot be transferred to adjacent tissue, so coagulation of the vessel wall will not occur. For example, there is a higher rate of bleeding during a peripheral iridotomy with a photodisruptive Nd:YAG laser compared to a photothermal argon or green laser.

Photochemical or Photostimulation

Photostimulation occurs when light is used to change or activate a biological process in a cell or tissue. This involves light serving as a trigger for a change in shape of a protein or the uncaging of a compound. The process of phototransduction in the retina is an excellent example of photostimulation. The opsins in the retina (rhodopsin, melanopsin, and the photopsins) are naturally sensitive to light. Upon being stimulated by light, the opsins change from an all-*cis* to an all-*trans* isomerization which begins the process of converting absorbed light energy into a signal to be sent to the brain. Verteporfin is an example of a pharmaceutical agent being photo-activated from an inactive to an active compound to help treat choroidal neovascular membranes.[16]

Selective Photothermolysis

Selective photothermolysis is similar to photostimulation in that it induces a biological response. However, selective photothermolysis has a slightly different mechanism of action. Instead of targeting a specific molecule or protein to cause a chemical change, a pigment in the tissue is targeted using a specific wavelength of light. The pigment alone absorbs the laser light energy and is photodisrupted. By applying the laser energy in a rapid pulse that is shorter than the thermal relaxation time of the tissue, the target is disrupted, but no heat is exchanged with the adjacent tissues. SLT targets TM melanosomes and fragments them.[9] This triggers an inflammatory response where macrophages are recruited to digest the pigment fragments. This process ultimately allows for better aqueous outflow. Tattoo removal is very similar. The pigment in the ink is selectively targeted, and a photodisruptive interaction results in ink fragmentation. Macrophages can digest fragmented ink particles and over time, the tattoo will fade.

Photoablation

Photoablation is a laser–tissue interaction that occurs exclusively with an excimer laser. The excimer emits rapid pulses with resultant high-power density similar to the photodisruptive mechanism, but since the emitted wavelength is UV (193 nm), there is also a photochemical component. A single photon with a 193-nm wavelength has enough energy to cleave a carbon–carbon bond, resulting in a photochemical interaction. The photoablative interaction with the corneal tissue allows for precision sculpting of the cornea (Photorefractive keratectomy and Laser *in situ* keratomileusis), resulting in optimal correction of refractive error.[17]

Laser–tissue interactions depend on wavelength, characteristics of the target tissue, and laser parameters, including spot size, pulse duration, and laser energy. To properly apply laser energy to an ocular tissue, all of these factors must be completely understood.

REFERENCES

1. Blumenkranz MS. The evolution of laser therapy in ophthalmology: A perspective on the interactions between photons, patients, physicians, and physicists: The LXX Edward Jackson Memorial Lecture. *Am J Ophthalmol.* 2014;158:12–25 e1.
2. Boettner EA, Wolter JR. Transmission of the ocular media. *Invest Ophth Visual.* 1962;1:776–783.
3. Boulnois JL. Photophysical processes in recent medical laser developments: A review. *Quantel.* 1986;BP 23:91941.
4. Boulton M, Docchio F, Dayhaw-Barker P, et al. Age-related changes in the morphology, absorption and fluorescence of melanosomes and lipofuscin granules of the retinal pigment epithelium. *Vision Res.* 1990;30:1291–1303.
5. Birngruber R, Hillenkamp F, Gabel VP. Theoretical investigations of laser thermal retinal injury. *Health Phys.* 1985;48:781–796.
6. Mainster MA. Wavelength selection in macular photocoagulation. *Ophthalmology.* 1986;93(7): 952–958.
7. Horecker BL. The absorption spectra of hemoglobin and its derivatives in the visible and near infra-red regions. *J Biol Chem.* 1943;148:173–183.
8. Milanowska J, Gruszecki WI. Heat-induced and light-induced isomerization of the xanthophyll pigment zeaxanthin. *J Photochem Photobiol B.* 2005;80:178–186.
9. Leahy KE, White AJ. Selective laser trabeculoplasty: Current perspectives. *Clin Ophthalmol.* 2015;9:833–841.
10. Paulus YM, Jain A, Gariano RF, et al. Healing of retinal photocoagulation lesions. *Invest Ophthalmol Vis Sci.* 2008;49:5540–5545.
11. Palanker D, Blumenkranz MS. Panretinal photocoagulation for proliferative diabetic retinopathy. *Am J Ophthalmol.* 2012;153:780–781; author reply 1–2.
12. van der Zypen E, Bebie H, Fankhauser F. Morphological studies about the efficiency of laser beams upon the structures of the angle of the anterior chamber. Facts and concepts related to the treatment of the chronic simple glaucoma. *Int Ophthalmol.* 1979;1:109–122.
13. Ritch R, Tham CC, Lam DS. Argon laser peripheral iridoplasty (ALPI): An update. *Surv Ophthalmol.* 2007;52:279–288.
14. Fankhauser F. [Physical and biological effects of laser radiation (author's transl)]. *Klin Monbl Augenheilkd.* 1977;170:219–227.
15. Niemz, MH. *Laser-Tissue Interactions: Fundamentals and Applications.* Berlin/Heidelberg. Springer Science & Business Media; 2007:126.
16. Woodburn KW, Engelman CJ, Blumenkranz MS. Photodynamic therapy for choroidal neovascularization: A review. *Retina.* 2002;22:391–405; quiz 527–528.
17. Munnerlyn CR, Koons SJ, Marshall J. Photorefractive keratectomy: A technique for laser refractive surgery. *J Cataract Refract Surg.* 1988;14:46–52.

5 Laser Hazards, Safety, and Injuries

Aaron B. Zimmerman • Neal Whittle

Laser light is highly monochromatic, is highly coherent, is highly directional, and has a high-power density. Each of these things makes lasers useful for a variety of applications, including ophthalmic surgery. However, each of these attributes also makes laser light hazardous to the eye. Recognizing these hazards and taking steps to reduce them is vital to ensure the safety of the physician, their staff, and their patients.

TYPES OF HAZARDS

Some powerful lasers can represent a fire hazard, as they can ignite flammable substances. This is especially true for lasers used for thermal purposes. Lasers used for surgical purposes often require large amounts of electricity to operate, and therefore they can pose an electrical hazard. Chemical and biological hazards also exist. The previously mentioned dye lasers have a liquid medium that is highly carcinogenic.[1] The tissue plume created by the excimer laser during laser *in situ* keratomileusis and photorefractive keratectomy can also contain harmful particles such as viruses (including human immunodeficiency virus), bacteria, carcinogens, and other toxic aerosols.[2]

High-powered lasers can pose skin hazards.[1] Depending on the wavelength, the skin can suffer from either a thermal injury or a photochemical injury. *Thermal injuries* occur when longer wavelength light (low-energy photons) causes a heat-based denaturation of the tissue's proteins. *Photochemical injuries* result from shorter wavelengths (high-energy photons) damaging the tissue's deoxyribonucleic acid (DNA) by introducing free radicals or directly damaging the DNA base pairs. Cell membranes are particularly susceptible to free radicals, so once introduced to a localized tissue, significant damage can occur. Higher-energy light can also directly damage the base pairs on cellular DNA, eventually leading to cellular apoptosis and cell death if the damage is sufficient.

Eyes are particularly prone to laser injuries. Depending on the laser's wavelength, laser light might be absorbed in the cornea, lens, or retina (Table 5.1).[3] Visible wavelengths are particularly hazardous, as they can pass freely through the eye and damage the retina, leading to permanent vision loss. Similar to the skin, the eye is susceptible to thermal and photochemical injuries. Photoreceptors

TABLE 5-1 A COMPARISON OF OCULAR AND SKIN PATHOLOGICAL EFFECTS FROM DIFFERENT WAVELENGTH BANDS OF LASER LIGHT

WAVELENGTH	OCULAR EFFECT	SKIN EFFECT
UV C (100–280 nm)	Photokeratitis	Sunburn, skin cancer
UV B (280–315 nm)	Photokeratitis	Accelerated skin aging, increased pigmentation
UV A (315–400 nm)	Photochemical UV cataract	Pigment darkening, skin burn
Visible light (400–780 nm)	Photochemical and thermal retinal injury	Photosensitivity, skin burn
Infrared A (780–1400 nm)	Cataract, retinal burns	Skin burn
Infrared B (1400–3000 nm)	Corneal burn, aqueous flare, infrared cataract	Skin burn
Infrared C (3000–10000 nm)	Corneal burn	Skin burn

Occupational Safety and Health Administration.
UV, ultraviolet.

contain large amounts of cell membrane, and therefore photochemical-free radical damage from visible laser light can quickly cause a retinal injury.

CATEGORY OF RISK

The degree of hazard does not just depend on the laser's power but also depends on several other factors that, when combined, determine the type and severity of the damage.[1] These factors include the pulse time, the beam size, beam divergence, and wavelength. The beam width and divergence change the power density of the beam. A smaller diameter beam would be more dangerous than a larger beam, as the energy is concentrated in a smaller area. The wavelength of the laser comes into play as well. For example, a person exposed to an infrared (IR) beam would not perceive the beam as visible. The individual would not blink or turn away due to this lack of sensitivity and would be at a greater thermal risk to the eye than a visible beam of equivalent power.

Lasers are grouped into four major categories based on the level of risk they present, particularly to the eye. There are two laser classification systems. The first system was developed in the 1970s and is still used today by the U.S. Food and Drug Administration (FDA). In 2002, the International Electrotechnical Commission (IEC) developed a revised classification system, which has been gradually phased in. The revised system's main purpose is taking the previous system and adding in the concept of maximum permissible exposure, which is the highest power density of laser light that is considered safe to the eye. Both the old and revised systems are currently accepted by the American National Standards Institute (ANSI) and the FDA. Both systems have four classifications, with the risk increasing with higher classes. Higher-risk lasers may damage the eye within the blink response time (0.25 s)[1], while

TABLE 5-2 COMPARISON OF FOOD AND DRUG ADMINISTRATION AND INTERNATIONAL ELECTROTECHNICAL COMMISSION CLASSES, LASER HAZARDS, AND CLASS EXAMPLES

FDA CLASS	IEC CLASS	LASER HAZARD	EXAMPLES
I	1, 1M	Considered nonhazardous	Blu-ray players, laser printers
II	2, 2M	Nonhazardous if viewed for times shorter than the blink response time; can cause damage at extreme exposure times (1000 s)	Barcode scanners
IIIa	3R	Low risk of injury at exposure times less than blink response time	Laser pointers
IIIb	3B	Exposure hazard from direct and specular reflection	Some Q-Switched Nd:YAG lasers
IV	4	Exposure hazard from direct, specular, and diffuse reflection	Most ophthalmic surgical lasers

FDA, Food and Drug Administration; IEC, International Electrotechnical Commission; Nd: YAG, neodymium yttrium aluminum garnet.

lower-risk lasers might require significantly more time. The FDA classification system uses Roman numerals (I–IV) while the revised IEC classification uses Arabic numerals (1–4).[4] Using the FDA classification system, examples of each laser class are found in the following section (Table 5.2):

Class I

Class I lasers are unable to emit a hazardous level of light under normal use. Class I laser devices can include lasers that might be classified as more hazardous but are enclosed in a way that they are not for viewing, such as a Blu-ray player or a laser printer.

Class II

Class II lasers are considered to be relatively safe. They are visible wavelength lasers (400–700 nm) that must be less than 1 mW. Any direct exposure shorter than the blink response time (0.25 s) will cause no damage to the retina. To produce retinal damage, the laser must be exposed to the retina for up to 1000 seconds, which is nearly 17 minutes.

Class III (IIIa and IIIb)

Class III lasers are divided into two subcategories, IIIa and IIIb. Class IIIa lasers are visible wavelength lasers of powers between 1 mW and less than 5 mW. They are considered "safe" when exposure is less than the blink response time but only safe in the sense that they will not cause injury to the retina. They may still cause temporary flash blindness by bleaching the photoreceptors. Most handheld laser pointers fall into this category.

Class IIIb lasers are visible lasers between 5 mW and 500 mW of power or any ultraviolet and IR laser 500 mW and below. These lasers represent a direct exposure hazard, meaning they can damage the retina within the blink response time if the beam is viewed directly or by specular reflection. Specific controls, such as protective filters, are recommended but not required by the Occupational Safety and Health Administration (OSHA) or the FDA. Some Q-Switched neodymium yttrium aluminum garnet (Nd:YAG) lasers used for capsulotomies and peripheral iridotomies are Class IIIb, but some are class IV.

Class IV

Class IV lasers are the most hazardous lasers in the classification system. They are lasers of any wavelength with a power greater than 500 mW. They can cause injury by direct viewing, specular reflection, and diffuse reflection. Most ophthalmic lasers fall into this category. Eye protection is required when operating class IV lasers.

LASER SAFETY REGULATIONS

There are several regulatory bodies that oversee the use of lasers in various settings, including ophthalmic surgery. In the United States, the development and use of laser safety standards is overseen by ANSI. Laser safety standards fall under ANSI Z136 and have several subcategories depending on what applications the laser will be used in, how to evaluate and protect against laser hazards, and the labeling and testing of protective equipment. The Z136.1 standard specifically covers the general use, hazards, and safety of lasers and serves as the parent document for all other ANSI laser standards. Z136.3 covers safe laser use in all health care fields, including ophthalmic use. It is a comprehensive resource that details laser hazards, non-beam hazards, training, administrative protocols, protective equipment, warning signage, and more. OSHA enforces laser safety standards to ensure employees' safety and well-being. Laser safety is covered in Section III: Chapter 6 of the OSHA Technical Manual, with specific control measures that are recommended (Class IIIb) or required (Class IV), depending on the class of laser being used.[1]

There are also regulatory bodies that oversee the manufacture and sale of lasers. The FDA regulates the sale of lasers in the United States, including those used in medical settings. Some lasers are exempt from FDA regulation if they are designed so that they are not for viewing under normal operation (e.g., a laser printer or DVD player). Lasers used for ophthalmic purposes are typically more hazardous. Therefore, they have stricter regulations such as keyed access, protective housings and interlocks, filters, shutters, a means of measuring laser output, and emergency stops. Each laser used for surgical or therapeutic purposes requires either FDA 510 k clearance or premarket approval.

SAFETY MEASURES

Safety control measures recommended by ANSI, OSHA, and the FDA either deal with how the laser is engineered or how the laser is used and labeled.

The FDA and OSHA require all of the following features to be present on Class IIIb or IV lasers to be sold in the United States: protective housing, safety interlocks, key control (Fig. 5.1), emission indicator, warning labels (Fig. 5.2), filters on viewing optics, and beam attenuators/shutters.[5] The protective housing prevents access to the internal parts of the laser. Safety interlocks are circuits that will not let the laser fire if certain conditions are not met, such as if the laser cavity is open or the central tower of the slit lamp is in the path of the beam. A key control to turn on the laser prevents unauthorized operation.

To properly measure the laser output, especially for ophthalmic surgery, all ophthalmic lasers will have some sort of display with both the current power/energy and the total cumulative power/energy to aid the physician in performing a laser

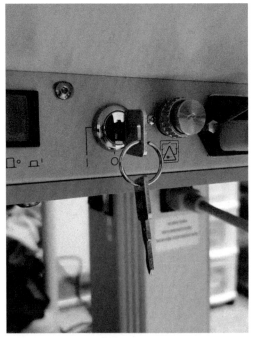

FIGURE 5-1 A key used to turn on the ophthalmic laser. It is unable to be removed in the "On" position.

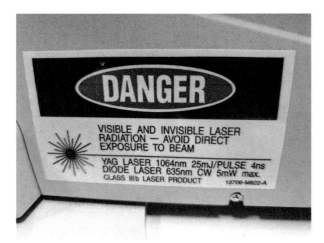

FIGURE 5-2 A warning label for a Class IIIb YAG laser showing the max energy per pulse, the pulse time, class, as well as the power of the aiming diode laser.
YAG, yttrium aluminum garnet.

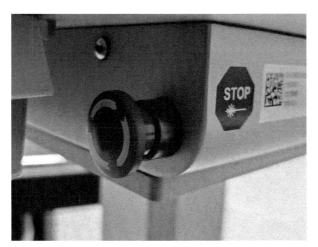

FIGURE 5-3 An emergency shutoff button on an ophthalmic laser.

procedure safely. All laser products have a warning label of some kind showing the degree of hazard presented by the laser and its class.

Laser light can be reflected from ocular media. Therefore, filters that filter out the laser's specific wavelength must be built into the laser's viewing oculars[5] therefore it is not necessary to wear laser safety goggles when viewing through the oculars.

Ophthalmic lasers must also have protective shutters that can be activated with an emergency shutoff switch or button (Fig. 5.3). This will instantly shut the laser down.

Besides the various engineering safety features that must be present on class IIIb and class IV lasers, there are also administrative and procedure controls to observe.[1]

The Laser Safety Officer (LSO) is "an individual designated by the employer with the authority and responsibility to effect the knowledgeable evaluation and control of laser hazards, and to monitor and enforce the control of such hazards."[6] A LSO is required for both class IIIb and class IV lasers. The LSO is responsible for maintaining safety standards, laser maintenance, education and training, investigation of accidents, and more.

Standard Operating Procedures are simply documents that detail how to safely interact with the laser, the possible hazards, and what to do during an emergency. They are recommended for class IIIb lasers and required for class IV.

Education and training are important for both the laser operators, the patient, and any support staff to minimize the risk of an accident. Also, area access must be limited to qualified or authorized personnel. In some cases, this means having the lasers locked in their own space with keyed or coded access. Appropriate warning signs (Fig. 5.4) relevant to each type of laser present must also be posted around the laser area.

The Nominal Hazard Zone (NHZ) must be determined and respected for each type of laser. The NHZ is the area around the laser in which there is a significant risk of eye injury. The size of the NHZ may be different for different lasers. For some lasers, it is the immediate area around the laser itself plus the beam's path. For others (particularly class IV), it is the size of the room that the laser is in.

Laser filters are among the most important safety measures to minimize the risk of eye damage from laser exposure. As previously stated, filters designed to absorb the specific wavelength that the laser produces are built into class IIIb and class IV lasers' oculars. Therefore, laser goggles are not necessary. However, there may be support staff, a student clinician, or a resident present in some cases, in which case laser safety goggles would be required.

Optical density (OD) is a measure of how well a filter blocks a particular wavelength. It is inversely proportional to transmission, which means that the higher the OD, the lower the transmission. An OD of zero is 100% transmission. OD is set on a logarithmic scale, such that each successive increase in OD decreases transmission by a factor of 10. Therefore, a filter with an OD of 1 has a 10% transmission, while an OD of 2 means transmission of 1%, and so on (Table 5.3).

The filters will have the OD and the wavelength they are designed to filter out printed on or engraved on the lens.[6] Some filters may have multiple optical densities for different wavelengths. Laser filters are a powerful safeguard against accidental laser injuries. However, there is no "one size fits all" laser filter. Each filter is designed with a particular laser in mind. A filter designed to block the IR wavelengths of the Nd:YAG laser would not protect someone from a 532-nm visible green wavelength (Fig 5.5).

In the ophthalmologic setting, there are two main reasons for laser-induced eye injuries:

1. Not using protective filter eyewear even when it is available.
2. Peeking around protective filter eyewear even when it is being used.

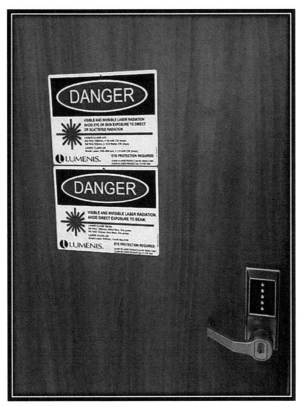

FIGURE 5-4 The door to a laser room with proper signage displaying the laser class as well as keyed and coded access to limit area access to qualified and authorized personnel.

TABLE 5-3 OPTICAL DENSITY AND PERCENT TRANSMISSION

OPTICAL DENSITY	PERCENT TRANSMISSION
0	100
1	10
2	1
3	0.1
4	0.01
5	0.001
6	0.0001
7	0.00001

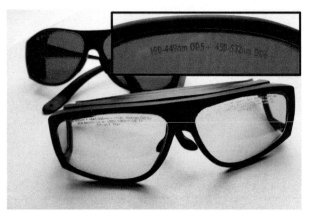

FIGURE 5-5 Laser safety glasses are optimized to filter out certain wavelengths of light. The orange glasses above are designed to filter out green light, while the green filters above are designed to filter out infrared light. Laser safety glasses can provide protection against multiple bandwidths. For example, the orange-colored glasses have an OD of 5+ for 190–499 nm and an OD of 6+ for 450–532 nm.
OD, optical density.

If you are operating a class IV laser, the safest place in the room is looking through the slit lamp viewing oculars, as they have filters built in that will block any reflected laser light. Do not look around the oculars when using an ophthalmic laser. If a person is in the room with a Class IV laser that is armed and is not performing the procedure, they are required by law to wear proper protective eyewear that is rated for that specific laser. Choose your protective eyewear accordingly and make sure to follow all safety protocols.

LASER INJURIES

Though laser ocular injuries may have occurred prior to 1964, Rathkey published the first detailed account of a retinal laser injury.[7] A student was adjusting a ruby laser when it accidentally misfired, resulting in a photocoagulative retinal lesion, which resulted in 20/200 visual acuity. Since lasers can be found in medicine, the military, entertainment, academia, industrial settings, and at home, any individual using or around a laser could suffer an injury.

As discussed previously, lasers emit a beam of concentrated light that, in certain circumstances, can deliver extremely high-power densities and be detrimental to ocular structures, not limited to, but most often, the retina. Depending on the offending laser's parameters and the distance from the laser, the ocular tissue can suffer photothermal, photodisruptive, or photochemical damage.[8] In addition to laser parameters, several factors can exacerbate or minimize the damage suffered from laser exposure. If an individual has a large physiologic pupil or is dilated or is exposed to a laser while using binoculars or a telescope, they will suffer a worse outcome. If an individual has an uncorrected refractive error or is accommodating when exposed, the laser image size will increase, which will result in a relatively better outcome.[8]

The location of the laser injury is also important. If the laser damages a non-foveal region, it may be detectable but generally will not cause visual impairment. If the fovea or parafoveal regions are involved, then instant vision loss can occur depending on the type of laser.[9]

Laser injuries can occur anywhere, and oftentimes the injury is an innocent mistake, though deliberate injuries can certainly occur. The military is a common occupation where individuals use lasers for various tasks, and improper training can lead to significant visual consequences. In 2003, Harris et al. reviewed military laser eye injuries.[8] In the military, lasers are used for range finding and guiding ordinance, among other applications. When laser injuries occur in the military, it is usually from poor device labeling, inadequate training, poorly engineered safety mechanisms, or accidental training exposures.[8] Lasers have also been intentionally used in conflicts to injure opposition soldiers, which has led to countries signing agreements to minimize lasers' intentional use to incapacitate adversaries.[10]

Other individuals generally at risk of laser exposure are airline pilots. The number of laser exposures suffered by commercial airline pilots is estimated to be around 3,000 per year[11] with a trend of increasing exposures.[12] Pilots have been exposed to lasers in military operations[13] but the typical exposures are likely due to individuals using a class IIIa or IIIb laser pointer. Laser exposures shined into the cockpit often result in dazzle or temporary blindness, but fortunately, most do not result in permanent ocular damage.[12] Due to the potential of a significant air disaster resulting from temporary blindness, there are significant penalties if an individual is caught shining a laser toward a plane.

The general public is not generally at risk of high-powered pulsed lasers, but rather handheld laser pointers. These laser pointers should be classified as an FDA IIIa with a laser output of less than 5 mW. Since the typical laser pointer should be less than 5 mW, then exposures of 250 ms or less should not result in permanent retinal injury. It is thought that 10 seconds of uninterrupted exposure is necessary to develop a retinal lesion.[14] Unfortunately, many laser pointers are manufactured with outputs far exceeding 5 mW and are obtained easily on the internet. Through a simple search on the internet, laser pointers up to 50,000 mW can be purchased for under $200.00.[15] These lasers are capable of causing retinal damage rapidly. A case report by Wyrsch et al. describes a 15-year-old boy who had access to a 150-mW laser pointer, which reflected off of a mirror and entered each of his eyes resulting in permanently impaired vision.[16] The laser pointer looked very similar to the typical 5-mW device and could not be differentiated without inspecting the labeled output. They concluded that individuals in possession of these laser pointers cannot distinguish a harmful one from a non-harmful one.[16]

Recently, Bhavsar et al. reviewed handheld laser pointer injuries.[11] They note that the first reported laser pointer macular injury was published in 1999. Since then, there are reports on 171 individuals with confirmed laser pointer retinal injuries. Individuals suffering from these injuries ranged from ages 6 to 46+ years, with 75% of the injuries occurring in individuals less than 20 years of age, and 80% were males. Most of the injuries occurred in the United States and Britain, and 85% of the cases involved high-powered lasers (i.e., those over 5 mW).[11]

If a laser injury occurs with a pulsed laser, for example, a Q-switched Nd:YAG-range finder, instant photodisruptive damage will occur to the retina. Depending on the proximity of the light–tissue interaction with retinal blood vessels, a vitreous, preretinal, intraretinal, or choroidal hemorrhage could develop. If a fluorescein angiography (FANG) is administered, the presence of a hemorrhage will initially result in a hypofluorescent signal. Much of the laser energy is absorbed by the retinal pigment epithelium (RPE), and the photoreceptors will suffer permanent structural and functional impairment. Following the resolution of a retinal hemorrhage, the resulting damage to the RPE will often result in FANG hyperfluorescence, or with autofluorescent imaging, a hypo-autofluorescent signal.[9] Significant retinal fibrosis can ultimately develop, causing hyper-reflective signals on optical coherence tomography (OCT). Exposure to a pulsed laser, such as a Q-switched Nd:YAG or pulsed ruby laser, would most often occur in military operations or academic or industrial settings. Typical reasons for these exposures are not wearing appropriate safety eyewear, poor equipment design, poor labeling, or attempting to align the beam without following safety protocols. Figure 5.6 is a laser injury that occurred when a laser was being adjusted.

The retinal findings associated with laser injuries suffered from handheld laser pointers range from mild mottling of the RPE to full-thickness macular holes and macular scars. The Bhavsar article reported that with OCT on initial presentation, 98% of the cases showed evidence of retinal disruption.[11] Over 50% of those cases had evidence of damage to the ellipsoid zone or the RPE. Macular holes were present in 21%, and vertical hyper-reflective bands extending from the outer segments to the outer plexiform were noted. At final evaluation, damage to the ellipsoid zone was the most common finding on OCT, with damage to the RPE the next most common. At resolution, macular holes were present in 7%. Contrary to pulsed lasers, retinal hemorrhages were only found in 8% of these reported cases. Final visual acuity following a laser pointer injury ranged from 20/32 to 20/630 with a median of 20/32.[11]

The clinical management of laser injuries includes acquiring a detailed history, running proper diagnostic tests, and providing appropriate treatment. Mainster et al. developed six criteria that should be met to diagnose a retinal laser injury properly.[9] (1) The first criterion is to evaluate ocular changes consistent with laser–tissue interactions. (2) If a possible laser injury is present, has it been assessed using diagnostic techniques such as FANG, fundus photos—including autofluorescence, and OCT? (3) Did the lesion evolve or heal in a manner consistent with a laser–retinal injury? (4) If such a lesion is present, are there significant vision complaints present? (5) Do those visual complaints objectively match the retinal findings? (6) If the offending laser can be obtained, are the laser parameters capable of producing the clinical

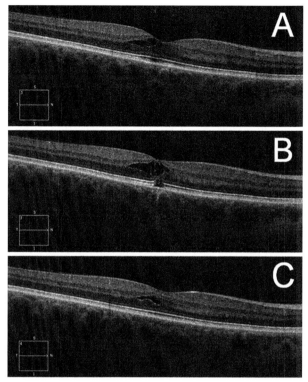

FIGURE 5-6 Laser eye injury that occurred 17 years prior to this five-line raster OCT scan. The individual remains 20/20 with minor Amsler grid metamorphopsia. In panel **A** (superior scan), a persistent intraretinal macular cyst is present with evidence of damage to the RPE. Panel **B** (middle scan) shows significant damage to the RPE, outer segments, myoid and ellipsoid zones, external limiting membrane, and the outer nuclear layer. Also present is the macular cyst. Panel **C** (inferior scan) shows no evidence of outer retinal or RPE damage.
OCT, optical coherence tomography; RPE, retinal pigment epithelium.

findings? As mentioned previously, if the laser can be obtained, the power output should be labeled on the device.

There is no single treatment for retinal laser injuries and no available proven therapy. Time is essential, particularly for the resolution of hemorrhages. Oral corticosteroids have been used with conflicting outcomes.[17,18] Surgical procedures to repair macular holes (Alsulaiman) in some cases have been demonstrated to improve outcomes.[19] The best treatment for a retinal laser injury is to prevent it in the first place. Increased regulation to limit both the production of and access to high-powered handheld lasers would help prevent serious injuries. Placing restrictions or clearer warnings on distributor websites and the devices themselves could educate the public and those who purchase the devices. In military, industrial, and academic/research settings, protocols should be established and strictly followed.

A patient of one of the authors was seen a few years ago for a routine exam. She had reported that she suffered a laser eye injury while adjusting the beam in her lab several years before. She said she knew better than to adjust the beam without safety glasses, but she neglected to wear them that moment in an effort to be efficient. She shared that since that day, whenever working in the lab, silently, she repeats to herself, "never look into or adjust the laser with your remaining good eye…".

REFERENCES

1. Occupational Safety and Health Administration. Laser Hazards, OSHA Technical Manual, Section III, Chapter 6 (n.d.) Retrieved from www.osha.gov/dts/osta/otm/otm_iii/otm_iii_6.html. Last Accessed September 1, 2020.
2. Bargman H. Laser-generated Airborne Contaminants. *J Clin Aesthet Dermatol.* 2011;4:56–57.
3. Boettner EA, Wolter JR. Transmission of the ocular media. *Invest Ophth Visual.* 1962;1:776–783.
4. US Food & Drug Administration. Laser products and instruments. Retrieved from https://www.fda.gov/radiation-emitting-products/home-business-and-entertainment-products/laser-products-and-instruments. Last Accessed September 1, 2020.
5. US Food & Drug Administration. Compliance guide for laser products (FDA 86-8260); 1992. Retrieved from https://www.fda.gov/regulatory-information/search-fda-guidance-documents/compliance-guide-laser-products-fda-86-8260. Last Accessed September 1, 2020.
6. American National Standards Institute. *Safe Use of Lasers (ANSI Z136.1).* Laser Orlando, FL: Institute of America; 2014.
7. Rathkey AS. Accidental laser burn of the macula. *Arch Ophthalmol.* 1965;74:346–348.
8. Harris MD, Lincoln AE, Amoroso PJ, et al. Laser eye injuries in military occupations. *Aviat Space Environ Med.* 2003;74:947–952.
9. Mainster MA, Stuck BE, Brown J Jr. Assessment of alleged retinal laser injuries. *Arch Ophthalmol.* 2004;122:1210–1217.
10. Seet B, Wong TY. Military laser weapons: Current controversies. *Ophthalmic Epidemiol.* 2001;8: 215–226.
11. Bhavsar KV, Michel Z, Greenwald M, Cunningham ET, Freund KB. Retinal injury from handheld lasers: A review. *Surv Ophthalmol.* 2021;66:231–260.
12. Palakkamanil MM, Fielden MP. Effects of malicious ocular laser exposure in commercial airline pilots. *Can J Ophthalmol.* 2015;50:429–432.
13. Barkana Y, Belkin M. Laser eye injuries. *Surv Ophthalmol.* 2000;44:459–478.
14. Sliney DH, Dennis JE. Safety concerns about laser pointers. *J Laser Appl.* 1994;6:159–164.
15. Laserpointerpro.com. Retrieved at https://www.laserpointerpro.com/50000mw-520nm-burning-high-power-green-laser-pointer-kits-gt-990-p-3906.html. Last Accessed September 1, 2020.
16. Wyrsch S, Baenninger PB, Schmid MK. Retinal injuries from a handheld laser pointer. *N Engl J Med.* 2010;363:1089–1091.
17. Lam TT, Takahashi K, Fu J, Tso MOM. Methylprednisolone therapy in laser injury of the retina. *Graefes Arch Clin Exp Ophthalmol.* 1993;231:729–736.
18. Schuschereba ST, Cross ME, Scales DK, et al. High dose methylprednisolone treatment of laser-induced retinal injury exacerbates acute inflammation and long-term scarring. *P Soc Photo-Opt Ins.* 1999;3591:430–447.
19. Alsulaiman SM, Alrushood AA, Almasaud J, et al. High-power handheld blue laser-induced maculopathy: The results of the King Khaled Eye Specialist Hospital Collaborative Retina Study Group. *Ophthalmology.* 2014;121:566–572 e1.

SECTION 2

Corneal Laser Procedures

6 Photorefractive Keratectomy

Karl Stonecipher • Andrew S. Whitley • Marguerite B. McDonald

The first introduction of the excimer (excited dimer) laser came to the forefront in the 1970s. The original work came from a laser utilizing a xenon dimer gas produced by Basov et al.[1] In 1976, Hoffman et al. published their work on a laser using an ultraviolet (UV) noble-gas halide laser. This work was followed by Burnham et al. using lasers that included xenon–fluoride, krypton–fluoride, and argon–fluoride gases.[2,3] It would not find its way to the cornea until the 1980s. Originally, Taboada et al. published work on the response of the corneal epithelium to krypton–fluoride excimer laser pulses (248 nm).[4] In another lab, Srinivasan et al. used an argon–fluoride excimer laser with a wavelength of 193 nm on organic tissue.[5,6] From the mid 1980s to early 1990s, multiple patents were filed and issued by Baron, Munnerlyn, Blum/Srinivasan, L'Esperance, Peyman, Bille, Warner, Telfair, Azema, Koziol, and Kohayakawa leading up to the Munnerlyn patent for photorefractive keratectomy (PRK) originally filed in 1987 and issued in 1992 after much legal debate[7–25] (Fig. 6.1).

Although multiple people are responsible for the development of PRK, everyone agrees it was in 1983 that Dr. Steven Trokel began research with Drs. Srinivasan, Wynne, Blum, Braren, Cotliar, Schubert, Mandel, Marshall, Rothery, Schubert, and Krueger. In 1985, Dr. Seiler et al. performed the first large area ablation for phototherapeutic keratectomy of a corneal dystrophy. The first human sighted eye to be enucleated was performed on March 25, 1988 by Marguerite McDonald, M.D. For a more detailed history, Reinstein et al. have published a more in-depth review of this topic.[26]

The procedure replaced incisional radial keratotomy (RK) as the leading refractive surgery in the early 1990s. It quickly gained popularity among surgeon's for the treatment of myopia, hyperopia, and astigmatism. In 1994, the Food and Drug Administration (FDA) panel recommended approval for phototherapeutic keratectomy and in 1995 finally approved the first excimer laser for phototherapeutic keratectomy.[27–30] In the following year, the Summit and VISX lasers were both approved for PRK.[31,32] Since its origin, there has been significant improvement in the PRK technique such as the inclusion of wave front technology, topographic technology, increased treatment zone diameter and blending, and enhanced epithelial removal techniques.

PRK corrects ametropia by a two-step method of epithelial removal and stromal photoablative resurfacing. Step 1 is epithelial removal and may be performed by three differing methods depending on the surgeon's choice. These methods of removal are

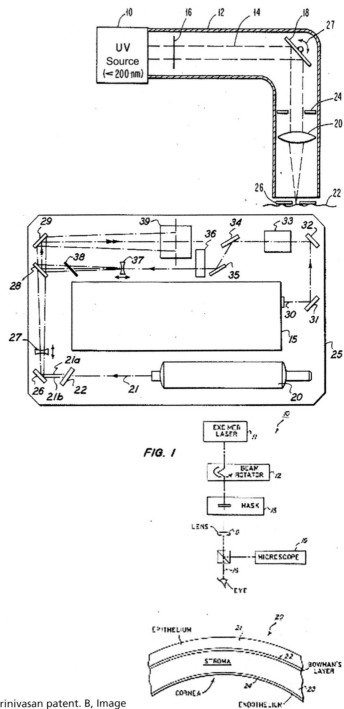

FIGURE 6-1 A, Image Srinivasan patent. B, Image Munnerlyn patent. C, Image Munnerlyn patent. UV, ultraviolet.

Munnerlyn Theoretical Exact Ablation Depth

$$= R_1 - \frac{R_1 \cdot (n-1)}{n-1+R_1 \cdot D}$$
$$- \sqrt{R_1^2 - \frac{OZ^2}{4}}$$
$$+ \sqrt{\left[\frac{R_1 \cdot (n-1)}{n-1+R_1 \cdot D}\right]^2 - \frac{OZ^2}{4}}$$

where n is the refractive index of the cornea (1,376) D is the correction in diopecers, and the other variables are illustrated in Figure 1.

FIGURE 6-2 Shown is the original Munnerlyn's formula.

mechanical, chemical, or laser. For step 2, PRK employs a 193-nm argon–fluoride excimer laser to photoablate the anterior corneal stroma and reshape the cornea, thus correcting the ametropia. The Munnerlyn's formula or algorithm was an adaptation from Barraquer's earlier formulas to calculate the ablation profile based on refractive error and zone diameter[33] (Fig. 6.2).

The PRK procedure required a longer healing period, which allowed laser-assisted in situ keratomileusis (LASIK) to surpass its total volume in the mid 1990s but never was PRK replaced entirely by LASIK. LASIK and PRK have proven to give comparable results in visual acuity, but LASIK's fast recovery time has placed it as the procedure of choice in many of the decisions for laser vision correction (LVC).[34,35] Despite PRK having a slower healing time, there are several long-term theoretical advantages of choosing PRK rather than LASIK. Some of these advantages include less tissue ablation, less risk to trauma, and avoidance of flap complications that may be seen with the LASIK procedure. Because of these perceived benefits, PRK remains a steady option for eyes that are unable to have LASIK due to patient/doctor preference, corneal thickness/integrity, or patient lifestyle needs.

INDICATIONS

Key Indications

- Myopia
- Hyperopia
- Astigmatism
- Therapeutic (topography-guided treatments in abnormal corneas)

Myopia is the most treated ametropia by PRK. There are multiple approved devices with treatments ranging from 0D to –13D of myopia, 0D to +5D of hyperopia, and 0D to 6D of astigmatism.[31] Dioptric limitations vary from study to study, but the generally accepted range for myopia is up to −8D with astigmatism up to 4D. Treating above these values increases the risk of corneal haze and has less predictability in refractive error outcomes. Most sources recommend treatment of astigmatism up to but not greater than 6D. Hyperopic treatments are less common, but most accepted guidelines recommend treatment from +0.75D to +3D. Most of the approved devices are for treating patients over the age of 18 but with appropriate consent and stable refractive errors less than 18 years of age can be considered on a case-by-case basis. It is also important to be aware of your device approval ranges as these vary from company to company and device to device.[35]

There has been significant success in using topography-guided PRK to treat beyond these parameters such as cases of extremely high refractive error, irregular astigmatism, posttransplant irregular corneas, and stable keratoconus.[36-38] Often, topography-guided PRK is the treatment of choice for corneal complications from prior refractive surgeries such as decentered ablations or small optical zones. Surface irregularities such as those seen in anterior corneal dystrophies may also be treated with excimer lasers in a stand-alone surface ablation without refractive correction Phototherapeutic Keratectomy (PTK), or with simultaneous correction of refractive error (PRK).

Wound healing has been described in both PRK and LASIK.[39] Some authors believe that because of trauma-induced flap complications, PRK is a better option than LASIK for any individual whose lifestyle places them at a higher risk for ocular trauma.[40,41]

ALTERNATIVES TO THE PHOTOREFRACTIVE KERATECTOMY PROCEDURE

There are several other alternatives for the correction of myopia and myopic astigmatism:

- Glasses or contact lenses
- Artificial lens implanted inside the eye
- Wave front–guided or corneal topography–assisted LASIK
- LASIK or refractive lenticule extraction using standard eye measurements

Each alternative has its own advantages and disadvantages and should be fully discussed with the patient before these alternatives should be considered and the patient should select the method that best meets their expectations and lifestyle.[42]

CONTRAINDICATIONS

PRK is an elective procedure and therefore strict screening protocols should be used to ensure that the patient is not put at risk. All absolute and relative contraindications should be found at the screening evaluation. It is worth noting that most contraindications to consider in PRK are even stronger concerns in LASIK because of reduced stromal bed thickness caused by LASIK flap creation.

Absolute Contraindications

Key Absolute Contraindications

- Visually significant cataract
- Unstable glaucoma
- Keratoconus, forme fruste keratoconus, and thin corneas
- Unstable refractive scenarios
- Deep corneal scar
- Active connective tissue disease (i.e., rheumatoid arthritis, systemic lupus)
- Severe dry eye disease (i.e., Sjögren's disease)
- Uncontrolled diabetes
- Active ocular diseases or inflammation (i.e., herpes simplex, herpes zoster)

Cataract

Eyes with visually significant cataracts or that have had cataract-induced refractive shifts should not be considered for LVC.[43]

Glaucoma

Because PRK can alter corneal thickness and hysteresis measurements, and therefore intraocular pressure (IOP) accuracy, it should be avoided in unstable glaucoma. However, many surgeon's have successfully performed PRK on glaucoma suspects and even those with controlled mild-to-moderate glaucoma. That is why most surgeon's believe PRK in controlled glaucoma is an option after informed consent.[44]

Keratoconus and Thin Corneas

The greatest consideration in LVC is that of corneal thickness and integrity. At-risk eyes due to thin corneas, forme fruste keratoconus, and keratoconus should be found in preoperative screening and excluded from candidacy. In therapeutic cases of stable keratoconus or eyes that have been cross-linked, PRK has been successfully done to alleviate some of the refractive error and treat the corneal irregularities. Although corneal ectasia and keratoconus are more likely to occur after LASIK, they have occurred after PRK. Thinner corneas, keratoconus, and forme fruste keratoconus can lead to complications after PRK surgery. These complications may result in the need for additional therapeutic surgery.[45–47]

Unstable Refractive Scenarios

Uncontrolled diabetes, pregnancy, nursing mothers, and certain medications such as amiodarone, isotretinoin, sumatriptan, and others can cause unstable refractive error, and therefore patients should not have PRK while on these medications or dealing with these conditions. In that regard, any unstable refractive error case should be advised against surgery.[48,49]

Deep Corneal Scars

PRK remains the best LVC option for many eyes, which have stable mild corneal scars from trauma, keratitis, or prior refractive surgical cuts like in RK. However, significant central corneal scars should not be lasered, especially if located in the posterior two thirds of the corneal stroma.[50–52]

Active Connective Tissue Disease

As early as 1992, Seiler et al. noted potential complications in patients with auto-immune disease and considered it an absolute contraindication. Any type of active connective tissue disease (e.g., rheumatoid arthritis), or active autoimmune disease (i.e., lupus), is not an option for an elective procedure like PRK. These conditions affect the body's ability to heal. However, inactive or controlled connective tissue disease is a controversial issue.[53,54]

Severe Dry Eye Disease

If patients have severely dry eyes, PRK may exacerbate this condition. This may or may not resolve with time and healing. Severe eye dryness may delay healing of the surgery. It may result in poor vision after PRK, which may be permanent.[55]

Uncontrolled Diabetes

Patients with poorly controlled diabetes can be a challenge prior to surgery in obtaining a stable refraction and after surgery have risk of poor healing and aberrant outcomes.[49,56]

Active Ocular Diseases or Inflammation

Patients with active eye infections or inflammation of the eye, such as recent herpes eye infections, should not be considered as candidates for an elective procedure like PRK.[57]

Relative Contraindications

Key Relative Contraindications

- Predispositions
- Connective tissue disease
- Immune compromise (systemic disease, i.e., human immunodeficiency virus [HIV] or pharmacological)
- Systemic medications (i.e., isotretinoin, sumatriptan, amiodarone)

- Keloids
- Mild corneal scars
- Herpes simplex keratitis or herpes zoster (inactive)
- Dry eye disease
- Ocular surface disease or abnormalities (i.e., anterior corneal dystrophies)
- Glaucoma
- Unstable or irregular topography or refractive error
- Amblyopia
- Monocular
- Binocular anomaly
- Age
- Psychological factors
- Pacemaker

Predispositions

The surgeon should consider systemic medications (i.e., Accutane or isotretinoin, Imitrex or sumatriptan, or Cordarone or amiodarone hydrochloride) the patient is taking. The surgeon should also consider any systemic or ocular condition that may predispose the eye to scarring or infection such as connective tissue disease, keloid formers, prior herpes simplex keratitis (HSK), ocular rosacea, and other causes of corneal neovascularization. If the patient's vision has not been stable and they have signs of increasing or unstable nearsightedness, eye disease, eye abnormality, previous eye surgery, or injury in the treatment area of the eye, PRK should not be considered an option. With refractive error that is outside the range of the surgeon's laser-approved range, it is not known if PRK is safe and effective outside those limits. Some surgeon's consider reducing but not elimination of refractive error as an option in select patients with appropriate informed consent. Re-treatments carry additional risks and should be discussed with the patient. It is possible following PRK treatment that patients can have reduced contrast sensitivity and will find it more difficult to see in conditions such as very dim light, rain, snow, fog, or glare from bright lights at night. A patient with a family history of thinning of the cornea or other degenerative corneal disease (i.e., keratoconus, pellucid marginal degeneration, Fuchs corneal dystrophy, granular corneal dystrophy (Types 1 and 2), and lattice corneal dystrophy) may not be a good candidate for PRK.[58,59]

Connective tissue disease

If the patient has a systemic disease that may affect wound healing, such as uncontrolled autoimmune or connective tissue disease, or uncontrolled diabetes, then it is imperative for the physician and the patient to acknowledge and document those risks and document those discussions and the potential risks and the issues with outcomes with the patient.

Immune compromise

If the patient has an immunocompromised status or takes medications that may result in a weakened immune system, such as antimetabolites, which can increase the risk of infection, then discussion and education to the patient need to be taken prior to surgical intervention.[60]

Isotretinoin (Accutane)

If a patient is taking or has taken the drug isotretinoin (Accutane), this can increase the risk of dry eye and may affect wound healing. While not an absolute contraindication, it does need to be documented as to the risks before proceeding.[61]

History of keloid formation

Keloid formers were once thought to be absolute contraindications, but recent studies have shown selective treatment of these patients with PRK can be considered with appropriate informed consent and considered on a case-by-case basis.[62,63]

Herpes simplex or herpes zoster (inactive)

Herpes simplex or herpes zoster infection that has affected a patient's eyes may be at higher risk for reactivation of the disease. Prior HSK cases may be considered for surgery with informed consent and prophylactic oral antiviral therapy on a case-by-case basis.[57]

Glaucoma (controlled)

Controlled glaucoma does not predispose the patient to additional risks; however, uncontrolled glaucoma is considered an absolute contraindication as mentioned earlier.[44,64]

Dry eye disease

If the patient has mild-to-moderate dry eye, PRK may increase the risk of worsening dry eye. Hyperopic treatments may create more issues than myopic treatments; however, both have been shown to exacerbate ocular surface disease.[55,65–67]

The ocular surface

Ocular surface health should be closely examined to diagnose significant dry eye disease, corneal warpage from contact lenses, and other surface irregularities like epithelial basement membrane dystrophy. PRK is an option for those with controlled dry eye disease. Theoretically, because less tissue is removed than with LASIK, less corneal nerve disruption occurs, and therefore less dry eye effects have been suggested. However, research has shown the two procedures to be more equal in dry eye outcomes than previously thought. This study, however, only observed the first 3 months after surgery and did not look at long-term outcomes. Other transient and permanent causes of unstable or irregular topography such as contact lens warpage and anterior corneal dystrophies should be diagnosed and managed well before scheduling PRK surgery.[67]

Amblyopia, monocular, and binocularity

Amblyopes may consider PRK but should be appropriately informed and consented to the possibility of a complication, which may cause them to become solely dependent on the amblyopic eye. Similarly, monocular patients can proceed with PRK, but only after thorough counseling and informed consent about the relative risks and benefits. The patient with binocular anomalies requiring prism must be advised that they will still need prism correction after PRK.[68]

Age and psychological factors

Patients should be at least 18 years of age with a stable refractive error and realistic goals for surgery. As mentioned before, patients under the age of 18 may be considered for surgery as an off-label procedure and on a case-by-case basis. PRK has been successfully done on children in anisometropic conditions and other circumstances. The patient's personality and visual goals should be strongly considered to ensure they do not expect more than the surgery can provide for them. If they have never been satisfied with the visual performance of glasses or contacts, then there is a likelihood that they will not be pleased with the outcome of PRK.[69–73]

Pacemaker

Despite labeling in the patient information booklet, there have been various opinions on the risk of pacemakers interfering with laser instrumentation. However, the National Institute of Health (NIH) released in 2019 that the current body of evidence and our concomitant experiences illustrate a low risk of complications in patients with cardiac implantable electronic devices during refractive surgery. For this reason, most surgeon's do not deter these patients from proceeding with surgery. However, it is still worth discussing with your patient and their primary care provider because of the labeling issues.[74]

PREOPERATIVE CARE

Patient Candidacy

Patient candidacy is key in the preoperative consultation process. There have been multiple studies through the years discussing candidacy and stability of treatment outcomes with low levels of risk. At least all the following bulleted items presented in the following section should be considered before recommending the procedure.[75–82]

Prior contact lens usage

Contact lens–induced corneal warpage can be resolved by discontinuing contact lens wear before preoperative examination. The FDA preoperative guidelines recommend that soft contact lens wearers discontinue lens wear for at least 2 weeks before examination and treatment. Typically, toric and rigid gas permeable (RGP) lenses take longer to establish stability after discontinuing and therefore the surgeon may have extended criteria for these lenses.[83]

Health history and medications

A thorough health history should be taken to ensure that the patient is not at increased risk for surgery based on current health diagnoses, past family medical and ocular history, current and past medications, or any allergies to medications.[84]

Examination Elements

Visual acuity

Uncorrected visual acuity (UCVA) and best corrected visual acuity (BCVA) should be recorded to prove that the surgery is warranted. This also shows documentable proof of the potential for improved uncorrected acuity after surgery.

Pachymetry

Although controversial, corneal thickness readings should be high enough to allow for a postoperative residual stromal bed of at least 250 μm, according to the most widely accepted guidelines. A residual thickness of 250 μm is a customary target; however, there is no substantive scientific evidence to support that single number. To that point, eyes with more than 250 μm of residual stromal bed have developed ectasia after LASIK while eyes with much less have remained stable.[11] Most lasers remove approximately 15 to 18 μm of tissue per diopter of ametropia. The thickness map, as imaged by Orbscan or Pentacam, should also be uniform throughout the cornea to ensure that there are not thin areas, which could increase the risk of iatrogenic keratoectasia. Abnormally thick corneas could indicate corneal edema and potential for unrecognized disease. More recently, Santhiago has suggested evaluation of the percent tissue altered in LVC.[85–87]

Keratometry

Keratometry values should be measured so that PRK does not excessively flatten or steepen postoperatively. For myopic treatments, laser ablation flattens the keratometry value at a rate of 0.7D per each 1D of myopia. Hyperopic treatments steepen at a 1:1 ratio. Most sources recommend postoperative keratometry values not to be flattened less than 36.0D or steepened greater than 48.0D. However, again with appropriate informed consent, keratometry readings post-PRK outside these ranges can be considered on a case-by-case basis.[88]

Corneal topography

Assessing the front and back surface corneal topography by either the Orbscan or Pentacam has become the standard of care in refractive surgery evaluations. Corneal topography, along with the magnitude of the refractive error, is important in determining whether corneal laser surgery (LASIK/PRK/laser epithelial keratomileusis [LASEK]) will lead to abnormally steep or abnormally flat postoperative corneal curvature, which can affect the quality of postoperative visual acuity.[49,89]

Slit lamp examination

Standard slit lamp examination for screening is recommended in all patients.

Intraocular pressure

Accurate preoperative IOP readings are crucial as they can be altered by thinning from the laser ablation. If the patient has a family history of glaucoma, a more detailed analysis such as optical coherence tomography (OCT) of the optic nerve should be considered prior to surgical intervention.[90–92]

Corneal hysteresis

Corneal hysteresis is one option that has been suggested as a screening tool in glaucoma suspects and can serve as a predictive factor in keratoconus and postsurgical ectasia.[93]

Manifest refraction

A careful manifest refraction with binocular balance is essential for the best outcomes in refractive surgery.

Cycloplegic refraction

Cycloplegic refraction is designed to rule out any accommodation that may skew the manifest refraction. Note that it is best to have topography and keratometry done before cycloplegia as the drops may induce surface changes. Cycloplegic refractions are not required but suggested in those patients with more accommodative amplitudes such as younger patients, patients with hyperopia, hyperopia with astigmatism, high myopia, high myopia with astigmatism, and mixed astigmatism.[94]

Vertex measurement

The vertex distance must also be measured carefully since surgical alterations of the corneal refraction are necessarily performed at the corneal plane. Fortunately, this information is usually incorporated into the laser system software and does not typically have to be measured at each preoperative examination. Once established in a refractive lane and standardized throughout the clinic, those parameters should remain constant.[57]

Eye dominance and monovision

Most surgeon's elect to do both eyes on the same day. There can be reasonable arguments on which eye to do first based on eye dominance. Eye dominance is important in patients for whom the surgeon chooses monovision as an option as this can reduce the potential for re-treatment when monovision fails. Females tend to prefer monovision over males, and the preferred eye is the dominant eye for distance in most patients; however, some patients prefer their dominant eye to be corrected for near. Contact lens trials are beneficial in determining patient preference because patients vary over which should be targeted as the reading eye based on eye dominance, habits, and hobbies.[95–101]

Pupil size and higher-order aberrations

Various technologies have been utilized to measure the pupil and higher-order aberrations (HOA) prior to refractive surgery. Significant advances in refractive surgery outcomes have resulted from wave front systems that measure dynamic pupil changes and HOA. Before this technology, most of the postoperative night vision complaints, glare, and halos were due to uncorrected HOAs and large pupils. Current technology has improved the ablation profiles to minimize HOA and induced dysphotopsias.[102–106]

Preoperative drops and perioperative hygiene

Many surgeon's decrease bacterial load on the eyes by having the patient start topical prophylaxis and discontinuance of all facial products and cosmetics for at least one day prior to surgery. Lid scrub use is also a potential strategy especially with patients who have lid margin disease.[107,108]

Vitamin C has proven in studies to prevent postoperative haze and enhance healing. This may be added to the preoperative regimen, however some physicians choose to initiate this option postoperatively.[109,110]

Omega 3 supplements, topical cyclosporine or lifitegrast, or punctal plugs may be added before treatment to enhance the ocular surface prior to surgery or considered postoperatively.[111]

Counseling Discussion Points

The patient should be given adequate opportunity to visit with the surgery team and the surgeon to set realistic expectations and ensure that PRK is the best option for their short- and long-term visual goals. Patients should also understand the sequence of events during surgery and what they might expect to feel, see, smell, or hear. Doing this prior to surgery will serve to reduce patient's anxiety over what to expect. They should be advised that visual acuity during the postoperative period is variable, especially for the first week. If their work schedule does not allow for an estimated 3 to 5 days of epithelial healing, they may want to consider other refractive options. Although pain is less common in the postoperative period with newer methodology, the patient should still be cautioned that pain control may be needed for the first 1 to 4 days. The need for reading glasses in presbyopia should always be discussed. Written instructions for postoperative medications should always be given.[34]

INFORMED CONSENT CONSIDERATIONS

Key consent discussion points should be verbalized to the patient and repeated on the written consent form. The written consent should include more detailed information that may not be verbally discussed.[112] Key consent items include the following:

Possible Short-Term Effects

1. Discomfort or pain
2. Infection
3. Corneal swelling
4. Double vision
5. Ghost images
6. Light sensitivity
7. Tearing
8. IOP elevation

Possible Long-Term Effects

1. Haze
2. Glare or halos
3. Loss of best vision
4. Corneal ectasia

Catastrophic Events Include the Following:

1. Blindness
2. Loss of eye
3. Severe allergic reactions
4. Severe infection
5. Death

Following are Some Free Consent Form Resources with More Detailed Information:

1. https://www.omic.com/prk-consent-forms/
2. https://www.omic.com/prk-bilateral-simultaneous/
3. https://www.omic.com/prk-off-label/

Informed Consent of the Patient

- Consent documents received by the patient
- Consent documents reviewed by the patient
- Surgeon discussion with the patient
- Risks and benefits of the procedure reviewed with the patient
- Questions answered for the patient
- Consent signed and placed in the chart

It is mandatory to discuss the procedure in detail, the benefits of the procedure, and the alternatives to the procedure including no surgery at all. The risks of the procedure should also be discussed and they include blindness, failure of the procedure, risk of loss of the eye or eyes, infection, and even death as a potential complication. Explaining and detailing the contents of the informed consent document to the patient is imperative. The patient should have an opportunity to ask questions and to have them answered in an understandable format. The patient and the doctor should verbally confirm that they understand what is about to take place and that they have agreed to proceed with the planned procedure. Personally, the authors believe this discussion is a legally binding contract between the patient and the doctor and is the surgeon's responsibility to undertake control of the informed consent process and should not be delegated. If co-management is to be part of the process, the patient must be informed of the individual duties of the comanaging clinician versus the surgeon, and follow-up procedures must be discussed in detail and agreed upon by the patient prior to surgery.

PROCEDURE

1. **Pre-Op Oral Medications**
   To alleviate patient anxiety and movement before and during PRK, most surgeon's choose a mildly sedating oral medication, such as alprazolam (Xanax) or lorazepam (Ativan).

2. **Pre-Op Lid Sterilization**
   The eyelid and periorbital area should be thoroughly cleaned with povidone-iodine or alcohol. If allergies exist, commercial nonallergenic eyelid scrubs can be utilized.[113,114]

3. **Pre-Op Drops**
   Newer generation topical fluoroquinolone antibiotics such as gatifloxacin or moxifloxacin are recommended prior to surgery. Individual surgeon protocols exist but most begin the antibiotics and steroids for 1 to 2 days prior to surgery at 3 to 4 times per day. Alternative antibiotics such as polymyxin B/trimethoprim or gentamicin eye drops should be considered in patients who have had a preexisting exposure to methicillin-resistant *Staphylococcus aureus* infection. Allergies must always be documented prior to any topical treatment.

In addition, to reduce postoperative pain, an ophthalmic nonsteroidal anti-inflammatory drug (NSAID) such as bromfenac or ketorolac is often used. With regard to NSAID, many surgeon's have started using this drop 1 to 2 days prior to surgery as part of the preoperative regimen to help control pain postoperatively. Many recommend NSAID use for only 24 to 48 hours after surgery because prolonged use can lead to delayed reepithelialization. Proparacaine or tetracaine used 3 to 4 times over 5-minute intervals before surgery is a helpful strategy to aid in softening the epithelium for chemical or mechanical removal and to provide appropriate anesthesia.[115–117]

4. **Positioning and Alignment**
Proper patient comfort and positioning can decrease the chance of movement during the surgery. Patient attention and fixation can be aided by a covering or tape over the eye that is not immediately being lasered. A gauze pad placed between the eye and adjacent ear will prevent fluid runoff. An eyelid speculum should be placed so that lids and lashes will not interfere with surgery (Fig. 6.3). Use of a 3M tegaderm drape is an option.

5. **Epithelial Removal**
The epithelium can be removed by chemical, mechanical, or laser methods. Whichever method is used, the surgeon needs to be sure to remove the tissue wider than the laser ablation zone. A sponge can be used to remove all the epithelial fragments clear of the treatment zone to avoid islands of untreated tissue. The exposed stroma should be smoothed prior to photoablation. Uneven hydration can cause surface irregularities, which can affect outcomes.[118,119]

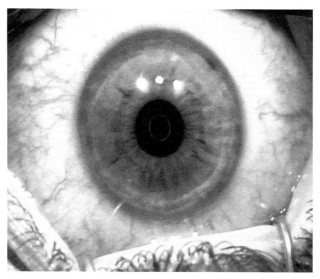

FIGURE 6-3 The eye is prepped and ready to go for PRK surgery. Notice the eyelid speculum holding the eyelids open. PRK, photorefractive keratectomy.

Methods of Epithelial Removal

Chemical (chemical PRK video and Video 6.1 description)

Chemical epithelial removal is the routine method performed by surgeon's. A diluted ethanol solution applied to the corneal epithelium for 10 to 30 seconds in a well (Figs. 6.4 and 6.5) or on a corneal light shield, followed by a thorough irrigation with balanced salt solution (BSS), will allow easy debridement with a spatula or microsponge (Figs. 6.6–6.8). This technique has led to many varieties of chemical epithelial removal. LASEK uses alcohol and a trephine (or a mechanical device) to create a hinged epithelial flap, which is then moved aside for stromal treatment. Next, the epithelium is repositioned before bandage contact lens addition. These more advanced techniques aim at retaining the epithelium to aid in the healing process. However, this step adds additional steps for the surgeon and has shown equivocal results in postoperative comparisons.[48,120,121]

Mechanical (Epi-Bowman keratectomy video and Video 6.2 description)

Mechanical methods include scraping, brush scrubbing, or Epi-Bowman keratectomy (EBK). Mechanical scraping using a blade or spatula was the first epithelial removal technique to be used. This method was time-consuming and often caused Bowman's nicking. An Amoils epithelial scrubber or Pallikaris brush incorporates a

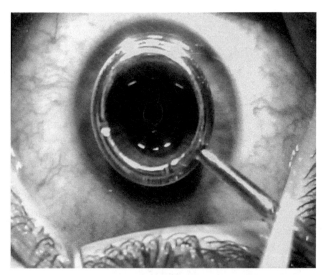

FIGURE 6-4 A well is placed onto the cornea and is ready for a diluted ethanol solution to be dripped into the well for epithelial softening prior to debridement. In this case, an 8 mm well was used.

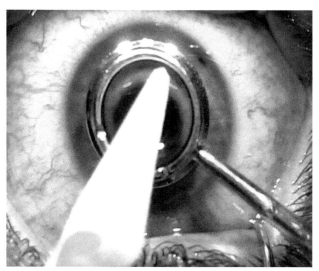

FIGURE 6-5 Following approximately 30 seconds of diluted ethanol in the well, a dry surgical sponge is used to soak up the ethanol in the well.

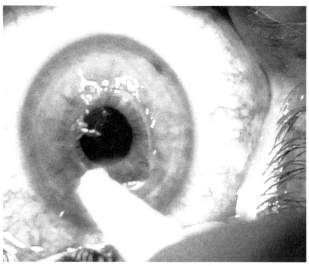

FIGURE 6-6 Following removal of the well and rinsing of the eye, epithelial debridement occurs. Epithelial debridement is illustrated here. In this case, the tip of a dry surgical sponge is being used to debride the loosened epithelium.

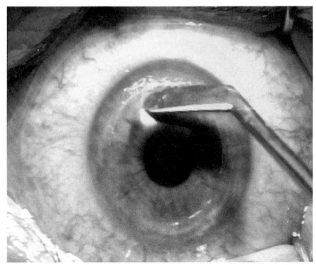

FIGURE 6-7 Nearing the completion of epithelial debridement. Illustrated here is a PRK spatula, also known as the Maloney's "hockey stick", which can be used to remove any remaining stubborn islands of epithelium and smooth the stromal bed getting it ready for laser ablation.
PRK, photorefractive keratectomy.

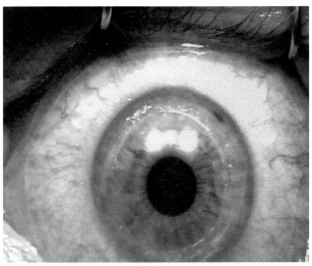

FIGURE 6-8 Epithelial debridement is now complete in this case, and the cornea is ready for laser treatment. Notice the nice, clean, circular, 8-mm debridement area.

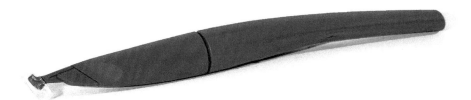

FIGURE 6-9 Illustrated here is the EBK device. It is a specially designed, multiblade polymer epikeratome that is used to mechanically remove the epithelium as opposed to a traditional blade or scalpel.
EBK, Epi-Bowman keratectomy.

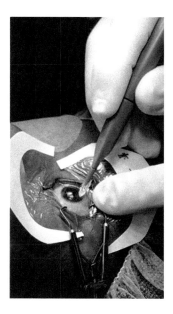

FIGURE 6-10 Illustrated here is mechanical removal of the epithelium with the Epi-Clear epikeratome. Epithelial removal is nearly complete in this image.

rotary brush to remove the epithelium out to 9.5 mm. EBK is a novel mechanical technique that implements the Epi-Clear epikeratome (ORCA Surgical) (Figs. 6.9 and 6.10) to collect epithelial tissue while leaving Bowman's membrane completely intact. Vingopoulos et al. have reported rapid reepithelialization with EBK when compared to alcohol removal.[122–124]

Laser removal (transepithelial photorefractive keratectomy video and Video 6.3 description)

The excimer laser may be used to ablate the epithelium in a technique that is known as transepithelial PRK (T-PRK). The procedure may be done in two steps (laser epithelium removal followed by stromal ablation) or a single-step continuous laser method of epithelium and stromal removal. T-PRK is less commonly done because not all lasers are approved for this treatment technique. As newer laser ablation profiles now include epithelial removal using epithelial mapping, T-PRK as a treatment option is increasing.[125]

Excimer Laser

1. *Fixation and eye tracking*

   Fixation and eye tracking vary from laser to laser. The patient information booklets for each FDA-approved laser system have details on the individual laser parameters. Fixation light colors vary, and the surgeon should discuss immediately prior to surgery what the patient is to expect and where they should focus their line of site for the procedure. The surgeon must manually align the laser reticule over the pupil and engage the eye-tracking system (Fig. 6.11). The eye is now ready for laser treatment.[126–129]

2. *Communication before and during laser*

   Communication to the patient is essential as they are expected to maintain fixation and remain motionless throughout the procedure. Surgeon's should regularly encourage the patient to relax and inform the patient when and what to expect. Other distractions should be minimized, as both the patient and surgeon may become distracted.[34]

3. *Stromal laser treatment*

   Once all tracking and fixation is engaged, the surgeon begins the laser stromal photoablation (Fig. 6.12). The surgeon should understand that moving the

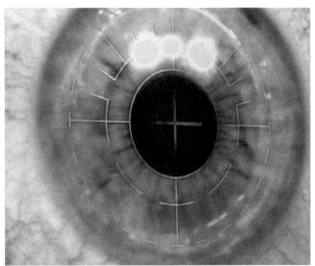

FIGURE 6-11 Fixation and eye tracking are complete, and the laser reticule is perfectly centered within the pupil and ready for laser treatment.

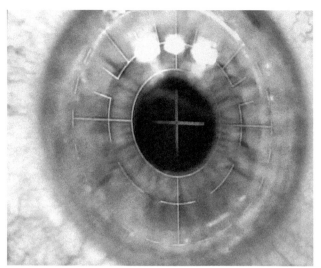

FIGURE 6-12 Right in the middle of PRK excimer laser ablation treatment. Notice the white plume of ablated tissue in the superior aspect of the pupil.
PRK, photorefractive keratectomy.

manual controls will correct the alignment of the laser reticule and this should be closely monitored during the treatment. The built-in automated tracking system will adjust for any small x, y, z movement or micro-saccades that occur. Large movements will result in a pause in the laser process, which may be resumed once the tracking is reengaged. These descriptions apply to modern laser units, and older systems may vary in tracking ability.

4. *Mitomycin C*
   A 10- to 30-second application of mitomycin C (MMC) 0.02% soaked into a surgical sponge has proven to reduce the occurrence of postoperative corneal haze (Fig. 6.13). There are various opinions on the concentration, duration, and dioptric range of use for mitomycin. Some surgeon's use it for all PRK cases, but most reserve its use for higher myopic cases over 4D. A thorough rinsing with saline solution after the MMC should be applied to avoid toxicity from overexposure.[34,130–133]

5. *Therapeutic contact lens*
   In the final step, a soft bandage contact lens should be applied to promote epithelial healing and decrease pain. FDA-approved lenses for use after PRK include Air Optix Night and Day, Acuvue Oasys, and PureVision.[134] One head-to-head study comparing senifilcon to lotrifilcon has shown that senifilcon lenses provided more comfort during the postoperative period, but slower healing than lotrifilcon.[135,136]

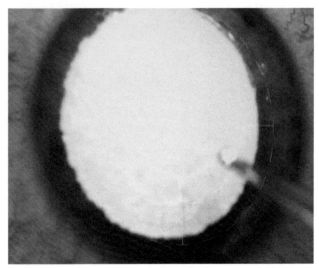

FIGURE 6-13 Mitomycin C 0.02% soaked in a surgical sponge is placed on the cornea for 10 to 30 seconds to help reduce postoperative corneal haze. After 10 to 30 seconds, the sponge is lifted off the cornea with forceps, and the eye is rinsed thoroughly with sterile saline. The final step would then be placement of the bandage contact lens on the eye and removal of the eyelid speculum.

POSTOPERATIVE CARE/CO-MANAGEMENT (FOLLOW-UP SCHEDULE)

Follow-Up Schedule

Follow-up schedule is per the physician's protocol (postoperative regimens vary dramatically) ranging from 1 to 7 days until the epithelium is fully healed and the bandage contact lens is removed. Many will see the patient daily until the bandage contact lens is removed, which typically is on postoperative days 4 to 7. The suggested patient schedule is then usually 1 to 2 weeks, 1 month, 3 months, 6 months, and 1 year. With new COVID-19 guidelines, newer follow-up treatment guidelines and telemedicine follow-ups have been utilized with success. On average, the epithelial defect is healed between days 2 and 5. Visual acuity is often good on the first day after PRK, between 20/20 and 20/40 is not uncommon. As the epithelium migrates centrally on days 2 to 5, the vision drops down and can vary. Some may experience worse vision during this time while the central epithelium begins to clear and reorganize. Average vision at one week is usually between 20/20 and 20/40. Under the bandage contact lens, the epithelial healing edge can be seen and measured with a bright slit lamp beam turned off-axis and scanned over the central cornea. By day 4, the epithelial defect is usually closed, and the bandage contact lens may be removed. There will be various levels of central haze, punctate epithelial erosions, and a healing line for the first 1 to 2 weeks after the contact lens removal. For these reasons, it may be beneficial to leave the contact on for an extended period based on vision. By 2 weeks, the cornea should be clear with minimal to no residual refractive error. Healing is variable from patient to patient. It is best to counsel the patient that there is much variation for a few weeks and that refractive error will be measured at 1 to 3 months after surgery. Diagnostics and their postoperative timing vary from surgeon to surgeon.[137,138]

Bandage Contact Lens

The contact lens should be examined at each postoperative exam to ensure proper position and minimal movement. The contact lens may be changed in the first few days if there is a lens defect or a problem with the fit. Keep in mind that the insertion and removal process often cause some epithelial disruption and may delay healing. For these reasons, it is best not to change the lens unless needed. The contact lens material may affect the healing rate and discomfort level. Contact lens materials and base curves have shown to affect epithelial healing rate and patient pain postoperatively. As contact lenses continue to improve, so too will their effectiveness in use postoperatively.[139]

Topical Antibiotics

Topical antibiotics are used prior to and at the time of the surgery and continued until reepithelialization. The timing of antibiotics is controversial, but most surgeon's now begin the antibiotics 24 to 48 hours prior to surgery. The 4th generation broad-spectrum fluoroquinolone are the current commonly used drops, dosed at three to four times daily. Variable wound healing has been reported with these medications. It is best for the surgeon to consult local antibiograms to insure they are using the most effective antibiotic for their postoperative prophylaxis as this can change as bacteria respond to continued use of these medications. Besifloxacin is often discouraged as it has an association with delayed epithelial healing when instilled prior to bandage contact lens placement immediately after surgery.[140–144]

Steroid

Topical corticosteroids are essential after PRK to minimize corneal edema, pain, haze, and sterile infiltrates. Some surgeon's start these prior to surgery, and others begin at the time of surgery at three to four times daily with a slow taper for 1 to 3 months. Since they are maintained for weeks to months, one should choose an option that has less penetration resulting in less effect on IOP and cataract formation. Effective examples of this include loteprednol, fluorometholone, and prednisolone phosphate. Prednisolone acetate and dexamethasone are also popular and effective options but do require closer IOP monitoring. Difluprednate after PRK is not well studied. Newer regimens have decreased duration and application of the steroid as medications improve.[145–148]

Lubrication

It is recommended to use preservative-free artificial tears until the epithelium is closed and then continuing as needed for weeks to months postoperatively based on individual patient healing. This treatment can aid in epithelial healing. Lubrication can prevent the bandage contact lens (BCL) from adhering to the epithelium and improve healing and avoid complications. Ointments are discouraged because they can lead to the BCL becoming dislodged or falling out. After epithelial closure, frequent lubrication is helpful to ongoing healing in PRK. Long-term artificial tears, punctal plugs, or topical cyclosporine is instituted based on varying healing among patients.[149,150]

Nonsteroidal Anti-Inflammatory Drugs

Topical NSAIDs are an option to reduce pain as the cornea reepithelializes. Studies vary on corneal wound healing and the use of NSAIDs postoperatively. Bromfenac twice daily or ketorolac up to four times daily has proven to be safe and equally effective in providing pain relief with no difference in epithelial healing time. Newer surgeon regimens have the patients using the NSAIDs 1 to 2 days before surgery. Once the epithelium is closed and pain is gone, the NSAID may be stopped.[118,151]

Pain Management

Pain or discomfort in the postoperative period has improved significantly in recent years with use of ocular NSAIDs, heavy lubrication, and newer epithelial removal methods that do not use alcohol, such as EBK and T-PRK. However, it is necessary to outline some ways for patients to combat breakthrough pain, if needed. Alternating oral acetaminophen and ibuprofen may provide enough analgesic effect. Another option is to use a topical dilution of 0.5% to 1% tetracaine or 0.05% proparacaine as needed for pain.[85] Compounding medications should be done as dictated by state law and varies from state to state. Oral narcotics such as tramadol, codeine, or hydrocodone and sedatives such as zolpidem or Benadryl are effective at reducing corneal pain when other measures are insufficient. With current restrictions, surgeon's are looking to alternative methods to reduce pain.[152–156]

Vitamin C

One study has shown that oral vitamin C 1000 mg may be used for up to 6 months postoperatively to aid in haze prevention. Vitamin C levels are reduced after PRK, and supplementation is presumed to restore adequate levels and decrease the harmful effects of free radicals created by the excimer laser. For these reasons, many surgeon's start vitamin C therapy a week or more before the surgery. Again, the use of vitamin C and its duration vary from surgeon to surgeon.[109,110]

Shield

A protective shield may be worn through the night for 1 week following surgery to prevent epithelial disruption from eye rubbing or bedding. However, many surgeon's do not use protective shields postoperatively. As with other regimens, using a shield or not is based on surgeon preference.

Ultraviolet Protection

UV-blocking sunglasses should be worn when outdoors for the first 3 to 6 months postoperatively to prevent keratocyte activation, which can induce haze.[157]

POTENTIAL COMPLICATIONS AND THEIR TREATMENT

Infection

Infection after PRK is extremely rare at a rate of 0.019% as reported by Wroblewski et al. but remains the most serious possible complication after PRK.[158] Known HIV patients are at higher risk with PRK with a rate of 6.3% as reported by Tisdale et al.[159] Infection risk is highest early after surgery with a compromised epithelium and a BCL in place. There have been reports of sterile infiltrate formation when using topical NSAID concomitantly with or without corticosteroids. Sterile infiltrates such as these are typically quick to resolve with intervention. Infectious ulcers should be caught early and treated by discontinuing the steroid and applying vigorous fluoroquinolone drops every 1 to 2 hours, and if unresponsive, fortified vancomycin (or cefazolin) and an aminoglycoside should be added to the regimen, alternating at once per hour. Less common etiologies such as mycobacterial, fungal, herpes simplex type 1, or acanthamoeba should be considered if the presentation is atypical or infection is not clearing with the previously mentioned measures.[48,160]

Haze

Subepithelial haze is a possible late complication that may appear 1 to 2 months postoperatively. It is present in 1% of myopic cases between –1D and –6D. This increases to 7% in the range of –6D to –10D. Haze is caused by activation of keratocytes and migration of wound healing response materials. UV exposure can increase the level of haze encountered. Mitomycin C 0.02% application during surgery significantly reduces the incidence of haze. Topical steroid, such as prednisolone phosphate 1%, can be used to resolve the haze and should be used 4 to 6 times daily, tapered over

1 to 3 months. If unresolved with topical steroid treatment, then treatment with topical MMC alone, superficial keratectomy, or PTK with or without MMC are all options.[34,161]

Undercorrection/Overcorrection/Regression

The number of cases of residual refractive error from overcorrection or undercorrection may vary from surgeon to surgeon. Main causal factors include incorrect original refraction, incomplete epithelial removal, or improper hydration before stromal ablation.[162] Overcorrection is common in the first few weeks and months and often resolves. Extended wear of a therapeutic contact lens combined with topical NSAID can promote regression and resolve some of the refractive error. Re-treatment with PRK or LASIK should not be offered until refractive stabilization, which typically occurs 3 to 6 months postoperatively depending on the type of refractive error and the level of refractive error. This allows adequate time for self-resolution or stability of refraction. Randleman et al. reported that the percentage of patients that need re-treatment after PRK myopic correction with an excimer laser is 6.3% (a range from 3.8% to 20.8% has been reported.)[163] Regression is a common long-term complication of PRK. It can occur months or years after successful PRK. Early regression is often caused by corneal edema and can be improved by topical steroids. Late regression (>6 months) in unsatisfied patients will need to be addressed with a possible enhancement procedure.[97,164,165]

Ocular Surface Disease

Dry eye disease is a common side effect of LVC procedures. At 3 months, dry eye symptoms are as common in PRK as in LASIK, and some reports have been up to 50% of the patient population. However, at 6 months and beyond, studies show better Schirmer and osmolarity testing for PRK compared to LASIK. Punctate epithelial erosions and recurrent corneal erosions are also sometimes seen in the short- or long-term follow-up of PRK. For the first 6 months, unresolving cases may need treatment such as heavy topical lubrication, omega 3 supplements, warm compresses, temporary or permanent punctal plugs, or topical cyclosporine or lifitegrast. Some patients may require long-term therapy.[55,66,67,166]

Central Islands

Precise etiology is unknown and is likely multifactorial. Several theories have been put forward to explain the development of central islands after refractive surgery. A central island is a type of irregular astigmatism that occurs after laser refractive surgery. It is generally defined as a central area of steeper corneal tissue having increased refractive power, as seen on topography, which is surrounded by a flattened corneal region with reduced refractive power. A central island is a localized elevated area within the corneal treatment ablation zone >1.5 mm in diameter and over 3D. The causes are many and include larger ablation zones, corneal tissue hydration, type of laser, vortex plume, inherent laser defects, or degraded optics. The incidence of central islands following PRK has significantly decreased with the advent of new technology specifically designed to prevent their formation. Central islands tend to disappear with epithelial remodulation but may be treated by topographic-guided laser if they persist and are symptomatic.[34,57,167–173]

Irregular Astigmatism

Irregular astigmatism may occur because of a central island, treatment decentration, ectasia, form-fruste keratoconus, or irregular healing. Irregular astigmatism is the most common cause of loss of best spectacle-corrected visual acuity (BSCVA) and is associated with symptoms of glare, halos, starburst, diplopia, and decreased contrast acuity. This rare complication of PRK can almost always be avoided with the rigid preoperative screening protocol that will rule out any corneal deformities. If irregular astigmatism is presumed to be the cause of reduced vision, a diagnostic contact lens evaluation can show improvement in visual acuity and help in the diagnosis. Topography-guided PRK is often needed in more pronounced cases, such as treatment zone decentration.[57,174–177]

Ectasia

One of the advantages of PRK over LASIK is that PRK has an almost nonexistent risk for ectasia. However, ectasia can still occur after PRK. The incidence in LASIK patients is estimated to be between 0.04% and 0.6%. Ectasia following PRK is considered extremely rare and has been described previously in only a few case reports and small case series. The Randleman ectasia risk scoring system can be used to identify more at-risk eyes.[178–181]

VIDEOS OF THE PROCEDURES

Video 6.1—This PRK procedure is done using chemical epithelial removal. An 8-mm lens well is held centrally on the cornea, and a diluted ethanol solution is dripped into the well and held inside the well for approximately 30 seconds to help soften and prepare the epithelium for debridement. Following removal of the ethanol within the well with a Weck-Cel sponge, the eye is rinsed with cool, sterile BSS. The tip of a dry Weck-Cel sponge is then used along with a PRK spatula (AKA Maloney's hockey stick) to debride the central 8 mm of the epithelium. A fairly clean, circular debridement zone is seen in this video. Special attention is taken to ensure the stromal bed is smooth and dry with no islands of epithelium remaining prior to excimer laser stromal ablation. Eye tracking and alignment is performed followed by laser ablation treatment. In this case, laser treatment lasted approximately 22 seconds. Immediately following laser treatment, mitomycin C soaked in a surgical sponge is laid on the central cornea for approximately 25 seconds. Another bottle of cool, sterile BSS is used to thoroughly rinse the eye. Lastly, a bandage contact lens is placed on the cornea, a round of postoperative drops are instilled, and the lid speculum is removed.

Video 6.2—Mechanical removal of the epithelium has been the standard with PRK since its inception. EBK is an improved way to remove the epithelium. The device is a single-use polymer epikeratome for removal of the surface cells atraumatically. With EBK, the edge of one blade creates a microepithelial elevated fold, while the second blade removes the epithelium a layer at a time and pulls the epithelium into the receptacle for complete removal from the surface without coming into contact with Bowman's layer and basal membrane. As with traditional PRK, first the surgeon will place a tegaderm drape to create a sterile field. Prior to surgery, aggressive addition of a topical anesthetic (proparacaine or tetracaine) and a topical NSAID (ketorolac or bromfenac) helps with epithelial removal, intraoperative pain, and postoperative pain. Next, the epithelium is removed with the Epi-Clear device. The refractive error is treated in this case with a topography-guided scanning spot laser. Mitomycin C 0.02% is applied for 12 seconds. Chilled BSS is applied to remove the residual mitomycin C. Pharmaceuticals are applied as per the surgeon's protocol usually consisting of a topical corticosteroid, antibiotic, and NSAID. A silicone hydrogel or hydrogel bandage contact lens with a high oxygen permeability (DK) is placed, and the procedure is complete.

Video 6.3—The current technology for T-PRK is available on multiple platforms outside the United States but only available on the VISX platform in the United States. Typically, the treatment is divided in two parts (epithelial folder and treatment folder). Prior to treatment, topical anesthetic typically is applied with proparacaine or tetracaine.

The epithelial folder is performed first and consists of a 6.0-mm phototherapeutic keratectomy with a 0.5-mm transition zone out to 6.5 mm with a –0.66 offset and an ablation depth of 70 microns. However, 58–60 microns is the typical amount used based on the epithelial thickness. The surgeon judges when to stop the ablation by looking at the epithelial fluorescence as seen in the video. A novice surgeon may begin with a maximum of 60 microns depth to make sure that removal of the epithelium does not lead in fact to stromal ablation. The surgeon then waits with the pedal in position one to dry the surface. It is a "no touch" technique. Next, the laser automatically converts to the PRK mode after prompting. The refractive treatment is performed. Mitomycin C is applied for 12 seconds. Pharmaceuticals are applied as per the surgeon's protocol usually consisting of a topical corticosteroid, antibiotic, and NSAID. A bandage contact lens is placed, and the procedure is complete.

EFFICACY

Short- (3–6 months) and long-term (10 years) outcomes of PRK for mild-to-moderate myopia and astigmatism are good and statistically equal to those of LASIK. Hyperopic treatment is also successful, but results are more variable in PRK compared to LASIK.

Short Term

The following early data are helpful for understanding PRK efficacy at the 6-month mark. The study included 150 eyes in a range from –1.50D to –6.50D.

- 80% achieved uncorrected acuity of 20/20.
- 100% achieved 20/25.
- 98.6% achieved ± 0.5D.
- 100% achieved ±1.00.
- 0.7% lost one line of BCVA.
- 0% had re-treatment.

Regarding hyperopia, a similar study looked at PRK cases ranging from +1.50D to +4.00D. As mentioned previously, this data represent outcomes at 6 months after PRK but included only 40 eyes.

- 70% achieved uncorrected acuity of 20/20.
- 90% achieved 20/40.
- 100% achieved ±1.00D.
- 17.5% lost one line of BCVA.
- 12.5% lost two lines of BCVA.
- 0% had re-treatment.

In three studies of PRK to correct astigmatism with 6 months of follow-up, less than 2% of patients lost two or more lines of BCVA. In these reports, 63% to 86% of patients were within 1.00D of their intended correction, and 82% to 94% had an UCVA of 20/40 or better.[48,182,183]

Long Term

Looking at a recent study from a contralateral eye study of topography-guided customized ablation treatment (TCAT) versus wavefront-optimized (WFO) PRK, Faria-Correia et al. showed in this small series that in both groups, 96% of eyes achieved an uncorrected distance visual acuity (UDVA) of 20/20 or better at 12 months. The corrected distance visual acuity (CDVA) remained stable in 46.2% and 53.9% of the eyes in the TCAT and WFO groups, respectively. Compared to the preoperative CDVA, 19.2% of eyes gained one or more lines of postoperative UDVA at 12 months in both groups. Regarding the spherical equivalent refractive accuracy, the percentage of eyes within ±0.50D was 81% in the WFO group and 85% in the TCAT group. Both types of ablation presented a similar stability during the 12-month follow-up.[184]

If we compare recent data using three laser systems with LASIK, the mean post-operative UDVA at 12 months was 20/19.25 ± 8.76, 20/16.59 ± 5.94, and 20/19.17 ± 4.46 for VISX iDESIGN, Alcon Contoura, and Nidek CATz, respectively. In at least 90% of treated eyes at 3 months and 12 months, all three lasers showed either no change or a gain of CDVA. Mesopic contrast sensitivity at 6 months showed a clinically significant increase of 41.3%, 25.1%, and 10.6% for eyes using VISX iDESIGN, Alcon Contoura, and Nidek CATz, respectively. Photopic contrast sensitivity at 6 months showed a clinically significant increase of 19.2%, 31.9%, and 10.6% for eyes using VISX iDESIGN, Alcon Contoura, and Nidek CATz, respectively. The total percentage of eyes that had postoperative UDVA equal to or greater than preoperative CDVA at 3 months were 69%, 89%, and 79% for VISX iDESIGN, Alcon Contoura, and Nidek CATz, respectively. The same comparison at 12 months was 65%, 89%, and 81% for VISX iDESIGN, Alcon Contoura, and Nidek CATz, respectively. Nidek CATz obtained a postoperative UDVA of two lines or better than preoperative CDVA in 13% and 18% of treated eyes at both postoperative time intervals, respectively, a value larger than the other two platforms. In at least 90% of treated eyes at 3 months and 12 months, all three lasers showed either no change or a gain of CDVA.[185]

It is accurate to counsel patients that myopic PRK has great long-term outcomes, only needing re-treatments approximately 5% to 10% of the time in the first 10 years.[164] One large study showed the need for 6.3% to have re-treatment in the first year.[163] Also notable is that 99% of mild-to-moderate myopic treatments retain as good or better BCVA after PRK as they had prior to treatment. In other words, less than 1% lose at least one line compared to their preoperative BCVA. This number is closer to 5% with hyperopic treatments from +1D to +3.50D.[183]

A meta-analysis study compared the visual outcomes of common forms of PRK (Traditional PRK, Trans-Epi PRK, LASEK, and Epi-LASIK) and found no statistical difference in treatment method. The surface under the cumulative ranking curve (SUCRA) ranking (from best to worst) was femtosecond LASIK, T-PRK, LASEK, PRK, LASIK, and Epi-LASIK. There were no statistically significant differences in the safety profiles.[185] Multiple studies have been performed with newer technologies, newer diagnostics, and newer platforms and have been listed in the references.[163,167,186–195]

CODING/BILLING AND MODIFIERS

LVC is not covered under medical insurances. Billing strategies are determined by individual surgery centers.

REFERENCES

1. Basov NG, Prokhorov AM. Application of molecular beams to the radio spectroscopic study of the rotation spectra of molecules. *Zhurnal Eksperimental'noi I Teoreticheskoi Fiziki*. 1954;274(4): 431–438.
2. Hoffman JM, Hays AK, Tisone GC. High powered UV noble-gas halide lasers. *Appl Phys Lett*. 1976;28(9):538–539.
3. Burnham R, Djeu N. Ultraviolet-preionized discharge-pumped lasers in XeF, KrF, and ArF. *Appl Phys Lett*. 1976;29(11):707–709.

4. Taboada J, Mikesell GW Jr, Reed RD. Response of the corneal epithelium to KrF excimer laser pulses. *Health Phys*. 1981;40(5):677–683.
5. Srinivasan R, Wynne JJ, Blum SE. Ablative photodecomposition of organic polymer films by far-UV excimer laser irradiation. Presented at: Conference on Lasers and Electro-Optics; May 17–20, 1983. Baltimore, MD.
6. Srinivasan R, Wynne JJ, Blum SE. Far-UV photoetching of organic material. *Laser Focus*. 1983:62–66.
7. Baron Patent 4461294. July 24, 1984.
8. Munnerlyn Patent 4561436. December 31, 1985.
9. L'Esperance Patent 4665913. May 19, 1987.
10. L'Esperance Patent 4669466. June 2, 1987.
11. L'Esperance Patent 4718418. January 12, 1988.
12. L'Esperance Patent 4729372. March 8, 1988.
13. L'Esperance Patent 4732148. March 22, 1988.
14. L'Esperance Patent 4770172. September 13, 1988.
15. L'Esperance Patent 4773414. September 27, 1988.
16. L'Esperance Patent 4798204. January 17, 1989.
17. Peyman Patent 4840175. June 20, 1989.
18. Bille Patent 4901718. February 20, 1990.
19. Warner Patent 4901718. February 27, 1990.
20. Bille Patent 4907586. March 13, 1990.
21. Telfair patent 4911711. March 27, 1990.
22. Azema Patent 4973330. November 27, 1990.
23. Kozioi 5074859. December 24, 1991.
24. Kohayakawa 5090798. December 24, 1991.
25. Munnerlyn Patent 5163934. November 17, 1992.
26. Reinstein DZ, Archer TJ, Gobbe M. The history of LASIK. *J Refract Surg*. 2012;28(4):291–298. doi: 10.3928/1081597X-20120229-01
27. Thompson V, Durrie DS, Cavanaugh TB. Philosophy and technique for excimer laser phototherapeutic keratectomy. *Refract Corneal Surg*. 1993;9(2 Suppl):S81–S85. PMID: 8499386.
28. Seiler T, Wollensak J. Myopic photorefractive keratectomy with the excimer laser: One-year follow-up. *Ophthalmology*. 1991 Aug;98(8):1156–1163. doi:10.1016/s0161-6420(91)32157-2. PMID: 1923351.
29. Starr M, Donnenfeld E, Newton M, Tostanoski J, Muller J, Odrich M. Excimer laser phototherapeutic keratectomy. *Cornea*. 1996 Nov;15(6):557–565. PMID: 8899266.
30. Ritu N, Maharana PK, Roop P, et al. Phototherapeutic keratectomy. *Surv Ophthalmol*. 2020;65(1): 79–108. doi:10.1016/j.survophthal.2019.07.002
31. U.S. Food & Drug Administration. FDA-approved lasers for PRK and other refractive surgeries. 2019. Available at: https://www.fda.gov/medical-devices/lasik/fda-approved-lasers-prk-and-other-refractive-surgeries
32. Premarket approval of Summit Technology. FDA. 1995. Available at: https://www.accessdata.fda.gov/cdrh_docs/pdf/p930034.pdf
33. Munnerlyn CR, Koons SJ, Marshall J. Photorefractive keratectomy: A technique for laser refractive surgery. *J Cataract Refract Surg*. 1988;14(1):46–52.
34. Somani SN, Moshirfar M, Patel BC. Photorefractive Keratectomy (PRK). In: Abai B, ed. Stat Pearls. Treasure Island, FL: Stat Pearls Publishing; June 26, 2020.
35. Bethke W, ed. Refractive surgery trends of the ISRS. Review of ophthalmology. 2016. Available at: https://www.reviewofophthalmology.com/article/refractive-surgery-trends-of-the-isrs
36. Koller T, Iseli HP, Donitzky C, et al. Topography-guided surface ablation for forme fruste keratoconus. *Ophthalmology*. 2006;113(12):2198–2202.
37. Kanellopoulos AJ, Binder P. Collagen cross-linking (CCL) with sequential topography guided PRK: A temporizing alternative for keratoconus to penetrating keratoplasty. *Cornea*. 2007;26(7):891–895.
38. Kanellopoulos AJ, Asimellis G. Keratoconus management: Long-term stability of topography-guided normalization combined with high-fluence CXL stabilization (the Athens Protocol). *J Refract Surg*. 2014;30(5):342–346.

39. Tuft SJ, Gartry DS, Rawe IM, Meek KM. Photorefractive keratectomy: Implications of corneal wound healing. *Br J Ophthalmol.* 1993;77(4):243–247. doi:10.1136/bjo.77.4.243

40. Ambró sio R Jr, Wilson S. LASIK vs LASEK vs PRK: Advantages and indications. *Semin Ophthalmol.* 2003 Mar;18(1):2–10. doi:10.1076/soph.18.1.2.14074. PMID: 12759854.

41. IDESIGN Refractive Studio-Driven Wavefront-Guided Photorefractive Keratectomy (PRK) Procedure using the STAR S4 IR Excimer Laser System: Patient Information Booklet.

42. https://www.accessdata.fda.gov/cdrh_docs/pdf/P930016S057C.pdf

43. Yoon SC, Jung JW, Sohn HJ, Shyn KH. Cataract and refractive surgery in; a survey of KSCRS members from 1995-2006. *Korean J Ophthalmol.* 2009 Sep;23(3):142–147. doi:10.3341/kjo.2009.23.3.142. Epub September 8, 2009. PMID: 19794938; PMCID: PMC2739965.

44. Osman E. Laser refractive surgery in glaucoma patients. *Saudi J Ophthalmol.* 2011 Apr;25(2):169–173. doi:10.1016/j.sjopt.2010.04.003. Epub April 21, 2010. PMID: 23960918; PMCID: PMC3729399.

45. Khakshoor H, Razavi F, Eslampour A, Omdtabrizi A. Photorefractive keratectomy in mild to moderate keratoconus: outcomes in over 40-year-old patients. *Indian J Ophthalmol.* 2015 Feb;63(2):157–161.

46. Al-Mohaimeed MM. Combined corneal CXL and photorefractive keratectomy for treatment of keratoconus: A review. *Int J Ophthalmol.* 2019 Dec 18;12(12):1929–1938. doi:10.18240/ijo.2019.12.16. PMID: 31850179; PMCID: PMC6901893.

47. Kohlhaas M. Iatrogene Keratektasie – eine Übersicht [Iatrogenic Keratectasia: A Review]. *Klin Monbl Augenheilkd.* 2015 Jun;232(6):765–772. German. doi:10.1055/s-0035-1545737. Epub April 8, 2015. PMID: 25853948.

48. Vasaiwala R, Bruce Jackson W, Azar DT, Al-Muammar A. Excimer laser surface treatment: Photorefractive keratectomy, Chapter 161. In: Krachmer JH, ed. *Cornea.* New York: Mosby; October 2010:1793–1816.

49. Sonmez B, Bozkurt B, Atmaca A, Irkec M, Orhan M, Aslan U. Effect of glycemic control on refractive changes in diabetic patients with hyperglycemia. *Cornea.* 2005;24(5):531–537.

50. Kanellopoulos AJ. The management of cornea blindness from severe corneal scarring, with the Athens Protocol (transepithelial topography-guided PRK therapeutic remodeling, combined with same-day, collagen cross-linking). *Clin Ophthalmol.* 2012;6:87–90. doi:10.2147/OPTH.S27175. Epub February 8, 2012. PMID: 22347790; PMCID: PMC3280100.

51. Wilson SE, Marino GK, Medeiros CS, Santhiago MR. Phototherapeutic keratectomy: Science and art. *J Refract Surg.* 2017 Mar 1;33(3):203–210. doi:10.3928/1081597X-20161123-01. PMID: 28264136.

52. Oliveira RF, Ferreira GA, Ghanem VC, Corrêa-Dantas PE, Ghanem RC. Transepithelial surface ablation with mitomycin C for the treatment of chronic central corneal scars following adenoviral keratoconjunctivitis. *J Refract Surg.* 2020 Jan 1;36(1):55–61. doi:10.3928/1081597X-20191203-01. PMID: 31917852.

53. Seiler T, Wollensak J. Komplikationen der Laserkeratomileusis mit dem Excimerlaser (193 nm) [Complications of laser keratomileusis with the excimer laser (193 nm)]. *Klin Monbl Augenheilkd.* 1992 Jun;200(6):648–653. German. doi:10.1055/s-2008-1045850. Erratum in: Klin Monatsbl Augenheilkd. 1992 Aug;201(2):145. PMID: 1507787.

54. Cua IY, Pepose JS. Late corneal scarring after photorefractive keratectomy concurrent with development of systemic lupus erythematosus. *J Refract Surg.* 2002 Nov–Dec;18(6):750–752. PMID: 12458872.

55. Sambhi RS, Sambhi GDS, Mather R, Malvankar-Mehta MS. Dry eye after refractive surgery: A meta-analysis. *Can J Ophthalmol.* 2020 Apr;55(2):99–106. doi:10.1016/j.jcjo.2019.07.005. Epub August 20, 2019. PMID: 31712000.

56. Simpson RG, Moshirfar M, Edmonds JN, Christiansen SM. Laser in-situ keratomileusis in patients with diabetes mellitus: A review of the literature. *Clin Ophthalmol.* 2012;6:1665–1674. doi:10.2147/OPTH.S36382. Epub October 12, 2012. PMID: 23109803; PMCID: PMC3474268.

57. Salz J, Trattler W. Excimer laser surface treatment: Photorefractive keratectomy, Chapter 159. In: Krachmer JH, ed. *Cornea.* New York: Mosby; October 2010:1767–1779.

58. Sher NA, Hardten DR, Fundingsland B, et al. 193-nm excimer photorefractive keratectomy in high myopia. *Ophthalmology.* 1994 Sep;101(9):1575–1582. doi:10.1016/s0161-6420(94)31135-3. PMID: 8090459.

59. Spadea L, Giovannetti F. Main complications of photorefractive keratectomy and their management. *Clin Ophthalmol.* 2019 Nov 27;13:2305–2315. doi:10.2147/OPTH.S233125

60. Alió JL, Artola A, Belda JI, et al. LASIK in patients with rheumatic diseases: A pilot study. *Ophthalmology.* 2005 Nov;112(11):1948–1954. doi:10.1016/j.ophtha.2005.06.022. Epub September 15, 2005. PMID: 16168484.

61. Ortega-Usobiaga J, Llovet-Osuna F, Djodeyre MR, et al. Outcomes of laser in situ keratomileusis and photorefractive keratectomy in patients taking isotretinoin. *Am J Ophthalmol.* 2018 Aug;192:98–103. doi:10.1016/j.ajo.2018.05.009. Epub June 1, 2018. PMID: 29772222.

62. Tanzer DJ, Isfahani A, Schallhorn SC, LaBree LD, McDonnell PJ. Photorefractive keratectomy in African Americans including those with known dermatologic keloid formation. *Am J Ophthalmol.* 1998;126(5):625–629.

63. Girgis R, Morris DS, Kotagiri A, Ramaesh K. Bilateral corneal scarring after LASIK and PRK in a patient with propensity to keloid scar formation. *Eye.* 2007 Jan;21(1):96–97. doi:10.1038/sj.eye.6702180. Epub December 2, 2005. PMID: 16327796.

64. Schallhorn JM, Schallhorn SC, Ou Y. Factors that influence intraocular pressure changes after myopic and hyperopic LASIK and photorefractive keratectomy: A large population study. *Ophthalmology.* 2015 Mar;122(3):471–479. doi:10.1016/j.ophtha.2014.09.033. Epub November 14, 2014. PMID: 25444636.

65. Albietz JM, Lenton LM, McLennan SG. Effect of laser in situ keratomileusis for hyperopia on tear film and ocular surface. *J Refract Surg.* 2002 Mar–Apr;18(2):113–123. PMID: 11934197.

66. Bower KS, Sia RK, Ryan DS, Mines MJ, Dartt DA. Chronic dry eye in photorefractive keratectomy and laser in situ keratomileusis: Manifestations, incidence, and predictive factors. *J Cataract Refract Surg.* 2015 Dec;41(12):2624–2634. doi:10.1016/j.jcrs.2015.06.037. PMID: 26796443; PMCID: PMC5702539.

67. Schallhorn JM, Pelouskova M, Oldenburg C, Teenan D, Hannan SJ, Schallhorn SC. Effect of gender and procedure on patient-reported dry eye symptoms after laser vision correction. *J Refract Surg.* 2019 Mar 1;35(3):161–168. doi:10.3928/1081597X-20190107-01. PMID: 30855093.

68. Autrata R, Krejčířová I, Griščíková L, Doležel Z. Refrakční chirurgie při myopické anizometropické amblyopii u dětí a srovnání s konzervativní léčbou kontaktními čočkami [Refractive Surgery in Children with Myopic Anisometropia and Amblyopia in Comparison with Conventional Treatment by Contact Lenses]. *Cesk Slov Oftalmol.* 2016 spring;72(2):12–19. Czech. PMID: 27341094.

69. Drack AV, Nucci P. Refractive surgery in children. *Ophthalmol Clin North Am.* 2001 Sep;14(3):457–466. doi:10.1016/s0896-1549(05)70244-3. PMID: 11705146.

70. Astle WF, Huang PT, Ells AL, Cox RG, Deschenes MC, Vibert HM. Photorefractive keratectomy in children. *J Cataract Refract Surg.* 2002;28(6):932–941.

71. Daoud YJ, Hutchinson A, Wallace DK, Song J, Kim T. Refractive surgery in children: Treatment options, outcomes, and controversies. *Am J Ophthalmol.* 2009 Apr;147(4):573–582.e2. doi:10.1016/j.ajo.2008.12.028. PMID: 19327445.

72. Fecarotta CM, Kim M, Wasserman BN. Refractive surgery in children. *Curr Opin Ophthalmol.* 2010 Sep;21(5):350–355. doi:10.1097/ICU.0b013e32833c5d19. PMID: 20601878.

73. Magli A, Forte R, Gallo F, Carelli R. Refractive surgery for accommodative esotropia: 5-year follow-up. *J Refract Surg.* 2014 Feb;30(2):116–120. doi:10.3928/1081597X-20140120-07. PMID: 24763477.

74. J Shah T, Moshirfar M, C Hoopes P. Safety of the excimer laser in LASIK and PRK for patients with implantable cardiac devices: Our clinical experience in the past two decades. *J Ophthalmic Vis Res.* 2019 Oct 24;14(4):530–531. doi:10.18502/jovr. v14i4.547

75. Goes FJ. Photorefractive keratectomy for myopia of –8.00 to –24.00 diopters. *J Refract Surg.* 1996 Jan–Feb;12(1):91–97. PMID: 8963825.

76. Consultation section. What is your current method of treating myopia of –2.00, –4.00, –8.00, –12.00, –16.00, and –20.00 diopters? *J Cataract Refract Surg.* 1997 Jan–Feb;23(1):19–26. PMID: 9100102.

77. Piovella M, Camesasca FI, Fattori C. Excimer laser photorefractive keratectomy for high myopia: Four-year experience with a multiple zone technique. *Ophthalmology.* 1997 Oct;104(10):1554–1565. doi:10.1016/s0161-6420(97)30096-7. PMID: 9331191.

78. Rajan MS, Jaycock P, O'Brart D, Nystrom HH, Marshall J. A long-term study of photorefractive keratectomy; 12-year follow-up. *Ophthalmology.* 2004 Oct;111(10):1813–1824. doi:10.1016/j.ophtha.2004.05.019. PMID: 15465541.

79. Alió JL, Muftuoglu O, Ortiz D, et al. Ten-year follow-up of photorefractive keratectomy for myopia of less than-6 diopters. *Am J Ophthalmol.* 2008 Jan;145(1):29–36. doi:10.1016/j.ajo.2007.09.007. PMID: 18154752.

80. Alió JL, Muftuoglu O, Ortiz D, et al. Ten-year follow-up of photorefractive keratectomy for myopia of more than-6 diopters. *Am J Ophthalmol.* 2008 Jan;145(1):37–45. doi:10.1016/j.ajo.2007.09.009. PMID: 18154753.

81. Vestergaard AH, Hjortdal JØ, Ivarsen A, Work K, Grauslund J, Sjølie AK. Long-term outcomes of photorefractive keratectomy for low to high myopia: 13 to 19 years of follow-up. *J Refract Surg.* 2013 May;29(5):312–319. doi:10.3928/1081597X-20130415-02. PMID: 23659229.

82. Vestergaard AH. Past and present of corneal refractive surgery: A retrospective study of long-term results after photorefractive keratectomy and a prospective study of refractive lenticule extraction. *Acta Ophthalmol.* 2014 Mar;92 Thesis 2:1–21. doi:10.1111/aos.12385. PMID: 24636364.

83. McKernan AL, O'Dwyer, Mannion LS. The influence of soft contact lens wear and two weeks cessation of lens wear on corneal curvature. Lloyd McKernan, Aoife et al. *Contact Lens and Anterior Eye.* 2014;37(1):31–37.

84. Chao-Shern C, Me R, DeDionisio LA, et al. Post-LASIK exacerbation of granular corneal dystrophy type 2 in members of a Chinese family. *Eye.* 2018 Jan;32(1):39–43. doi:10.1038/eye.2017.265. Epub December 1, 2017. PMID: 29192679; PMCID: PMC5770725.

85. Kim SW, Byun YJ, Kim EK, Kim TI. Central corneal thickness measurements in unoperated eyes and eyes after PRK for myopia using Pentacam, Orbscan II, and ultrasonic pachymetry. *J Refract Surg.* 2007 Nov;23(9):888–894. PMID: 18041241.

86. Wu W, Wang Y, Xu L. Meta-analysis of Pentacam vs. ultrasound pachymetry in central corneal thickness measurement in normal, post-LASIK or PRK, and keratoconic or keratoconus-suspect eyes. *Graefes Arch Clin Exp Ophthalmol.* 2014 Jan;252(1):91–99. doi:10.1007/s00417-013-2502-5. Epub November 12, 2013. PMID: 24218039.

87. Santhiago MR. Percent tissue altered and corneal ectasia. *Curr Opin Ophthalmol.* 2016 Jul;27(4):311–315. doi:10.1097/ICU.0000000000000276. PMID: 27096376.

88. Böhm A, Kohlhaas M, Lerche RC, Hjortdal JO, Ehlers N, Draeger J. Biomechanische Untersuchung der Hornhautstabilität nach photorefraktiver Keratektomie [Biomechanical study of corneal stability after photorefractive keratectomy]. *Ophthalmologe.* 1997 Feb;94(2):109–113. German. doi:10.1007/s003470050090. PMID: 9156634.

89. Lombardo M, Lombardo G, Ducoli P, Serrao S. Long-term changes of the anterior corneal topography after photorefractive keratectomy for myopia and myopic astigmatism. *Invest Ophthalmol Vis Sci.* 2011 Sep 1;52(9):6994–7000. doi:10.1167/iovs.10-7052. PMID: 21791596.

90. Busool Y, Mimouni M, Vainer I, et al. Risk factors predicting steroid-induced ocular hypertension after photorefractive keratectomy. *J Cataract Refract Surg.* 2017 Mar;43(3):389–393. doi:10.1016/j.jcrs.2016.12.030. PMID: 28410723.

91. De Bernardo M, Capasso L, Caliendo L, Vosa Y, Rosa N. Intraocular pressure evaluation after myopic refractive surgery: A comparison of methods in 121 eyes. *Sem Ophthalmol.* 2016;31:233–242.

92. De Bernardo M, Salzano FA, Rosa N. Steroid-induced ocular hypertension after photorefractive keratectomy. *J Cataract Refract Surg.* 2018 Jan;44(1):118. doi:10.1016/j.jcrs.2017.10.048. PMID: 29502607.

93. Shimmyo M, Fry K, Hersh PS, Taylor D, Hayashi NI. Eyes at risk of ectasia: Corneal hysteresis and corneal resistance factor in keratoconus, pre-and post-LASIK eyes. *Invest Ophthalmol Vis Sci.* 2007;48(13):2361.

94. Naderi M, Sabour S, Khodakarim S, Daneshgar F. Studying the factors related to refractive error regression after PRK surgery. *BMC Ophthalmol.* 2018 Aug 14;18(1):198. doi:10.1186/s12886-018-0879-y. PMID: 30107828; PMCID: PMC6092795.

95. Sippel KC, Jain S, Azar DT. Monovision achieved with excimer laser refractive surgery. *Int Ophthalmol Clin.* 2001 Spring;41(2):91–101. doi:10.1097/00004397-200104000-00009. PMID: 11290924.

96. Cox CA, Krueger RR. Monovision with laser vision correction. *Ophthalmol Clin North Am.* 2006 Mar;19(1):71–75, vi. doi:10.1016/j.ohc.2005.10.002. PMID: 16500529.

97. Braun EH, Lee J, Steinert RF. Monovision in LASIK. *Ophthalmology.* 2008 Jul;115(7):1196–1202. doi:10.1016/j.ophtha.2007.09.018. Epub December 3, 2007. PMID: 18061266.

98. Zhou J, Feng L, Lin H, Hess RF. On the maintenance of normal ocular dominance and a possible mechanism underlying refractive adaptation. *Invest Ophthalmol Vis Sci.* 2016 Oct 1;57(13):5181–5185. doi:10.1167/iovs.16-19696. PMID: 27699413.

99. Feng L, Lin H, Chen Y, et al. The effect of Lasik surgery on myopic anisometropes' sensory eye dominance. *Sci Rep.* 2017 Jun 15;7(1):3629. doi:10.1038/s41598-017-03553-8. PMID: 28620156; PMCID: PMC5472567.

100. Zarei-Ghanavati S, Eslampour A, Shokouhirad S, et al. The effect of eye dominancy on patients' cooperation and perceived pain during photorefractive keratectomy. *J Curr Ophthalmol.* 2019 Jul 23;31(4):373–376. doi:10.1016/j.joco.2019.07.003. PMID: 31844785; PMCID: PMC6896458.

101. Ooi TL, He ZJ. Sensory eye dominance: Relationship between eye and brain. *Eye Brain.* 2020 Jan 20;12:25–31. doi:10.2147/EB. S176931. PMID: 32021530; PMCID: PMC6980844.

102. Kezirian GM, Stonecipher KG. Subjective assessment of mesopic visual function after laser in situ keratomileusis. *Ophthalmol Clin North Am.* 2004 Jun;17(2):211–224, vii. doi:10.1016/j.ohc.2004.03.004. PMID: 15207563.

103. Netto MV, Ambrósio R Jr, Wilson SE. Pupil size in refractive surgery candidates. *J Refract Surg.* 2004 Jul–Aug;20(4):337–342. PMID: 15307395.

104. Salz JJ, Trattler W. Pupil size and corneal laser surgery. *Curr Opin Ophthalmol.* 2006 Aug;17(4):373–379. doi:10.1097/01.icu.0000233958.96133.02. PMID: 16900031.

105. Linke SJ, Baviera J, Munzer G, Fricke OH, Richard G, Katz T. Mesopic pupil size in a refractive surgery population (13,959 eyes). *Optom Vis Sci.* 2012 Aug;89(8):1156–1164. doi:10.1097/OPX.0b013e318263c165. PMID: 22773178.

106. Myung D, Schallhorn S, Manche EE. Pupil size and LASIK: A review. *J Refract Surg.* 2013 Nov;29(11):734–741. doi:10.3928/1081597X-20131021-02. PMID: 24203804.

107. Albietz JM, Lenton LM. Management of the ocular surface and tear film before, during, and after laser in situ keratomileusis. *J Refract Surg.* 2004 Jan–Feb;20(1):62–71. PMID: 14763473.

108. Chen KJ, Yu T, Pan J, Liu LN, Lang M, Bai J. [Effect of different medication time prior to corneal refractive surgery on tear film stability]. *Zhonghua Yan Ke Za Zhi.* 2018 Oct 11;54(10):744–747. Chinese. doi:10.3760/cma.j.issn.0412-4081.2018.10.005. PMID: 30347561.

109. Bilgihan A, Bilgihan K, Toklu Y, et al. Ascorbic acid levels in human tears after photorefractive keratectomy, transepithelial photorefractive keratectomy, and laser in situ keratomileusis. *J Cataract Refract Surg.* 2001 Apr;27(4):585–588. doi:10.1016/s0886-3350(00)00877-4

110. Stojanovic A, Ringvold A, Nitter T. Ascorbate prophylaxis for corneal haze after photorefractive keratectomy. *J Refract Surg.* 2003 May–Jun;19(3):338–343. PMID: 12777030.

111. Ong NH, Purcell TL, Roch-Levecq AC, et al. Epithelial healing and visual outcomes of patients using omega-3 oral nutritional supplements before and after photorefractive keratectomy: A pilot study. *Cornea.* 2013 Jun;32(6):761–765. doi:10.1097/ICO.0b013e31826905b3. PMID: 23132445.

112. Abbott RL. Medical malpractice predictors and risk factors for ophthalmologists performing LASIK and PRK surgery. *Trans Am Ophthalmol Soc.* 2003;101:239–274. PMID: 14971582; PMCID: PMC1358993.

113. Speaker MG, Menikoff JA. Prophylaxis of endophthalmitis with topical povidone-iodine. *Ophthalmology.* 1991 Dec;98(12):1769–1775. doi:10.1016/s0161-6420(91)32052-9. PMID: 1775308.

114. Carrim ZI, Mackie G, Gallacher G, Wykes WN. The efficacy of 5% povidone-iodine for 3 minutes prior to cataract surgery. *Eur J Ophthalmol.* 2009 Jul–Aug;19(4):560–564. doi:10.1177/112067210901900407. PMID: 19551669.

115. Rajpal RK, Cooperman BB. Analgesic efficacy and safety of ketorolac after photorefractive keratectomy. Ketorolac Study Group. *J Refract Surg.* 1999 Nov–Dec;15(6):661–667. PMID: 10590004.

116. Ram J, Kaushik S, Brar GS, Taneja N, Gupta A. Prevention of postoperative infections in ophthalmic surgery. *Indian J Ophthalmol.* 2001 Mar;49(1):59–69. PMID: 15887720.

117. Sher NA, Golben MR, Bond W, Trattler WB, Tauber S, Voirin TG. Topical bromfenac 0.09% vs. ketorolac 0.4% for the control of pain, photophobia, and discomfort following PRK. *J Refract Surg.* 2009 Feb;25(2):214–220. doi:10.3928/1081597X-20090201-07. PMID: 19241773.

118. Lee HK, Lee KS, Kim JK, Kim HC, Seo KR, Kim EK. Epithelial healing and clinical outcomes in excimer laser photorefractive surgery following three epithelial removal techniques: Mechanical, alcohol, and excimer laser. *Am J Ophthalmol.* 2005 Jan;139(1):56–63. doi:10.1016/j.ajo.2004.08.049. PMID: 15652828.

119. Shapira Y, Mimouni M, Levartovsky S, et al. Comparison of three epithelial removal techniques in PRK: Mechanical, alcohol-assisted, and transepithelial laser. *J Refract Surg.* 2015 Nov;31(11):760–766. doi:10.3928/1081597X-20151021-05. PMID: 26544564.

120. Ghoreishi M, Attarzadeh H, Tavakoli M, et al. Alcohol-assisted versus mechanical epithelium removal in photorefractive keratectomy. *J Ophthalmic Vis Res.* 2010 Oct;5(4):223–227. PMID: 22737365; PMCID: PMC3381083.

121. Li SM, Zhan S, Li SY, et al. Laser-assisted subepithelial keratectomy (LASEK) versus photorefractive keratectomy (PRK) for correction of myopia. *Cochrane Database Syst Rev.* 2016 Feb 22;2:CD009799. doi:10.1002/14651858.CD009799.pub2. PMID: 26899152; PMCID: PMC5032141.

122. Pallikaris IG, Karoutis AD, Lydataki SE, Siganos DS. Rotating brush for fast removal of corneal epithelium. *J Refract Corneal Surg.* 1994 Jul–Aug;10(4):439–442. PMID: 7528616.

123. Amoils SP. Photorefractive keratectomy using a scanning-slit laser, rotary epithelial brush, and chilled balanced salt solution. *J Cataract Refract Surg.* 2000 Nov;26(11):1596–1604. doi:10.1016/s0886-3350(00)00542-3. PMID: 11084266.

124. Vingopoulos F, Kanellopoulos AJ. Epi-Bowman blunt keratectomy versus diluted EtOH epithelial removal in myopic photorefractive keratectomy: A prospective contralateral eye study. *Cornea.* 2019;38(5):612–616. doi:10.1097/ICO.0000000000001863

125. Adib-Moghaddam S, Soleyman-Jahi S, Sanjari Moghaddam A, et al. Efficacy, and safety of transepithelial photorefractive keratectomy. *J Cataract Refract Surg.* 2018 Oct;44(10):1267–1279. doi:10.1016/j.jcrs.2018.07.021. Epub August 29, 2018. PMID: 30172569.

126. Krueger RR. In perspective: Eye tracking and autonomous laser radar. *J Refract Surg.* 1999 Mar–Apr;15(2):145–149. PMID: 10202709.

127. Mrochen M, Eldine MS, Kaemmerer M, Seiler T, Hütz W. Improvement in photorefractive corneal laser surgery results using an active eye-tracking system. *J Cataract Refract Surg.* 2001 Jul;27(7):1000–1006. doi:10.1016/s0886-3350(00)00884-1. PMID: 11489567.

128. Gharaee H, Ghanavati SZ, Rad SS, Omidtabrizi A, Naseri H. Effectiveness of Technolas torsional eye tracking system on visual outcomes after photorefractive keratectomy. *J Curr Ophthalmol.* 2016 Feb 3;27(3–4):82–86. doi:10.1016/j.joco.2015.11.007. PMID: 27239583; PMCID: PMC4881233.

129. Khakshoor H, McCaughey MV, Vejdani AH, Daneshvar R, Moshirfar M. Use of angle kappa in myopic photorefractive keratectomy. *Clin Ophthalmol.* 2015 Jan 29; 9:193–195. doi:10.2147/OPTH.S70690. PMID: 25678767; PMCID: PMC4322872.

130. Thornton I, Xu M, Krueger RR. Comparison of standard (0.02%) and low dose (0.002%) mitomycin C in the prevention of corneal haze following surface ablation for myopia. *J Refract Surg.* 2008 Jan;24(1):S68–S76. doi:10.3928/1081597X-20080101-13. PMID: 18269154.

131. Sia RK, Ryan DS, Edwards JD, Stutzman RD, Bower KS. The U.S. Army Surface Ablation Study: Comparison of PRK, MMC-PRK, and LASEK in moderate to high myopia. *J Refract Surg.* 2014 Apr;30(4):256–264. doi:10.3928/1081597X-20140320-04. PMID: 24702577.

132. Majmudar PA, Schallhorn SC, Cason JB, et al. Mitomycin-C in corneal surface excimer laser ablation techniques: A report by the American Academy of Ophthalmology. *Ophthalmology.* 2015 Jun;122(6):1085–1095. doi:10.1016/j.ophtha.2015.01.019. Epub March 18, 2015. PMID: 25795477.

133. Carlos de Oliveira R, Wilson SE. Biological effects of mitomycin C on late corneal haze stromal fibrosis following PRK. *Exp Eye Res.* 2020 Nov;200:108218. doi:10.1016/j.exer.2020.108218. Epub September 6, 2020. PMID: 32905844; PMCID: PMC7655619.

134. Mathew J. Contact lens practice pearls newer uses for silicone hydrogel contact lenses. Contact Lens Spectrum. Available at: https://www.clspectrum.com/issues/201/august-2014/contact-lens-practice-pearls

135. Sánchez-González JM, López-Izquierdo I, Gargallo-Martínez B, De-Hita-Cantalejo C, Bautista-Llamas MJ. Bandage contact lens use after photorefractive keratectomy. *J Cataract Refract Surg.* 2019 Aug;45(8):1183–1190. doi:10.1016/j.jcrs.2019.02.045. Epub 2019 Jun 15. PMID: 31213328.

136. Taylor KR, Caldwell MC, Payne AM, et al. Comparison of 3 silicone hydrogel bandage soft contact lenses for pain control after photorefractive keratectomy. *J Cataract Refract Surg.* 2014 Nov;40(11): 1798–1804. doi:10.1016/j.jcrs.2014.02.040. Epub September 10, 2014. PMID: 25217073.

137. Azar DT, Chang JH, Han KY. Wound healing after keratorefractive surgery: Review of biological and optical considerations. *Cornea.* 2012 Nov;31 Suppl 1(1):S9–S19. doi:10.1097/ICO.0b013e31826ab0a7. PMID: 23038040; PMCID: PMC3682490.

138. Stonecipher KG. COVID: Before and after. Corneal Visual Summit; December 2020.

139. Duru Z, Duru N, Ulusoy DM. Effects of senofilcon A and lotrafilcon B bandage contact lenses on epithelial healing and pain management after bilateral photorefractive keratectomy. *Cont Lens Anterior Eye.* 2020 Apr;43(2):169–172. doi:10.1016/j.clae.2019.08.008. Epub September 5, 2019. PMID: 31495762.

140. Solomon R, Donnenfeld ED, Perry HD, Wittpenn JR, Greenman H, Stein J. Effect of gatifloxacin 0.3% and moxifloxacin 0.5% on corneal epithelial wound healing after photorefractive keratectomy. *Invest Ophthalmol Vis Sci.* 2005;46(13):4895.

141. Shin JH, Lee HB, Park HY. Comparison of the effects of fourth-generation fluoroquinolones on epithelial healing after photorefractive keratectomy. *Cornea.* 2010 Nov;29(11):1236–1240. doi:10.1097/ICO.0b013e3181d5d955. PMID: 20697276.

142. Talamo JH, Hatch KM, Woodcock EC. Delayed epithelial closure after PRK associated with topical besifloxacin use. *Cornea.* 2013 Oct;32(10):1365–1368. doi:10.1097/ICO.0b013e31829e1e8c. PMID: 23974887.

143. Yee R, Setabutr P, Foltermann M, Sami M, Chuang A. The effects of topical moxifloxacin 0.5% ophthalmic solution and gatifloxacin 0.3% solution on corneal healing after bilateral photorefractive keratectomy. *Cornea.* 2006;25:S8–S11. doi:10.1097/01.ico.0000176607.17871.6e

144. Asbell PA, Pandit RT, Sanfilippo CM. Antibiotic resistance rates by geographic region among ocular pathogens collected during the ARMOR surveillance study. *Ophthalmol Ther.* 2018 Dec;7(2):417–429. doi:10.1007/s40123-018-0141-y. Epub August 9, 2018. PMID: 30094698; PMCID: PMC6258574.

145. Baek SH, Chang JH, Choi SY, Kim WJ, Lee JH. The effect of topical corticosteroids on refractive outcome and corneal haze after photorefractive keratectomy. *J Refract Surg.* 1997 Nov–Dec;13(7): 644–652. PMID: 9427202.

146. Shokoohi-Rad S, Daneshvar R, Jafarian-Shahri M, Rajaee P. Comparison between betamethasone, fluorometholone and loteprednol etabonate on intraocular pressure in patients after keratorefractive surgery. *J Curr Ophthalmol.* 2017 Dec 7;30(2):130–135. doi:10.1016/j.joco.2017.11.008. PMID: 29988925; PMCID: PMC6033780.

147. Karimian F, Faramarzi A, Fekri S, et al. Comparison of loteprednol with fluorometholone after myopic photorefractive keratectomy. *J Ophthalmic Vis Res.* 2017 Jan–Mar;12(1):11–16. doi:10.4103/2008-322X.200161. PMID: 28299001; PMCID: PMC5340049.

148. Mifflin MD, Betts BS, Frederick PA, et al. Efficacy and safety of a 3-month loteprednol etabonate 0.5% gel taper for routine prophylaxis after photorefractive keratectomy compared to a 3-month prednisolone acetate 1% and fluorometholone 0.1% taper. *Clin Ophthalmol.* 2017 Jun 12;11:1113–1118. doi:10.2147/OPTH.S138272. PMID: 28652697; PMCID: PMC5476723.

149. Albietz JM, McLennan SG, Lenton LM. Ocular surface management of photorefractive keratectomy and laser in situ keratomileusis. *J Refract Surg.* 2003 Nov–Dec;19(6):636–644. PMID: 14640428.

150. Beheshtnejad AH, Hashemian H, Kermanshahani AM, Mahmoudi A, Johari MK. Evaluation of tear osmolarity changes after photorefractive keratectomy. *Cornea.* 2015 Dec;34(12):1541–1544. doi:10.1097/ICO.0000000000000649. PMID: 26488623.

151. Gogri P, Parkar M, Bhalerao SA. Visual outcomes of sterile corneal infiltrates after photorefractive keratectomy. *Indian J Ophthalmol.* 2020 Dec;68(12):2956–2959. doi:10.4103/ijo.IJO_1300_20. PMID: 33229677.

152. O'Doherty M, Kirwan C, O'Keeffe M, O'Doherty J. Postoperative pain following epi-LASIK, LASEK, and PRK for myopia. *J Refract Surg.* 2007 Feb;23(2):133–138. PMID: 17326352.

153. Woreta FA, Gupta A, Hochstetler B, Bower KS. Management of post-photorefractive keratectomy pain. *Surv Ophthalmol.* 2013 Nov–Dec;58(6):529–535. doi:10.1016/j.survophthal.2012.11.004. PMID: 24160728.

154. Faktorovich EG, Melwani K. Efficacy and safety of pain relief medications after photorefractive keratectomy: Review of prospective randomized trials. *J Cataract Refract Surg.* 2014 Oct;40(10): 1716–1730. doi:10.1016/j.jcrs.2014.08.001. PMID: 25263042.

155. Fay J, Juthani V. Current trends in pain management after photorefractive and phototherapeutic keratectomy. *Curr Opin Ophthalmol.* 2015 Jul;26(4):255–259. doi:10.1097/ICU.0000000000000170. PMID: 26058021.

156. Golan O, Randleman JB. Pain management after photorefractive keratectomy. *Curr Opin Ophthalmol.* 2018 Jul;29(4):306–312. doi:10.1097/ICU.0000000000000486. PMID: 29708926.

157. Al-Sharif EM, Stone DU. Correlation between practice location as a surrogate for UV exposure and practice patterns to prevent corneal haze after photorefractive keratectomy (PRK). *Saudi J Ophthalmol.* 2016 Oct–Dec;30(4):213–216. doi:10.1016/j.sjopt.2016.11.004. Epub November 10, 2016. PMID: 28003777; PMCID: PMC5161811.

158. Wroblewski KJ, Pasternak JF, Bower KS, et al. Infectious keratitis after photorefractive keratectomy in the United States army and navy. *Ophthalmology.* 2006 Apr;113(4):520–525. doi:10.1016/j.ophtha.2005.09.038. Epub February 17, 2006. PMID: 16488012.

159. Tisdale CS, Justin GA, Wang X, et al. Refractive surgery in the HIV-positive U.S. Military Natural History Study Cohort: Complications and risk factors. *J Cataract Refract Surg.* 2019 Nov;45(11): 1612–1618. doi:10.1016/j.jcrs.2019.06.017. Epub October 1, 2019. PMID: 31585850; PMCID: PMC6842682.

160. Shortt AJ, Allan BD, Evans JR. Laser-assisted in-situ keratomileusis (LASIK) versus photorefractive keratectomy (PRK) for myopia. *Cochrane Database Syst Rev.* 2013 Jan 31;(1):CD005135. doi:10.1002/14651858.CD005135.pub3. PMID: 23440799.

161. Stojanovic A, Nitter TA. Correlation between ultraviolet radiation level and the incidence of late-onset corneal haze after photorefractive keratectomy. *J Cataract Refract Surg.* 2001 Mar;27(3):404–410. doi:10.1016/s0886-3350(00)00742-2. PMID: 11255052.

162. George Stan P, Johnson Donald G. Photorefractive keratectomy retreatments, comparison of two methods of excimer laser epithelium removal. *Ophthalmology.* 1999;106:1469–1480. doi:10.1016/S0161-6420(99)90439-6

163. Randleman JB, White AJ Jr, Lynn MJ, et al. Incidence, outcomes, and risk factors for retreatment after wavefront-optimized ablations with PRK and LASIK. *J Refract Surg.* 2009;25:273–276. doi:10.3928/1081597X-20090301-06

164. Shojaei A, Mohammad-Rabei H, Eslani M, Elahi B, Noorizadeh F. Long-term evaluation of complications and results of photorefractive keratectomy in myopia: An 8-year follow-up. *Cornea.* 2009;28(3):304–310. doi:10.1097/ICO.0b013e3181896767

165. Kanellopoulos AJ, Pe LH. Wavefront-guided enhancements using the wave-light excimer laser in symptomatic eyes previously treated with LASIK. *J Refract Surg.* 2006;22:345–349. doi:10.3928/1081-597X-20060401-08

166. Lee JB, Ryu CH, Kim J-H, Kim EK, Kim HB. Comparison of tear secretion and tear film instability after photorefractive keratectomy and laser in situ keratomileusis. *J Cataract Refract Surg.* 2000 Sep;26(9):1326–1331. doi:10.1016/S0886-3350(00)00566-6

167. Puliafito CA, Stern D, Kruger RR, Mandel ER. High-speed photography of excimer laser ablation of the cornea. *Arch Ophthalmol.* 1987;105:1255–1259.

168. Kruger RR, Campos M, Wang W, et al. Corneal surface morphology following excimer laser ablation with humidified gases. *Arch Ophthalmol.* 1993;111:1131–1137.

169. Kruger RR, Saedy NF, McDonell PJ. Clinical analysis of steep central islands after excimer laser photorefractive keratectomy. *Arch Ophthalmol.* 1996;114:377–381.

170. Noack J, Tonnies R, Hohla K, et al. Influence of ablation plume dynamics on the formation of central islands in excimer laser photorefractive keratectomy. *Ophthalmology.* 1997;104:823–830.

171. Abbas UL, Hersh PS. Natural history of corneal topography after excimer laser photorefractive keratectomy. *Ophthalmology.* 1998;105:2197–2206.

172. Rachid MD, Yoo SH, Azar DT. Phototherapeutic keratectomy for decentration and central islands after photorefractive keratectomy. *Ophthalmology*. 2001;108:545–552.
173. https://eyewiki.aao.org/Central_Islands_After_Laser_Refractive_Surgery
174. Stojanovic A, Suput D. Strategic planning in topography-guided ablation of irregular astigmatism after laser refractive surgery. *J Refract Surg*. 2005 Jul–Aug;21(4):369–376. PMID: 16128335.
175. Allan BD, Hassan H. Topography-guided transepithelial photorefractive keratectomy for irregular astigmatism using a 213 nm solid-state laser. *J Cataract Refract Surg*. 2013 Jan;39(1):97–104. doi:10.1016/j.jcrs.2012.08.0156. Epub November 14, 2012. PMID: 23158680.
176. Ghoreishi M, Peyman A, Koosha N, Golabchi K, Pourazizi M. Topography-guided transepithelial photorefractive keratectomy to correct irregular refractive errors after radial keratotomy. *J Cataract Refract Surg*. 2018 Mar;44(3):274–279. doi:10.1016/j.jcrs.2017.12.015. Epub March 30, 2018. PMID: 29610024.
177. Reinstein DZ, Archer TJ, Dickeson ZI, Gobbe M. Transepithelial phototherapeutic keratectomy protocol for treating irregular astigmatism based on population epithelial thickness measurements by artemis very high-frequency digital ultrasound. *J Refract Surg*. 2014,30(6):380–387. doi:10.3928/1081597X-20140508-01
178. Sorkin N, Kaiserman I, Domniz Y, Sela T, Munzer G, Varssano D. Risk assessment for corneal ectasia following photorefractive keratectomy. *J Ophthalmol*. 2017;2017, Article ID 2434830:10 pages. doi:10.1155/2017/2434830
179. Ghadhfan F, Al-Rajhi A, Wagoner MD. Laser in situ keratomileusis versus surface ablation: Visual outcomes and complications. *J Cataract Refract Surg*. 2007 Dec;33(12):2041–2048. doi:10.1016/j.jcrs.2007.07.026. PMID: 18053901.
180. Randleman JB, Stulting RD. Ectasia after photorefractive keratectomy [letter]. *Ophthalmology*. 2007;114:396. doi:10.1016/j.ophtha.2006.09.008
181. Randleman JB, Woodward M, Lynn MJ, Stulting RD.Risk assessment for ectasia after corneal refractive surgery. *Ophthalmology*. 2008;115:37–50. doi:10.1016/j.ophtha.2007.03.073
182. Wen D, McAlinden C, Flitcroft I, et al. Postoperative efficacy, predictability, safety, and visual quality of laser corneal refractive surgery: A network meta-analysis. *Am J Ophthalmol*. 2017;178:65–78. doi:10.1016/j.ajo.2017.03.013
183. American Academy of Ophthalmology Preferred Practice Pattern Refractive Management/Intervention Panel. Refractive errors & refractive surgery preferred practice pattern. *Ophthalmology*. 2018;125(1):P1–P104. doi:10.1016/j.ophtha.2017.10.003g
184. Faria-Correia F, Ribeiro S, Lopes BT, Salomão MQ, Ambrósio R Jr. Outcomes comparison between wavefront-optimized and topography-guided PRK in contralateral eyes with myopia and myopic astigmatism. *J Refract Surg*. 2020 Jun 1;36(6):358–365. doi:10.3928/1081597X-20200416-01. PMID: 32521022
185. Moshirfar M, Tirth S, Skanchy D, Linn S, Kang P, Durrie D. Comparison and analysis of FDA reported visual outcomes of the three latest platforms for LASIK: Wavefront guided Visx iDesign, topography guided WaveLight Allegro Contoura, and topography guided Nidek EC-5000 CATz. *Clin Ophthalmol*. 2017;11:135–147. doi:10.2147/OPTH.S115270
186. Wen D, Tu R, Flitcroft I, et al. Corneal surface ablation laser refractive surgery for the correction of myopia: a network meta-analysis. *J Refract Surg*. 2018;34(11):726–735. doi:10.3928/1081597X-20180905-01
187. Schallhorn SC, Venter JA, Hannan SJ, Hettinger KA. Wavefront-guided photorefractive keratectomy with the use of a New Hartmann-Shack Aberrometer in patients with myopia and compound myopic astigmatism. *J Ophthalmol*. 2015;2015:514837. doi:10.1155/2015/514837. Epub October 4, 2015. PMID: 26504595; PMCID: PMC4609463.
188. Murray A, Jones L, Milne A, et al. A systemic review of the safety and efficacy of elective photorefractive surgery for the correction of refractive error. Aberdeen, Scotland: Health Services Research Unit, University of Aberdeen; 2005. Available at: www.sheffield.ac.uk/polopoly_fs/1.43792!/file/Photorefractive-IPP.pdf. Accessed September 29, 2017.
189. Gershoni A, Mimouni M, Livny E, Bahar I. Z-LASIK and Trans-PRK for correction of high-grade myopia: Safety, efficacy, predictability, and clinical outcomes. *Int Ophthalmol*. 2019 Apr;39(4):753–763. doi: 10.1007/s10792-018-0868-4. Epub March 12, 2018. PMID: 29532217.

190. Mifflin MD, Betts BS, Nguyen J, Pouly S. High myopic photorefractive keratectomy outcomes with the Alcon Wavelight EX500 excimer laser. *Clin Ophthalmol.* 2018 Jun 6;12:1041–1048. doi:10.2147/OPTH.S164110. PMID: 29922033; PMCID: PMC5995275.

191. Jun I, Kang DSY, Reinstein DZ, et al. Clinical outcomes of SMILE with a triple centration technique and corneal wavefront-guided transepithelial PRK in high astigmatism. *J Refract Surg.* 2018 Mar 1;34(3):156–163. doi:10.3928/1081597X-20180104-03. PMID: 29522224.

192. Jun I, Kang DSY, Arba-Mosquera S, Kim EK, Seo KY, Kim TI. Clinical outcomes of transepithelial photorefractive keratectomy according to epithelial thickness. *J Refract Surg.* 2018 Aug 1;34(8):533–540. doi:10.3928/1081597X-20180618-02. PMID: 30089183.

193. Seven I, Lloyd JS, Dupps WJ. Differences in simulated refractive outcomes of photorefractive keratectomy (PRK) and laser in-situ keratomileusis (LASIK) for myopia in same-eye virtual trials. *Int J Environ Res Public Health.* 2019 Dec 31;17(1):287. doi:10.3390/ijerph17010287. PMID: 31906169; PMCID: PMC6982132.

194. Ganesh S, Brar S, Patel U. Comparison of ReLEx SMILE and PRK in terms of visual and refractive outcomes for the correction of low myopia. *Int Ophthalmol.* 2018 Jun;38(3):1147–1154. doi:10.1007/s10792-017-0575-6. Epub May 27, 2017. PMID: 28551832.

195. Jun I, Yong Kang DS, Arba-Mosquera S, et al. Clinical outcomes of mechanical and transepithelial photorefractive keratectomy in low myopia with a large ablation zone. *J Cataract Refract Surg.* 2019 Jul;45(7):977–984. doi:10.1016/j.jcrs.2019.02.007. Epub April 24, 2019. PMID: 31029476.

7 Laser In Situ Keratomileusis

Karl Stonecipher • Jessica Mathew • Stephen Brint

Laser in situ keratomileusis (LASIK) is the combination of using the excimer laser with a device used for making a flap of corneal tissue. More than 60 years ago, Jose I. Barraquer, M.D., created the initial concept of in situ keratomileusis (cornea/carving), which really consisted of adding, removing, or altering corneal tissue to modify the refractive power of the eye.[1] Keratomileusis in situ initially started over 50 years ago with the creation of a corneal lamellar disc (surface), also called lamellar keratoplasty, with a device called a keratome. By 1962, Dr. Barraquer looked at addition, subtraction, or modification of the corneal tissue. Initially, this started with the development of the cryolathe where he would freeze the removed lamellar disc and alter its shape to reduce the refractive error of the patient. However, this was fraught with complications including but not limited to corneal scarring and irregular astigmatism.[2-10] Fast forward to the late 1980s and early 1990s when Pallikaris started animal studies using an excimer laser combined with a microkeratome with both Pallikaris and Burrato doing the early human trials and Peymon patenting what is known as LASIK today (Fig. 7.1).[11-20] A more detailed history of LASIK can be found in an article by Reinstein et al.[21]

INDICATIONS

- Myopia
- Hyperopia
- Myopic astigmatism
- Hyperopic astigmatism
- Mixed astigmatism
- Presbyopic treatments

Laser vision correction was designed to reduce or eliminate refractive errors of essentially normal corneas. However, there are more advanced laser vision correction options now available that can also reduce or eliminate higher-order aberrations. The primary goal of LASIK is to allow the patient to see postoperatively equal to or better than their present refractive correction (glasses, contact lens, etc.) while providing a safe procedure with low to no complications or repeat procedures, known commonly as enhancements.

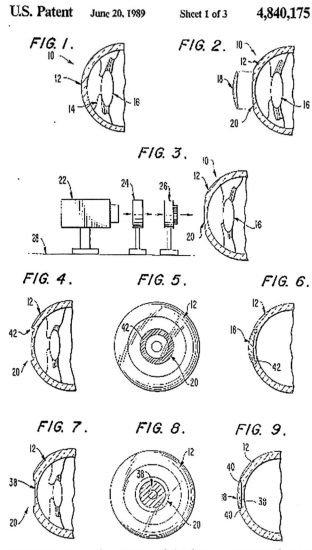

FIGURE 7-1 Copy of an image of the first U.S. Patent of LASIK in 1989.

CONTRAINDICATIONS FOR LASER IN SITU KERATOMILEUSIS

- Keratoconus
- Corneal scarring or opacification
- Pellucid marginal degeneration

- Corneal ectasia
- Various corneal dystrophies
- Unstable refraction
- Contact lens warpage
- Uncontrolled ocular surface disease
- Uncontrolled systemic diseases (i.e., diabetes, thyroid, etc.)
- Uncontrolled connective tissue disease
- Uncontrolled intraocular inflammation (i.e., uveitis, etc.)

The screening process for LASIK continues to evolve. Initially, the screening process consisted primarily of a routine eye examination to include manifest refraction, cycloplegic refraction, and topography. Today, additional diagnostics are included, such as tomography, corneal hysteresis, corneal aberrometry, corneal pachymetry, ray tracing, and others are added to the mix but not necessarily all inclusive. Standard of care ranges from country to country but basics include a refraction, corneal thickness, corneal topography, and/or corneal tomography as an addition to a routine eye exam.

PATIENT-INFORMED CONSENT PROCESS

Following are some free consent form resources with more detailed information:

1. https://www.omic.com/lasik-consent-forms/
2. https://www.omic.com/lasik-bilateral-simultaneous/
3. https://www.omic.com/lasik-off-label/
4. https://www.omic.com/lasik-assumption-of-post-op-care/

Informed Consent of the Patient

- Consent documents received by the patient
- Consent documents reviewed by the patient
- Surgeon discussion with the patient
- Risks and benefits of the procedure reviewed with the patient
- Questions answered for the patient
- Consent signed and placed in the chart

It is mandatory to discuss the procedure in detail, the benefits of the procedure, the alternatives to the procedure including no surgery at all.[22] The risks of the procedure should also be discussed and include blindness, failure of the procedure, risk of loss of the eye or eyes, infection, and even death as a potential complication. Explaining and detailing the contents of the informed consent document to the patient is imperative. The patient should have an opportunity to ask questions and to have them answered in an understandable format. The patient and the doctor should verbally confirm that they understand what is about to take place and that they have agreed

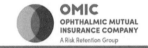

OMIC
OPHTHALMIC MUTUAL
INSURANCE COMPANY
A Risk Retention Group

Customize to your practice before using this document.
1. Remove this banner and replace with your letterhead on the
first page of the consent form.
2. Keep each section together on same page: move as needed.
3. Change font size for large print.

Sample Informed Consent Document

Consent for planned comanagement after eye surgery

Patient Name:_____

Dr. _____ (name of surgeon) will be performing _____ (type of surgery)

on me. Because of _____ (state reason), I would like Dr. _____ (name of

comanaging optometrist) to perform my postoperative follow-up care. I have discussed this

postoperative selection with my surgeon.

I understand that my comanaging optometrist Dr. _____ (name of comanaging

optometrist) will contact my surgeon immediately if I experience any complications related to my eye

surgery.

I understand that I may contact Dr. _____ (name of surgeon) at any time after the

surgery.

Patient:_____ Date: _____

FIGURE 7-2 Sample informed consent created by Ophthalmic Mutual Insurance Company.

to proceed with the planned procedure. Personally, the authors believe this discussion is a legally binding contract between the patient and the doctor and is the surgeon's responsibility to undertake control of the informed consent process and should not be delegated.[22–24] If co-management is to be part of the process, the patient must be informed of the individual duties of the comanaging clinician versus the surgeon, and follow-up procedures must be discussed in detail and agreed upon by the patient prior to surgery (Fig. 7.2).[25]

PREOPERATIVE PREPARATION FOR LASER IN SITU KERATOMILEUSIS

- Medical history
- Allergies
- Medication history

- Past medical history
- Ocular history
- Surgical history
- Ocular surface disease assessment and treatment
- Contact lens discontinuation prior to evaluation

A full ocular examination, complete with medical history, current medications, and allergies, is performed prior to the procedure. Patients will be documented in the chart as candidates or noncandidates. Confirmation that the patient's refraction is stabilized is imperative. This requires that contact lens wear be discontinued for an appropriate amount of time. Typically, soft single vision contact lenses should be discontinued for one week, while soft toric/astigmatic and multifocal contact lenses should be discontinued for two weeks. Rigid gas permeable lens wear can cause more of a challenge for reaching stability of the patient's refraction due to reshaping of the corneal surface. On average, about one month per decade of lens wear is generally needed for the cornea to return to its original shape and for the refraction to reach stabilization. It goes without saying that ocular surface disease, glaucoma, and retinal diseases must be evaluated and treated prior to surgery, and patients must understand their candidacy or noncandidacy depends on this diagnostic work-up. The diagnostic devices and the refraction used for treatment depend on stabilization of the afore-mentioned for stable outcomes.[26–28]

As already mentioned, risks and benefits of the operation must be discussed in depth with each patient as well as quality of life after surgery. It is of utmost importance to appropriately set patient expectations prior to LASIK.[29] In most patients, LASIK is overwhelmingly successful; however, postoperative refractive error including astigmatism, myopia, and hyperopia following LASIK can occur depending on individual patient healing and/or laser data entry errors.[30]

SETTINGS AND PROCEDURE

- Sedation
- Pre-procedure preparation
- Flap preparation
- Flap lift
- Laser ablation
- Flap repositioning
- Flap assessment at the end of the procedure and post-procedure prior to patient departure for position confirmation

The LASIK procedure consists of flap creation with a mechanical keratome or a femtosecond laser.[31] Data from the previously measured refraction and diagnostic devices, along with the aid of a nomogram, are utilized to determine the amount of refractive error needed to treat lower- and, possibly, higher-order aberrations. The laser shot file is then transferred to the excimer laser. After making a flap with a mechanical microkeratome or a femtosecond laser, the stromal bed is treated with the patient-specific treatment profile created by the inputted data in a conventional fashion (Figs. 7.3–7.7).

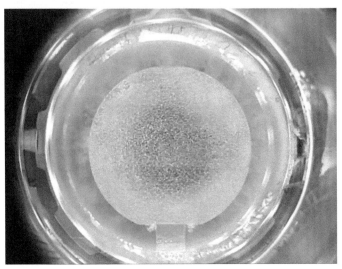

FIGURE 7-3 Creation of a 100 micron flap, which is 9 mm in diameter and has been created in 9 seconds.

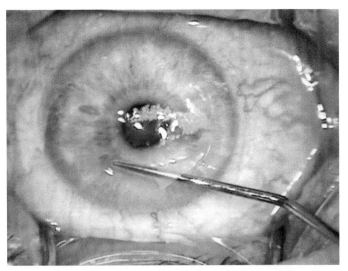

FIGURE 7-4 The surgeon in this figure is lifting the flap that was just created to prepare for excimer laser ablation of the stromal bed.

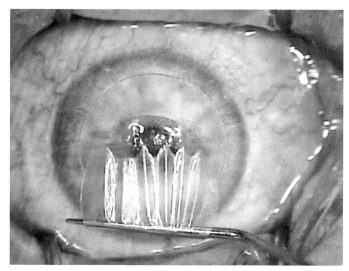

FIGURE 7-5 The flap is hinged and the flap is being lifted by the surgeon in this figure.

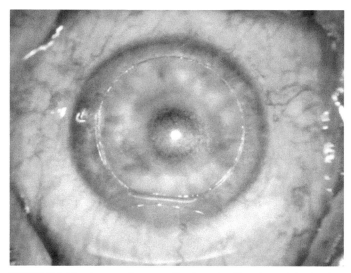

FIGURE 7-6 The laser pulses are fired on to the stromal bed using either a topography-guided profile, an aberrometry-guided profile or wave front–optimized profile.

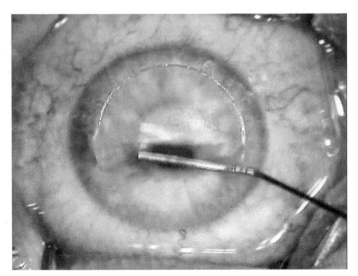

FIGURE 7-7 The flap is replaced to its original anatomical position, and pharmaceuticals are applied as per the surgeon's protocol.

POSTOPERATIVE CARE/CO-MANAGEMENT (FOLLOW-UP SCHEDULE)

- Postoperative day 1
- Postoperative week 1 (in person or telemedicine)
- Postoperative month 1 (in person or telemedicine)
- Postoperative months 3 (in person for data point for future nomogram development)
- Postoperative year 1 (some include a six-month visit if indicated by the three-month exam)

Postoperative examinations are performed either by the surgeon or the comanaging doctor at 1 day, 1 week, and 1, 3, 6, and 12 months in most instances but vary based on surgeon or comanaging doctor preference.[32] With current nuances with COVID-19, telemedicine has been included as part of the option to care and co-manage these patients to allow for reduced exposure of both the staff and the patients.[33]

POTENTIAL COMPLICATIONS AND THEIR TREATMENT

Complications for Laser In Situ Keratomileusis

Complications for LASIK can occur at any step (preoperative or postoperative) and vary based on timing, techniques, and technology used. The authors felt it was best to define the events in an easily regimented format using the Sentinel Article to define the complications as outlined below. The references referred to below provide the reader with more detailed discussion, description, prevention and potential treatment for each event listed.

Preoperative Events

- Refraction accuracy (manifest and cycloplegic)
  Stable refractions are mandatory prior to surgical intervention.

- Topographic issues:
  - Irregular astigmatism
  - Contact lens "warpage"[34]

- Tomography to evaluate posterior surface[35–37]

- Pupil size
  Pupil size is a debated issue. Some suggest counseling patients about the additional risks of postoperative dysphotopsias with pupils larger than 8 mm.[38]

- Corneal pachymetry
  The original limitations of 250 microns of the stromal bed were a theoretical assumption with keratomileusis procedures. Current thought surrounds the evaluation of the percent tissue altered as to judge the candidacy of a patient or lack thereof.[39]

- LASIK is contraindicated in granular corneal dystrophy type 2 (Avellino corneal dystrophy).

Intraoperative Events

- Suction loss
  Suction loss with a mechanical microkeratome can result in devastating complications; however, this issue is less of an event with the femtosecond laser.[40]

- Decentered flap
  Flap decentration was not uncommon early on with mechanical keratomes (especially those in which blind passes were made). With newer centration technology, decentration is a rare event. With highly astigmatic, short, and long eyes, the surgeon centration is more of a challenge and requires diligence in these eyes.[41]

- Opaque bubble layer (OBL)
  The creation of an OBL occurs when the expanding gases created by the femtosecond laser become trapped in the stroma. It is related to settings on the laser and poor venting of the expanding gases through the channel or pocket depending on the type of laser used.[42]

- Difficult flap lift/side cut tags
  During flap creation, poor separation of the corneal tissues by the laser can occur. The reasons are multifactorial and are rare occurrences with today's laser systems.[43]

- Gas bubbles in anterior chamber (AC bubbles)
  The presentation or migration of AC bubbles is a rare occurrence during flap creation with the femtosecond laser. The etiology is debated but may be anatomically related or laser setting related. Interference with tracking on the laser systems is an issue and waiting for resolution is recommended.[44]

- Gas breakthrough
  Gas breakthrough can be related to suction, anatomy (i.e., corneal scars), and thin flap settings of a variety of multifactorial issues. Depending on the severity, continuing the case must be managed on a case-by-case basis.[45]
  - Vertical gas breakthrough
  - Horizontal gas breakthrough

Postoperative Events

Day 1

Epithelial defects/desiccation

Epithelial defects and surface issues related to corneal dystrophy or ocular surface disease was not uncommon with mechanical keratomes. While still possible, the femtosecond laser has reduced the overall presentation of this complication. Management is on a case-by-case basis.[46]

Debris/foreign bodies in interface

Interface debris is related to foreign or organic matter. Inflammatory reactions to the debris or foreign bodies are the main issue, and surgeon's vary on their management of these cases.[47]

Flap slippage

The postoperative day-1 visit is imperative because flap slippage if caught early does not result in reduced outcomes. These can occur idiopathically or traumatically in the early postoperative period. Striae in the flaps are defined as visually significant or visually insignificant and management is on a case-by-case basis; however, with visually significant flap slippage, it is considered an urgent if not emergent intervention.[48]

Diffuse lamellar keratitis

Diffuse lamellar keratitis (DLK) is graded from 1 to 4 and grade 4 is considered a toxic event. Management is discussed at length in reference [49], and when present, it needs to be addressed urgently and followed diligently.[49]

Week 1

Dislocated flap (trauma)

As mentioned earlier, movement of the flap can occur traumatically. Surgical intervention is considered urgent if not emergent to warrant a good outcome without loss of best corrected visual acuity (BCVA). When a flap is lost completely, then a bandage contact lens (BCL) is placed and the patient is managed like a postoperative photorefractive keratectomy (PRK). With resolution and refractive stability, outcomes can be surprisingly good.[50]

Infectious keratitis

A complete book could be written on the etiology and management of infectious keratitis after any type of refractive surgery. Reference [51] is a nice summary of the options.[51]

Diffuse lamellar keratitis

This results from accumulation of inflammatory cells in the interface between the LASIK flap and corneal stroma and should be treated quickly. Management of this occurrence can be found in reference [49].

Refractive error

Retreatment or enhancements after refractive surgery have been reduced with better lasers, ablation profiles, diagnostics, and postoperative regimens. Retreatments should occur after refractive stability and only in patients with appropriate anatomy postoperatively.[52]

Months 1 to 12

Dislocated flap

Late flap dislocation should be treated as an ocular emergency and handled quickly. Blunt or penetrating trauma is usually the issue, and lateral damage to other ocular structure should be investigated and ruled out.[50]

Flap melt

Flap melting is related to severe inflammation or autoimmune disease. Screening prior to surgery will help reduce this postoperative risk.[53,54]

Late keratitis (fungal or mycobacterium species)

A complete book could be written on the etiology and management of infectious keratitis after any type of refractive surgery. Reference [51] is a nice summary of the options.[51]

Dry eye disease

Dry eye postoperatively is a debated and controversial topic. Screening prior to surgery is warranted, and despite careful screening, postoperative ocular surface disease can be an issue.[55]

Diffuse lamellar keratitis

DLK is graded from 1 to 4 and grade 4 is considered a toxic event. Management is discussed at length in reference [49], and when present, it needs to be addressed urgently and followed diligently.[49]

Central toxic keratitis

The present thought on grade 4 DLK is that it is a toxic keratopathy, and management is in fact different than that of DLK grades 1 to 3. Diligent follow-up and management of this complication is imperative.[56]

Epithelial ingrowth

Epithelial ingrowth intervention varies from surgeon to surgeon. However, when visual acuity or topographical changes, warrant intervention with lifting of the flap and removal is the standard procedure.[57,58]

Pressure-Induced Interlamellar Stromal Keratitis

Pressure-induced interlamellar stromal keratitis is a diagnosis easily missed because postoperative intraocular pressure (IOP) measurement following LASIK can be challenging. Proper reduction of the IOP will lead to resolution.[59]

Refractive error

If a retreatment is required for residual refractive error, it should occur after stability of the refraction is achieved, and only in patients with appropriate anatomy postoperatively.[52]

Transient light sensitivity

Transient light sensitivity is uncommon with newer laser designs. It is unique to the femtosecond laser but has been reported after mechanical keratomes.[60]

Iatrogenic keratectasia

This type of keratectasia occurs either due to too much corneal tissue being removed causing a weakness in the mechanical strength of an otherwise normal cornea or due to a missed diagnosis of form fruste keratoconus prior to surgery. Cases of patients with normal corneal findings during preoperative evaluation have gone on years later to show signs of frank keratoconus or keratoectasia. Cross-linking in these patients is an option.[61,62]

VIDEO OF PROCEDURE

Video 8.1—LASIK consists of two parts as you will see in video 8.1. Part one is making the flap in this case with the femtosecond laser made by Alcon, the WaveLight FS200. FS200. The femtosecond laser works at 10^{-15} of a second and works by the principle of photodisruption. Roughly 2–5 micron bubbles are created, which expand in a lamellar fashion to create the flap and are stacked to create the side cut. Femtosecond laser flaps on average are created between 100 and 120 microns. In this video, the surgeon is making a 100-micron flap. Following flap creation, the flap is laid back and the hinge protected to prevent any stray ablations onto the hinge itself. The laser used in the video is the excimer laser made by Alcon, the WaveLight EX500. The spot size is 0.95 mm and Gaussian. It cycles at 500 Hz and photoablates at 193 nm at a latency of 2 ms per pulse. It treats 1D in 1.9 s at 6.5 mm. The tracking system works at 1050 Hz synchronized to the 500-Hz laser. This excimer portion of the surgery recontours the stromal bed to correct myopia, hyperopia, and astigmatism either with topography-guided profiles, aberrometry-guided profiles or wavefront-optimized profiles. After laser photoablation, care is taken to place the flap in its original anatomical position. Topical pharmaceuticals are applied as per the surgeon's protocol, and the procedure is complete.

EVOLUTION OF LASER IN SITU KERATOMILEUSIS

This section discusses an overview of the evolution of conventional LASIK to its present-day form. Over the years, technologies have improved and so have refractive outcomes, complications, and enhancement rates. Treatment profiles continue to become more sophisticated as the technology improves but issues of individual patient healing still remain and so regimens preoperatively, intraoperatively, and postoperatively will need to continue to improve. Advanced diagnostic instruments have allowed for individual patient corneal measures to be obtained, which ultimately allows for more customized treatments and helps to improve postsurgical outcomes. In addition to the aforementioned, the use of nomograms has helped us to develop decision trees, which have then led to the development of analytic engines. In the future, and with enough data collection, the use of artificial

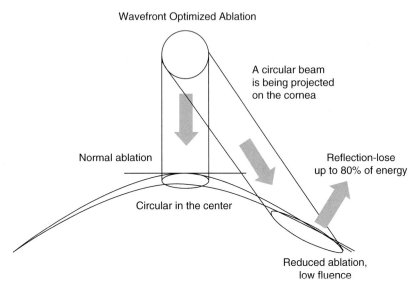

FIGURE 7-8 In order to compensate for reduce energy in the peripheral secondary to the "cosine effect", additional pulses are placed in order to maintain the natural aspheric shape of the eye.

intelligence will be possible and will allow for further improvement in the level of patient satisfaction.[63–75]

Enhancement rates, as published by one of the authors (KS), have gone from 4.5% to 0.22%. The hope is that, one day, enhancements will be eliminated altogether, and that all patients will see better than in their contact lenses or glasses from a quality and quantity standpoint after their laser vision correction.[76,77]

With early conventional profiles initially designed for PRK, higher-order aberrations were seen with the greatest of these being spherical aberration. With higher myopic levels, the spherical aberrations could increase by up to 20-fold. Drs. Mrochen and Seiler developed the initial wavefront-optimized profile to try to reduce these anomalies by increasing optical zone sizes, using aspheric ablation profiles and delivering more energy to the periphery to reduce the cosine effect (Fig. 7.8).[78] Also, the early profiles were designed for flat poly(methyl methacrylate) plates and did not consider curved corneal surfaces. This added to peripheral undercorrections related to beam ovalization toward the periphery, which resulted in a larger area of energy distribution for the same amount of energy thus lowering the energy per unit area (Fig. 7.8).[78]

The transition from a conventional treatment to the wavefront-optimized profile, in common use today, compensated for these effects, resulting in a corneal ablation that produced a more purely refractive change in the eye. This combined with larger optical zones, and more peripheral blend zones provided a large central area of the cornea that exhibited the required refractive change with minimal to no increase in spherical aberration. The goal of the wavefront-optimized profile was to maintain a similar relationship between the central and mid-peripheral curvatures of the anterior cornea, thereby reducing optical phenomena associated with a more abrupt transition zone. Further refinement of wavefront-optimized ablation profiles occurred based on data obtained during early research using wavefront-guided treatments.[78] Evaluation of preoperative and postoperative aberrometry suggested that standard myopic ablations resulted in significant increases in spherical aberration. The amount of spherical aberration within the treated area was a function of both the treatment magnitude and the preoperative spherical aberration of the eye being treated. To decrease the amount of induced spherical aberration, wavefront-optimized treatment profiles were designed to produce a more prolate postoperative result. With current wavefront-optimized profiles, in normal eyes, little spherical aberration is induced with treatments up to 6D. Beyond that range, there is insufficient corneal tissue to allow for complete correction of spherical aberration. However, the amount of spherical aberration induced with a wavefront-optimized profile in these eyes is lower than would be induced with a standard profile.

Minimizing the induction of spherical aberration at the time of laser refractive surgery is important because it is an aberration that can limit optical quality as the pupil size increases, such as in dim light. Patients may experience more glare and reduced contrast sensitivity, visual acuity, and visual quality in dim light. Subjective data collected in the course of studies conducted to obtain approval for WaveLight wavefront-optimized LASIK in the United States showed that, on average, patients experienced a decrease in glare symptoms after the procedure, a finding attributed to the prolate ablation profile. However, results for individual eyes varied. The specific reasons for higher levels of induced aberrations in some patients, particularly spherical aberration, appeared difficult to predict in any individual eye before the treatment is performed. As a result, wavefront-optimized ablation profiles were refined based on clinical experience.[79–83]

A more complicated ablation profile than the wavefront-optimized profile is the wavefront-guided profile. This profile is designed to correct the higher-order aberrations, including spherical aberration, measured in an individual patient's eye preoperatively. To be effective, the wavefront measurement and the wavefront-guided treatment must be precisely aligned, which requires some form of registration of the eye at the time of both measurement and treatment. Wavefront-guided treatments are calculated based on aberrometry data using Fourier or Zernike principles and are designed to treat all higher-order aberrations of a given eye. They have the additional potential to be used for a second treatment, to reduce induced aberrations from previous treatments. It is important to remember wavefront-guided treatments are centered on the line of sight whereas wavefront-optimized treatments are aligned on the pupil center.[79]

In addition to the previously mentioned treatments, topographic profiles have been utilized with several laser platforms for over 15 years. A procedure known as C-CAP (custom contour ablation pattern) was implemented on the Visx excimer laser platform (Johnson and Johnson, New Brunswick, NJ) and was designed to provide phototherapeutic keratectomy. A Humphrey topography unit provided the topographic data for integration with the laser. This early treatment modality was designed to correct irregular astigmatism on the anterior corneal surface, whether occurring naturally or in patients with previous refractive surgery that experienced an issue such as decentration.[84] The procedure suffered from poor reproducibility because of inaccurate topographic data, poor registration of the topographic and laser data, and limited ability to smooth the anterior corneal surface. The consequence was considerable variability in the refractive outcomes achieved.

Modern topography-guided procedures address these limitations. Topography-based profiles are designed by converting a height map of the anterior cornea to a Zernike or Fourier matrix, which is then used to generate the ablation profile for the laser. The treatment profiles help reduce higher-order aberrations from the cornea (not the entire eye) and reduce induced spherical aberration by compensating for cosine effect and by normalizing or "smoothing" the overall surface of the cornea to improve overall regularity. Since the treatment profiles are based on the specific topography of the cornea, tracking devices are used to align the treatment ablation to visible iris features (iris registration) to ensure proper placement of the treatment correction. The treatments are also centered on the corneal vertex or the point on the cornea through which the line of fixation passes (the central part of the cornea). These profiles are unaffected by lenticular or vitreous opacities because the measurement is from the anterior cornea only. Topography-guided treatments are not limited by pupil size, allowing for large treatment zones. This also allows for measurement and treatment of peripheral corneal irregularities, which can be responsible for visual disturbances in some patients. Further, the treatment profile is not necessarily derived purely from topographic data, as the sphere and cylinder components can be modified by the surgeon at their discretion. Another more simplified and standardized approach for current topography-guided surgical planning is to use a newly developed software application, Phorcides Analytic Engine. This software objectively calculates the exact treatment profile required without manual input from the surgeon. Further, it takes into account all structures that influence the optical path of light through the eye: anterior corneal astigmatism, topographic irregularities that create higher-order aberrations, posterior corneal astigmatism, and lenticular astigmatism.[93,98]

To summarize, there have been four general ablation profiles developed for LASIK. The first was the conventional profile developed by Dr. Charles Munnerlyn and colleagues that ignored corneal curvature effects; it is no longer in common use.[70] Wavefront-optimized profiles were then developed to compensate for corneal curvature effects to reduce induced spherical aberration. They were designed to produce a pure refractive change; they are centered on the pupil and based on the refractive error.[78] The third general profile type is the wavefront-guided profile, designed to minimize the preoperative measured aberrations in an individual eye.[79,85] Finally, topography-guided profiles include consideration of the shape of the anterior corneal surface.[86]

EFFICACY

Some early comparisons of these various treatment options have been made. Stonecipher et al. performed a single-eye study comparing eyes treated with a wavefront-optimized profile with those treated with a wavefront-guided profile.[77] Those with >0.3 μm root mean square (RMS); (higher-order aberrations) preoperatively were treated with wavefront-guided LASIK (approximately 20% of eyes) while the remaining eyes were treated with wavefront-optimized LASIK, since attempts to correct small wavefront errors have shown no clinical benefit. Results from this study showed that clinical outcomes were similar between groups and that eyes with significant amounts of preoperative higher-order aberrations (e.g., >0.3 μm RMS) did well with wavefront-guided LASIK and experienced an average reduction in their wavefront errors with treatments.[77–79] Stonecipher et al. also compared results from wavefront-optimized treatments with the WaveLight Allegretto laser to wavefront-guided treatments using the Visx CustomVue laser.[77] More recent comparisons of the various profiles are reviewed in the following section.[83]

The WaveLight EX500 excimer and Nidek 2000 EC-50000 excimer lasers are the only U.S.-approved topography-guided lasers using the LASIK approach. The prospective food and drug administration (FDA) study on normal eyes showed excellent visual outcomes after Contoura Vision, with uncorrected distance visual acuity (UDVA) of 20/20 or better in 92.6% of eyes and 20/16 or better in 64.8% of eyes, 20/12.5 or better in 34.4%, and 20/10 or better in 15.7% (at 12 months).[89] These results were achieved when the manifest refraction was used and in eyes where the difference between the topographic astigmatism and manifest refractive cylinder were nominal. Additionally, 30.9% of eyes gained one or more lines of UDVA compared with preoperative corrected distance visual acuity (CDVA). Visual acuity improvements from 3 to 12 months was also shown (Fig. 7.9).[89]

Study results listed in the following section include only those studies where Contoura Vision was used consistently with the approved FDA indications for use, where the manifest refraction was used for the surgical planning and where 20/15 visual outcomes were provided. In general, all treatments were equally effective at the 20/20 level, but differences at 20/15 and 20/10 were shown. Additionally, residual refractive error among all treatments was similar across the studies mentioned unless stated otherwise.

WaveLight WFO versus topography guided

Stonecipher et al.[90] conducted a large prospective study on 846 eyes comparing wavefront-optimized (WFO) (*n* = 430) to topography-guided Contoura Vision (*n* = 416) using manifest refraction for treatment planning.[90] The study showed that more patients achieved better than 20/20 vision with Contoura Vision than with WFO: 54.6% versus 45.0% had UDVA of 20/15 or better. These visual acuity percentages did not reach the levels seen in the FDA study. However, this study included all patients with normal corneal parameters and was not restricted by differences in

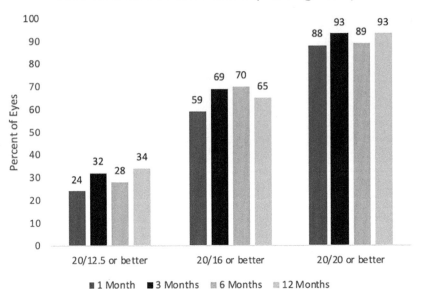

FIGURE 7-9 FDA clinical trial showing uncorrected distance visual acuity at each post-operative visit following Contoura Vision treatment.[89]

corneal and refractive astigmatism as was the case in the FDA study. They also found in this study that the postoperative spherical equivalent refraction and the residual cylinder were slightly worse in the wavefront-optimized group.[90]

A different study showed that the number of patients with postoperative UDVA was numerically higher at 20/16 with WFO (vs. Contoura Vision); however, this difference was reported as not being statistically significant.[91] They also showed that topography-guided LASIK with Contoura Vision induced fewer total corneal higher order aberrations (HOAs) ($p = 0.13$) and less coma ($p = 0.003$). Notably, this study was substantially smaller ($n = 86$ eyes) than the other studies reported here.[91]

WaveLight Contoura Vision: Manifest refraction versus Phorcides

Several retrospective analyses on Contoura Vision using manifest refraction versus Contoura Vision using the Phorcides software for treatment planning have recently been published. These studies show that the two treatment profiles are equivalent at 20/20. However, more patients can achieve 20/15 and 20/10 acuities with the use of Phorcides.[93,100] Lobanoff et al.[93] showed that a significantly higher percentage of patients reached 20/16 vision with Phorcides versus manifest refraction-based Contoura Vision (62.5% vs. 41.3%; $p < 0.001$).[93] The number of patients in this study with UDVA better than their preoperative CDVA was significantly higher in the Phorcides group (36.5% vs. 23.0%; $p < 0.001$), and significantly more eyes in the Phorcides group gained one or more lines of CDVA (42.7% vs. 30.3%; $p = 0.001$). Importantly, these studies showed 20/20, 20/15, and 20/10 results that are very similar to the percentages in the FDA study results, which selected for eyes with tight agreement between the manifest astigmatism and the measured anterior corneal astigmatism, whereas these studies were not selective in this way and represented the true clinical population better (Fig. 7.10).[93,100]

In addition to the studies already presented, there are several publications by Wallerstein et al. and others using a manifest refraction-based nomogram that also show that Contoura Vision treatment can be highly effective.[94–98] However, these studies did not provide direct head-to-head comparisons of their approach to either WFO or Phorcides.[94–98]

WFO and Contoura Vision treatments both provide excellent visual outcomes especially at the 20/20 level. While both treatments can also deliver 20/15 visual acuity (uncorrected), Contoura Vision has shown, overall, that a higher number of patients can achieve 20/15 or better.[93,100] Further, the use of the Phorcides Analytic Engine software has consistently delivered higher percentages of 20/15 (uncorrected) over the standard manifest refraction-based Contoura Vision planning, even in patients whose manifest and topography astigmatism do not match.[93,100]

While Contoura Vision has the potential for better visual outcomes and has been used successfully on a wide range of patients, there are a few instances where WFO treatments would be preferred.

1. When several good quality topography images are not obtainable, as this will limit the ability to accurately define the anterior corneal elevations.
2. When the clinical refraction is outside of the FDA-approved parameters for Contoura Vision (e.g., Hyperopia, myopia >8.00D, cylinder >3.00D, manifest refraction spherical equivalent (MRSE) >9.00D).

To summarize, WaveLight LASIK treatments, WFO and Contoura Vision are both effective at the 20/20 level; however, Contoura Vision, and specifically the use of the Phorcides Analytic Engine software, provides even better visual outcomes overall, with more patients reaching 20/15 and 20/10.[97,98] The Phorcides software helps surgeon's avoid the subjective nature of Contoura Vision that can require determining the right balance of cylinder magnitude and axis, and it provides a more objective, user-friendly approach that makes it more appealing to surgeon's.[101]

UPCOMING TREATMENT PROFILES

A newer ablation profile that is not yet available in the United States, is ray tracing. To improve the outcomes of custom excimer laser ablations for LASIK, an innovative treatment algorithm was developed, which takes into account all optically significant structures of the eye.[87] Current custom treatments are based on values generated using a single diagnostic technique such as corneal topography or ocular wave front

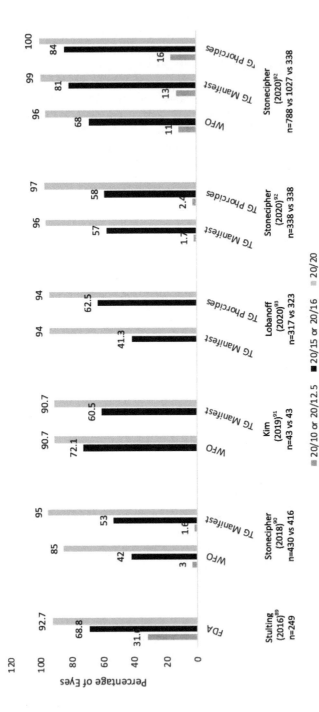

FIGURE 7-10 Visual acuity percentages among multiple studies where the manifest refraction was used for topography-guided treatment.
Post-op UDVA: Stulting[89] at 3 months; Stonecipher[90] at 1 day; Kim[91] at 3 months; Lobanoff[93] at 2 to 5 months; Stonecipher[92] at 1 day.

so that the treatment relies, to some degree, on approximations. The new optical ray-tracing algorithm uses data from a beam of light passing through the various refracting media of the eye to focus precisely on the fovea, contributing data to a highly individualized custom ablation profile. The addition of biometry readings, which considers keratometry, central corneal thickness, horizontal corneal diameter, anatomic anterior chamber depth, central lens thickness, retinal thickness, axial length, and pupillometry, provides critical data to the calculation and allows this treatment to be truly individualized.

CODING/BILLING MODIFIERS

Laser surgery is usually not covered by medical insurance. Some insurance companies will offer partial payments.

REFERENCES

1. Barraquer JI. Queratoplastia refractive. *Estudios Inform.* 1949;10:221.
2. Troutman RC. Artiphakia and aniseikonia. *Trans Am Ophthalmol Soc.* 1962;60:590–658.
3. Ainslie D. The surgical correction of refractive errors by keratomileusis and keratophakia. *Ann Ophthalmol.* 1976 Mar;8(3):349–367.
4. Troutman RC, Kelly S, Kaye D, Clahane AC. The use and preliminary results of the Troutman surgical keratometer in cataract and corneal surgery. *Trans Sect Ophthalmol Am Acad Ophthalmol Otolaryngol.* 1977;83(2):232–238.
5. Troutman RC, Swinger C. Refractive keratoplasty: keratophakia and keratomileusis. *Trans Am Ophthalmol Soc.* 1978;76:329–339.
6. Swinger CA, Barraquer JI. Keratophakia and keratomileusis--clinical results. *Ophthalmology.* 1981;88(8):709–715. doi:10.1016/s0161-6420(81)34958-6
7. Swinger CA, BarkerBA. Prospective evaluation of myopic keratomileusis. *Ophthalmology.* 1984;91:785–792.
8. Nordan LT, Fallor MK, Myopic keratomileusis: 74 consecutive cases with one-year follow-up. *J Refract Surg.* 1986;2:124–128.
9. Maguire LJ, Klyce SD, Sawelson H, McDonald MB, Kaufman HE. Visual distortion after myopic keratomileusis: computer analysis of keratoscope photographs. *Ophthalmic Surg.* 1987;18(5):352–356.
10. Barraquer C, Gutierrez AM, Espinosa A. Myopic keratomileusis: short-term results. *Refract Corneal Surg.* 1989;5(5):307–313.
11. Peymon, Gholam, US Patent 4,840,175, "METHOD FOR MODIFYING CORNEAL CURVATURE", granted June 20, 1989.
12. Barraquer JI. Basis of refractive keratoplasty—1967. *Refract Corneal Surg.* 1989;5:179–193.
13. Pallikaris IG, Papatzanaki ME, Georgiadis A, Frenschock O. A comparative study of neural regeneration following corneal wounds induced by an argon fluoride excimer laser and mechanical methods. *Laser Light Ophthalmol.* 1990;3(2):89–95.
14. Pallikaris IG, Papatzanaki ME, Stathi EZ, Frenschock O, Georgiadis A. Laser in situ keratomileusis. *Lasers Surg Med.* 1990;10:463–468.
15. Pallikaris IG, Papatzanaki ME, Siganos DS, Tsilimbaris MK. A corneal flap technique for laser in situ keratomileusis; human studies. *Arch Ophthalmol.* 1991;109:1699–1702.
16. Buratto L, Ferrari M, Rama P. Excimer laser intrastromal keratomileusis. *Am J Ophthalmol.* 1992;113:291–295.

17. Kezirian GK, Stonecipher KG. Comparison of the intralase femtosecond laser and mechanical keratomes for LASIK. *J Cataract and Refractive Surg.* 2004;30(4):803–810.
18. Stonecipher KG, Kezririan GK. How to develop your nomogram: A 10-year study of nomogram development for refractive surgery and refractive cataract surgery. *Supplement of the Journal of Cataract and Refractive Surgery,* April 2009.
19. Stonecipher KG. A 10-year study of nomogram development for refractive surgery and refractive cataract surgery: A review of over 30,000 cases. Presentation ESCRS September 2009.
20. Seiler T, Koufala K, Richter G. Iatrogenic keratectasia edema upon the smoothness of excimer laser ablation after laser in situ keratomileusis. *J Refract Surg.* 1998;14:312–317.
21. Reinstein DZ, Archer TJ, Gobbe M. The history of LASIK. *J Refract Surg.* 2012;28(4):291–298. doi: 10.3928/1081597X-20120229-01
22. Grady C, Cummings SR, Rowbotham MC, McConnell MV, Ashley EA, Kang G. Informed consent. *N Engl J Med.* 2017 Mar 2;376(9):856–867. doi:10.1056/NEJMra1603773. PMID: 28249147.
23. Abbott RL. Medical malpractice predictors and risk factors for ophthalmologists performing LASIK and PRK surgery. *Trans Am Ophthalmol Soc.* 2003;101:239–274. PMID: 14971582; PMCID: PMC1358993.
24. Menke AM, Briceland DJ. Comanagement of surgical patients. https://www.omic.com/comanagement-of-surgical-patients (Accessed October 18, 2020)
25. https://www.omic.com/comanagement-consent-form (Accessed October 18, 2020)
26. Albietz JM, Lenton LM. Management of the ocular surface and tear film before, during, and after laser in situ keratomileusis. *J Refract Surg.* 2004 Jan–Feb;20(1):62–71. PMID: 14763473
27. De Bernardo M, Cembalo G, Rosa N. Reliability of intraocular pressure measurement by Goldmann applanation tonometry after refractive surgery: a review of different correction formulas. *Clin Ophthalmol.* 2020;14:2783–2788. https://doi.org/10.2147/OPTH.S263856
28. Wilkinson CP. Interventions for asymptomatic retinal breaks and lattice degeneration for preventing retinal detachment. *Cochrane Database Syst Rev.* 2012;3(3):CD003170. Published March 14, 2021. doi:10.1002/14651858.CD003170.pub3
29. Wilkinson JM, Cozine EW, Kahn AR. Refractive eye surgery: helping patients make informed decisions about LASIK. *Am Fam Physician.* 2017 May 15;95(10):637–644. PMID: 28671403.
30. Stonecipher KG, Ignacio TI, Stonecipher MN. Advances in Refractive Surgery: Microkeratome and femtosecond laser flap creation in relation to safety, efficacy, predictability, and biomechanical stability. *Current Medical Opinion,* 2006.
31. Kezirian GK, Stonecipher KG. Comparison of the intralase femtosecond laser and mechanical keratomes for LASIK. *J Cataract and Refractive Surg.* 2004;30(4):803–810.
32. Callaway RF. Charting the perils of LASIK comanagement. https://www.omic.com/charting-the-perils-of-lasik-comanagement (Accessed October 18, 2020)
33. Stonecipher K. Virtual Poster Presentation American Academy of Ophthalmology, outcomes of planning topography-guided LASIK with new analytic software versus planning with manifest refraction in eyes with topography guided parameters. November 2020.
34. Vainer I, Mimouni M, Rabina G, Spierer O, Nemet AY, Shapira Y, Sela T, Kaiserman I. Age-and gender-related characteristics of corneal refractive parameters in a large Cohort study. *Am J Ophthalmol.* 2020 Jan;209:45–54. doi:10.1016/j.ajo.2019.09.007. Epub September 14, 2019. PMID: 31526796.
35. Luz A, Lopes B, Salomão M, Ambrósio R. Application of corneal tomography before keratorefractive procedure for laser vision correction. *J Biophotonics.* 2016 May;9(5):445–453. doi:10.1002/jbio.201500236. Epub April 15, 2016. PMID: 27079610.
36. Lopes BT, Ramos IC, Salomão MQ, et al. Enhanced tomographic assessment to detect corneal ectasia based on artificial intelligence. *Am J Ophthalmol.* 2018 Nov;195:223–232. doi:10.1016/j.ajo.2018.08.005. Epub August 9, 2018. PMID: 30098348.
37. Golan O, Hwang ES, Lang P, Santhiago MR, Abulafia A, Touboul D, Krauthammer M, Smadja D. Differences in posterior corneal features between normal corneas and subclinical keratoconus. *J Refract Surg.* 2018 Oct 1;34(10):664–670. doi:10.3928/1081597X-20180823-02. PMID: 30296327.

38. Kezirian GM, Stonecipher KG. Subjective assessment of mesopic visual function after laser in situ keratomileusis. *Ophthalmol Clin North Am.* 2004 Jun;17(2):211–224, vii. doi:10.1016/j.ohc.2004.03.004. PMID: 15207563.

39. Ong HS, Farook M, Tan BBC, Williams GP, Santhiago MR, Mehta JS. Corneal ectasia risk and percentage tissue altered in myopic patients presenting for refractive surgery. *Clin Ophthalmol.* 2019;13:2003–2015 https://doi.org/10.2147/OPTH.S215144

40. Santhiago MR, Kara-Junior N, Waring GO 4th. Microkeratome versus femtosecond flaps: accuracy and complications. *Curr Opin Ophthalmol.* 2014 Jul;25(4):270–274. doi:10.1097/ICU.0000000000000070. PMID: 24837579.

41. Tse SM, Farley ND, Tomasko KR, Amin SR. Intraoperative LASIK complications. *Int Ophthalmol Clin.* 2016 Spring;56(2):47–57. doi:10.1097/IIO.0000000000000110. PMID: 26938337.

42. Kanellopoulos AJ, Asimellis G. Essential opaque bubble layer elimination with novel LASIK flap settings in the FS200 Femtosecond Laser. *Clin Ophthalmol.* 2013;7:765–770. doi:10.2147/OPTH.S43723

43. Vesaluoma MH, Petroll WM, Pérez-Santonja JJ, et al. Laser in situ keratomileusis flap margin: wound healing and complications imaged by in vivo confocal microscopy. *Am J Ophthalmol.* 2000;130:564–573. doi:10.1016/S0002-9394(00)00540-7

44. Perez-Straziota C, Randleman JB. Femtosecond-assisted LASIK: Complications and management. *Int Ophthalmol Clin.* 2016 Spring;56(2):59–66. doi:10.1097/IIO.0000000000000105. PMID: 26938338.

45. Haft P, Yoo SH, Kymionis GD, Ide T, O'Brien TP, Culbertson WW. Complications of LASIK flaps made by the IntraLase 15-and 30-kHz femtosecond lasers. *J Refract Surg.* 2009 Nov;25(11):979–984. doi:10.3928/1081597X-20091016-02. Epub November 13, 2009. PMID: 19921765.

46. Dastgheib KA, Clinch TE, Manche EE, Hersh P, Ramsey J. Sloughing of corneal epithelium and wound healing complications associated with laser in situ keratomileusis in patients with epithelial basement membrane dystrophy. *Am J Ophthalmol* 2000;130:297–303.

47. Knorz MC. Flap and interface complications in LASIK. *Curr Opin Ophthalmol.* 2002 Aug;13(4):242–245. doi:10.1097/00055735-200208000-00010. PMID: 12165708.

48. Aslanides IM, Tsiklis NS, Ozkilic E, Coskunseven E, Pallikaris IG, Jankov MR. The effect of topical apraclonidine on subconjunctival hemorrhage and flap adherence in LASIK patients. *J Refract Surg.* 2006 Jun;22(6):585–588. PMID: 16805122.

49. Linebarger EJ, Hardten DR, Lindstrom RL. Diffuse lamellar keratitis: diagnosis and management. *J Cataract Refract Surg.* 2000;26:1072–1077.

50. Iskander NG, Peters NT, Anderson Penno E, Gimbel HV. Late traumatic flap dislocation after laser in situ keratomileusis. *J Cataract Refract Surg.* 2001;27(7):1111–1114.

51. Donnenfeld ED, Kim T, Holland EJ, Azar DT, Palmon FR, Rubenstein JB, Daya S, Yoo SH. Management of infectious keratitis following laser in situ keratomileusis. *J Cataract Refract Surg.* 2005 Oct;31(10):2008–2011. doi:10.1016/j.jcrs.2005.10.030. PMID: 16338575.

52. Pérez-Santonja JJ, Bellot J, Claramonte P, Ismail MM, Alió JL. Retreatment after laser in situ keratomileusis. *Ophthalmology.* 1999;106:21–28.

53. Castillo A, Diaz-Valle D, Gutierrez AR, Toledano N, Romero F. Peripheral melt of flap after laser in situ keratomileusis. *J Refract Surg.* 1998;14:61–63.

54. Smith RJ, Maloney RK. Laser in situ keratomileusis in patients with autoimmune diseases. *J Cataract Refract Surg.* 2006;32:1292–1295.

55. Nettune GR, Pflugfelder SC. Post-LASIK tear dysfunction and dysesthesia. *Ocul Surf.* 2010;8(3):135–145. doi:10.1016/s1542-0124(12)70224-0

56. Sonmez B, Maloney R. Central toxic keratopathy: description of a syndrome in laser refractive surgery. *Am J Ophthalmol.* 2007;143:420–427. doi:10.1016/j.ajo.2006.11.019

57. Wang MY, Maloney RK. Epithelial ingrowth after laser in situ keratomileusis. *Am J Ophthalmol.* 2000;129:746–751.

58. Friehmann A, Mimouni M, Nemet AY, Sela T, Munzer G, Kaiserman I. Risk Factors for epithelial ingrowth following microkeratome-assisted LASIK. *J Refract Surg.* 2018 Feb 1;34(2):100–105. doi:10.3928/1081597X-20180105-01. PMID: 29425388.

59. Tourtas T, Kopsachilis N, Meiller R, Kruse FE, Cursiefen C. Pressure-induced interlamellar stromal keratitis after laser in situ keratomileusis. *Cornea.* 2011 Aug;30(8):920–923. doi:10.1097/ICO. PMID: 21734483.

60. Stonecipher KG, Dishler JG, Ignacio TS, Binder PS. Transient light sensitivity after femtosecond laser flap creation: clinical findings and management. *J Cataract Refract Surg.* 2006 Jan;32(1):91–94. doi:10.1016/j.jcrs.2005.11.015. PMID: 16516785.

61. Seiler T, Koufala K, Richter G. Iatrogenic keratectasia after laser in situ keratomileusis. *J Refract Surg.* 1998;14:312–317.

62. Wolle MA, Randleman JB, Woodward MA. Complications of refractive surgery: ectasia after refractive surgery. *Int Ophthalmol Clin.* 2016 Spring;56(2):127–139. doi:10.1097/IIO.0000000000000102. PMID: 26938343; PMCID: PMC4780337.

63. Trokel SL, Srinivasan R, Braren B. Excimer laser surgery of the cornea. *Am J Ophthalmol.* 1983;96(6):710–715.

64. Srinivasan R. Kinetics of ablative photodecomposition of organic polymers in the far ultraviolet (193 nm). *J Vac Sci Tech.* 1983;1:923.

65. Garrison BJ, Srinivasan R. Microscopic model for the ablative photodecomposition of polymers by far-ultraviolet radiation (193 nm). *Appl Phys Lett.* 1984;44:849.

66. Dehm EJ, Puliafito CA, Adler CM, Steinert RF. Corneal endothelial injury following excimer laser ablation and 193 and 248 nm. *Arch Ophthalmol.* 1986;104(9):1364–1368.

67. Garrison BJ, Srinivasan R. Microscopic model for the ablative photodecomposition of polymers by far-ultraviolet radiation (193 nm). *Appl Phys Lett.* 1984;44:849.

68. Puliafito CA, Stern D, Krueger RR, Mandel ER. High-speed photography of the excimer laser ablation of the cornea. *Arch Ophthalmol.* 1987;105(9):1255–1259.

69. Puliafito CA, Wong K, Steinert RF. Quantitative and ultrastructural studies of excimer laser ablation of the cornea at 193 and 248 nanometers. *Lasers Surg Med.* 1987;7(2):155–159.

70. Munnerlyn CR, Koons SJ, Marshall J. Photorefractive keratectomy: a technique for laser refractive surgery. *J Cataract Refract Surg.* 1988 Jan;14(1):46–52. doi:10.1016/s0886-3350(88)80063-4. PMID: 3339547.

71. Fowler WC, Rowsey JJ, Nordquist RE, et al. Transmission electron microscopy (TEM) analysis of corneal wound healing in monkeys 28 months after excimer laser photorefractive keratectomy. *IOVS Supp.* 1991;32(4).

72. McDonald MB, Liu JC, Byrd TJ, et al. Central photorefractive keratectomy for myopia. Partially sighted and normally sighted eyes. *Ophthalmology.* 1991;98:1327–1337.

73. Krasin ski JS, Rudzewicz C, Krueger RR, et al. Experimental evidence of excimer laser plasma shielding and its dependence on pulse width. *IOVS Supp.* 1992;33(4).

74. Krueger RR, Krasinski JS, Radzewicz C, et al. High speed shadowgraphy of excimer laser excited shock wave: The effect of helium on propagation velocity. Supplement to Investigative Ophthalmology & Visual Science 1992;33(4).

75. Nguyen H, Stonecipher KG, Krueger RR. An analysis of refractive surgery with the excimer laser, Holmium: YAG laser and picosecond Nd: YAG laser by electron and light microscopy in the primate and cadaver cornea. *IOVS Supp.* 1992;33(4).

76. Stonecipher MN, Stonecipher KG. Influences on enhancement rates in laser vision correction. *US Ophthalmic Review.* 2016;9(2):2–4.

77. Stonecipher KG, Potvin R, Meyer JJ, Durrie D. Refractive surgery outcomes comparison-all Wavefront-guided versus a decision tree for selecting Wavefront-guided or Wavefront optimized. *US Ophthalmic Review.* 2012;5(1):14–17.

78. Mrochen M, Donitzky C, Wullner C, Loffler J. Wavefront-optimized ablation profiles: theoretical background. *J Cataract Refract Surg.* 2004;4:777–785.

79. Stonecipher KG, Kezirian GK. Wavefront-optimized versus Wavefront-guided LASIK for myopic astigmatism with the ALLEGRETTO WAVE: three-month results of a prospective FDA trial. *J. Refract Surg.* 2008;24: S424–S430.

80. Kezirian GK, Moore CR, Stonecipher KG. SurgiVision Consultants Inc WaveLight investigator group: four-year postoperative results of the US ALLEGRETTO WAVE clinical trial for the treatment of hyperopia. *J Refract Surg.* 24: S431–S438, 2008.

81. Stonecipher KG, Kezirian GK, Stonecipher MN. LASIK for-6.00 D to-10.00 D of myopia with up to 3.00 D of cylinder using the ALLEGRETTO wave: 3-and 6-month results with the 200-Hz and 400-Hz platforms. *J Refract Surg.* 2010;26(10):814–818.

82. Stonecipher KG, Kezirian GK, Stonecipher KG. LASIK for mixed astigmatism using the ALLE-GRETTO wave: 3-and 6-month results with the 200-Hz and 400-Hz platforms *J Refract Surg.* 2010;26(10):819–823.

83. Stonecipher KG, Potvin R, Meyer JJ, Durrie D, Stonecipher KG. Refractive surgery outcomes comparison-all Wavefront-guided versus a decision tree for selecting Wavefront-guided or Wavefront optimized. *US Ophthalmic Review.* 2012;5(1):14–17.

84. Lin DY, Manche EE. Custom-contoured ablation pattern method for the treatment of decentered laser ablations. *J Cataract Refract Surg.* 2004 Aug;30(8):1675–1684. doi:10.1016/j.jcrs.2003.12.052. PMID: 15313290.

85. Seiler T, Mrochen M, Kaemmerer M. Operative correction of ocular aberrations to improve visual acuity. *J Refract Surg.* 2000 Sep–Oct;16(5): S619–S622. PMID: 11019886.

86. Kohnen T. Classification of excimer laser profiles. *J Cataract Refract Surg.* 2006 Apr;32(4):543–544. doi:10.1016/j jcrs.2006.02.002. PMID: 16698450.

87. Mrochen M, Bueeler M, Donitzky C, Seiler T. Optical ray tracing for the calculation of optimized corneal ablation profiles in refractive treatment planning. *J Refract Surg.* 2008;24(4):S446–S451.

88. Cummings AB, Kelly GE. Optical ray tracing-guided myopic laser in situ keratomileusis: 1-year clinical outcomes. *Clin Ophthalmol.* 2013;7:1181–1191. doi:10.2147/OPTH.S44720

89. Stulting D, Fant, B, T-Cat Study Group (Stonecipher KG). Results of topography-guide LASIK custom ablation treatment with a refractive excimer laser. *J Cataract Refract Surg.* 2016;42(1):11–18.

90. Stonecipher K, Parrish J, Stonecipher M. Comparing wavefront-optimized, wavefront-guided and topography-guided laser vision correction: clinical outcomes using an objective decision tree. *Curr Opin Ophthalmol.* 2018;29(4):277–285, doi:10.1097/ICU.0000000000000495

91. Kim J, Choi SH, Lim DH, Yang CM, Yoon GJ, Chung TY. Topography-guided versus wavefront-optimized laser in situ keratomileusis for myopia: surgical outcomes. *J Cataract Refract Surg.* 2019 Jul;45(7):959–965. doi:10.1016/j.jcrs.2019.01.031. Epub June 2019, 10. PMID: 31196580.

92. Stonecipher K, Tooma T, Lobanoff M, Wexler S. Outcomes of planning topography-guided LASIK with new analytic software vs. planning with manifest refraction in eyes with T-CAT parameters. Virtual ASCRS Presentation, Boston, MA, 2020.

93. Lobanoff M, Stonecipher K, Tooma T, Wexler S, Potvin R. Clinical outcomes after topography-guided LASIK: comparing results based on a new topography analysis algorithm to those based on the manifest refraction. *J Cataract Refract Surg.* 2020;46(6):814–819.

94. Wallerstein A, Gauvin M, Cohen M. WaveLight Contoura topography-guided planning: contribution of anterior corneal higher-order aberrations and posterior corneal astigmatism to manifest refractive astigmatism. *Clin Ophthalmol.* 2018;12:1423–1426.

95. Wallerstein A, Caron-Cantin M, Gauvin M, Adiguzel E, Cohen M. Primary topography-guided LASIK: refractive, visual, and subjective quality of vision outcomes for astigmatism ≥2.00 diopters. *J Refract Surg.* 2019;35:78–86.

96. Wallerstein A, Gauvin M, Qi SR, Bashour M, Cohen M. Primary topography-guided LASIK: treating manifest refractive astigmatism versus topography-measured anterior corneal astigmatism. *J Refract Surg.* 2019;35:15–23.

97. Kanellopoulos AJ. Topography-modified refraction (TMR): adjustment of treated cylinder amount and axis to the topography versus standard clinical refraction in myopic topography-guided LASIK. *Clin Ophthalmol.* 2016;10:2213–2221.

98. Stulting D, Durrie D, Potvin R, Linn S, Krueger R, Lobanoff MC, Motwani M, Lindquist T, Stonecipher K. Topography-guided refractive astigmatism outcomes: predictions comparing three

different programming methods. *Clin Ophthalmol.* 2020;14:1091–1100. doi:10.2147/OPTH.S244079

99. Durrie D, Stulting RD, Potvin R, Petznick A. More eyes with 20/10 distance visual acuity at 12 months versus 3 months in a topography-guided excimer laser trial: Possible contributing factors. *J Cataract Refract Surg.* 2019 May;45(5):595–600. doi:10.1016/j.jcrs.2018.12.008. Epub February 25, 2019. PMID: 30819561.

100. Stonecipher KG. Outcomes of planning topography-guided LASIK with new analytic software vs. planning with manifest refraction in eyes with topography-guided parameters. Presented at American Academy of Ophthalmology 2020.

101. Mathew J, Stonecipher K. Wavefront optimized versus topography guided corneal ablations with Wavelight platform: A summary of visual outcomes. White Paper. 2020 Alcon Inc. 06/20 US-ALL-2000003.

8 Small-Incision Lenticule Extraction

D. Rex Hamilton

Cornea refractive surgery began in the late 1970s and early 1980s with radial keratotomy (RK) and moved into the laser arena with the introduction of excimer laser (193 nm) ablation in the 1990s. The Food and Drug Administration (FDA) approval of photorefractive keratectomy (PRK) in 1995 represented the first excimer laser technique for vision correction. The PRK procedure afforded many advantages over the incisional RK procedure: higher predictability, improved safety, and better long-term stability. While the technique is still used today, recovery time is quite long with PRK as the technique requires removal of the corneal epithelium, which must subsequently heal and stabilize. Patients can expect about a month before their vision stabilizes. Laser in situ keratomileusis (LASIK) was developed in the early 1990s with the FDA approval occurring in 1999. The stromal flap created as the first step of this procedure affords overnight recovery with outstanding vision on postoperative day 1. The second step of the procedure is the same as the PRK excimer ablation. The fast recovery, coupled with predictability, safety, and long-term stability equivalent to PRK, led to the ascension of LASIK as the procedure of choice for laser vision correction. To date, more than 40 million LASIK procedures have been performed worldwide.

Nevertheless, the penetration of laser vision correction amongst myopic patients throughout the world remains very low. In the United States, for example, in 2012, approximately 700,000 eyes were treated, representing only 1.2% of the population pool.[1] Despite the outstanding safety record of LASIK, fear remains the major barrier to entry for the majority of potential vision correction candidates. These fears revolve around the existence of the flap, concerns over complications, and simply the concept of having laser surgery on one's eyes.

The Small-Incision Lenticule Extraction (SMILE) procedure was developed in the late 2000s and utilizes a single femtosecond laser to create a lenticule-shaped piece of corneal stromal tissue, customized to a patient's refractive correction. The laser also creates a small surface incision through which the lenticule is extracted without the creation of a flap. The SMILE procedure was FDA approved for spherical myopic treatments in October 2016. In March 2018, the procedure was approved for myopic astigmatic treatments. At the time of publication, SMILE is gaining popularity throughout the world with more than 4 million procedures performed. SMILE may be an attractive alternative to LASIK for those patients fearful of laser surgery: no flap, no sound (excimer laser makes sound), no smell (odor of vaporized corneal tissue from excimer ablation), no pressure (negligible pressure associated with the VisuMax femtosecond laser), and shorter procedure time relative to LASIK. In addition, because there is no flap and the incision is so small, there are virtually no postoperative restrictions on lifestyle. There is also strong evidence that the severity and duration of dry eye symptoms is less with SMILE than LASIK.[2,3]

INDICATIONS

Key Indications

- *Myopia and myopic astigmatism:* –1.00D to –10.00D in spherical power with –0.75D to –3.00D in astigmatic power with manifest spherical equivalent of no more than –10.00D (FDA-approved ranges)

CONTRAINDICATIONS

Key Contraindications

- *Keratoconus or other corneal ectatic disorders:* Normal corneal tomography (and regular epithelial thickness maps if available) is essential for clearing patients for any corneal refractive surgery.
- *Previous herpes simplex keratitis:* Contraindicated if active disease within 1 year. If more than 1 year, check corneal sensitivity and use oral antiviral medication prophylaxis before and after surgery.
- *Active autoimmune disease:* Lupus, rheumatoid arthritis, Sjögren's syndrome
- *Severe aqueous deficient dry eye*
- *Pregnancy or nursing:* Vision can fluctuate during pregnancy. In addition, antibiotic eye drops are used for several days after surgery while steroid eye drops are used for 7 to 10 days following surgery. There may be some systemic absorption of these medications that could affect the fetus and/or be present in breast milk.
- *Current isotretinoin (Accutane) use*
- *Unrealistic expectations*

Relative Contraindications

- *Cataract:* Corneal refractive surgery is a good option for patients into their mid-50s with mild, nonprogressive cataract due to risk of retinal complications from refractive lens exchange. Progressive myopia and/or astigmatism changes on manifest that do not match corneal astigmatism usually indicate need for cataract surgery

- *Glaucoma:* If intraocular pressure (IOP) is well controlled with minimal visual field loss, SMILE surgery can be safely performed. It is important to take note of change in corneal thickness as this has an impact on IOP measurements: measured IOP will be lower than actual IOP following myopic corneal refractive surgery.[4] Intraoperative IOP elevation associated with VisuMax laser docking is the lowest of any femtosecond laser and is not a contraindication for patients with mild glaucoma.

- *Optic nerve head drusen or crowded optic nerve:* PRK is not associated with increased IOP as there is no suction ring required and it has been considered a safer option relative to LASIK in this setting. However, the VisuMax affords the lowest increase in IOP of any femtosecond laser or microkeratome at levels that are negligible.[5,6]

- *Epithelial or anterior stromal dystrophies:* PRK may be a more appropriate treatment as it has the therapeutic effect of removing opacities and/or increasing adherence of corneal epithelium in basement membrane disease. LASIK is contraindicated in granular corneal dystrophy type 2 (Avellino corneal dystrophy). There are no reports of SMILE in Avellino corneal dystrophy, but corneal opacities are a relative contraindication (see in the following section).

- *Fuchsendothelial dystrophy:* Endothelial cell count should be performed before surgery in patients with corneal guttata. Low endothelial cell count places the patient at risk of poor settling of the tissues on either side of the SMILE interface, leading to increased corneal back scatter and poor-quality vision.

- *Corneal opacity:* Any opacity can alter the efficacy of femtosecond laser cutting. Because the laser energies for SMILE are significantly lower than those used for a LASIK flap, care must be taken to identify any significant opacity that will fall within the lenticule zone as treatment can lead to an uncut area, making dissection and lenticule removal challenging.

- *Depression or anxiety conditions if not stabilized:* This is an important relative contraindication for all refractive surgical procedures.

- *Uncontrolled Diabetes:* These patients have a higher risk of infection and slower healing response. Of the corneal refractive procedures, SMILE has the smallest incision and, thus, has the quickest healing time, minimizing the infection risk relative to LASIK or PRK.

INFORMED CONSENT CONSIDERATIONS

Key Informed Consent Adverse Events

- Infection
- Glare, halos, starburst from irregular astigmatism (decentered treatment, retained lenticule fragment)
- Suction break requiring conversion to LASIK, PRK, or postponement of surgery
- Residual myopia and/or astigmatism
- Consecutive hyperopia and/or astigmatism
- Corneal ectasia

Informed consent should include a description of the procedure in plain language. For example, "A laser will be used to create a lens-shaped piece of tissue (lenticule) within the cornea (front window of the eye). This lenticule, customized to your prescription, will then be removed by your surgeon through a small surface incision, also created by the laser. By removing this lenticule, your cornea will be flatter and rounder, thus improving your vision without glasses or contact lenses."

Potential alternative treatments, such as LASIK, PRK, phakic intraocular lens implantation, glasses, and contact lenses, should be listed.

A note from the counseling physician should be included and phrased similar to, "I have counseled this patient as to the nature of the proposed procedure, the attendant risks involved, and the expected results." The patient's and doctor's name should be printed and signed with the date as well as with a witness (typically a staff member).

PREOPERATIVE CARE

Key Preoperative Considerations

- Medical history including diagnoses and medications
- Ophthalmic history including diagnoses, drops, and previous surgery
- Contact lens history (e.g., type of lens, wearing and cleaning habits, date of last use)
- Corneal tomography including back surface imaging
- Ocular dominance
- Pupils
- Cover testing at distance and near, with and without glasses, and ocular motility testing
- Confrontational fields testing
- Monocular and binocular uncorrected distance visual acuity (UDVA)

Key Preoperative Considerations

- Monocular and binocular uncorrected near visual acuity
- Lensometry of current spectacles and corrected distance visual acuity (CDVA)
- Distance-corrected near vision for myopic patients over 40
- Distance manifest refraction
- Slit-lamp examination including fluorescein staining, taking note of location, size, and depth of any corneal opacities
- Tear break-up time
- Goldmann applanation tonometry
- Cycloplegic refraction and CDVA (after dilation with 1.0% tropicamide)
- Dilated fundus examination using slit-lamp and binocular indirect ophthalmoscopy

As with all refractive surgical techniques, the manifest refraction is the cornerstone to a successful SMILE outcome. Consistency in refraction is critical and, therefore, it is desirable to have the same refractionist performing the measurements on all patients. Variations in refraction technique can account for differences in endpoints, which can lead to variability in outcomes. Binocular balance is important to reduce the possibility of postoperative anisometropia. Patients with spectacle- or contact lens–corrected vision rarely need to deal with anisometropia: the power of the spectacle lens or contact lens can be easily adjusted to bring both eyes to a plano endpoint. Since spectacle-/contact lens–corrected patients are not used to it, anisometropia following refractive surgery can be quite noticeable, particularly in the immediate postoperative period. Cycloplegic refraction is particularly important in younger patients who are susceptible to over-minusing. Care should be taken to identify amblyopia in patients with significant anisometropia, asymmetric astigmatism, and a history of strabismus. It is important to counsel amblyopic patients so that they understand the laser procedure cannot fix the "wiring of the eye to the brain", which limits the ultimate visual acuity.

PROCEDURE AND SETTINGS

 Video 8.1 shows the key steps of the SMILE procedure. There are two components:

1. Laser treatment
2. Lenticule dissection and removal

The VisuMax laser has two microscopes (laser and operating) one for each of these steps (Figure 8.1).

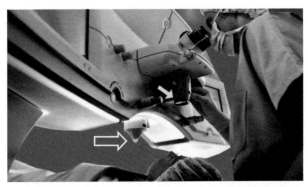

FIGURE 8-1 The VisuMax femtosecond laser (Carl Zeiss Meditec, Dublin, CA) includes two microscopes: A laser microscope (open white arrow) for visualization of the laser creation of the lenticule and an operating microscope (yellow arrow) for visualization of the cornea during lenticule dissection and removal. Image courtesy of Carl Zeiss Meditec.

Laser Treatment

Preparation of the Eye

Surgeon's may choose to premedicate the patient with an oral anxiolytic agent such as alprazolam 0.5 mg. One drop of proparacaine is placed in each eye of the patient in the preoperative area. Once the patient is positioned on the laser bed, a second drop of proparacaine is placed and the patient is asked if there was any stinging. While it is obviously important to anesthetize the eye, it is also important not to use too much proparacaine as this loosens the corneal epithelium. Because there is some pressure placed on the posterior edge of the surface incision during lenticule dissection, epithelial sloughing can occur. If this occurs, there is some risk of introducing epithelium into the interface, which can lead to epithelial proliferation (much like epithelial ingrowth with LASIK).

The skin surrounding the eye is prepped with betadine swabs. A drop of antibiotic is placed in the eye. The lashes are draped and a lid speculum is placed.

The corneal surface is wiped clean using a Weck-Cel sponge soaked in sterile balanced salt solution (BSS). It is very important to confirm there is no material (e.g., mucous) on the cornea or the patient interface prior to docking. Any material trapped between the interface and the cornea can block the laser shots, resulting in "black spots," which represent tissue that has not been cut by the laser, leading to inability to dissect the lenticule in that area.

Centration

In LASIK flap creation, the femtosecond laser is not performing the refractive correction. Thus, centration of the flap is important but not as critical as with SMILE where the laser

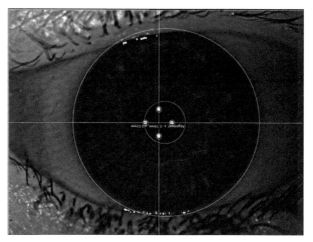

FIGURE 8-2 A verify image, such as this one from the Galilei G4 tomography system (Ziemer Ophthalmic, Port, Switzerland), is useful for the surgeon to confirm centration on the visual axis (cross hairs) when docking the laser to the patient's cornea prior to firing the laser.

is performing the refractive correction. Consequently, care must be taken to properly center the suction ring on the visual axis. Certain diagnostic systems (e.g., Galilei G4 Tomography system, Ziemer USA) take pictures of the iris and pupil with the position of the visual axis within the pupil identified with crosshairs (Figure 8.2). This picture can be printed and taken to the laser suite and used as a reference during docking. By noting the position of the visual axis relative to the pupil through the laser microscope, the surgeon can ensure the eye is appropriately centered during the docking procedure.

Docking

The VisuMax patient interface features a curved applanation glass that only touches the cornea (Figure 8.3). The pressure associated with docking is minimal. It feels like putting a contact lens in the eye of the patient. With no conjunctival touch, there is no subconjunctival hemorrhage with the VisuMax that is commonly seen with other femtosecond lasers that grab onto the conjunctiva.

Laser Treatment

Figure 8.4 shows the tissue planes that define the SMILE lenticule and the opening incision. The posterior aspect of the lenticule is cut first with the laser spiraling in from the periphery. The optical zone is 6.5 mm in the United States. This zone can be decreased to 6.0 mm in sphere-only treatments to remove less tissue. The depth of the posterior aspect of the lenticule is defined by the amount of refractive correction. Next, the lenticule side cut is created, followed by the cap cut (anterior

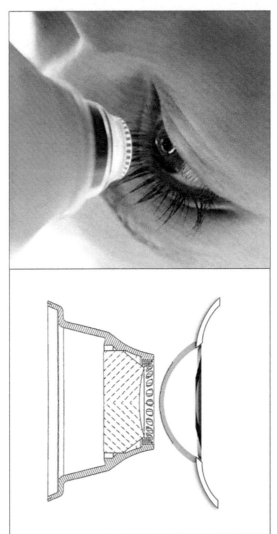

FIGURE 8-3 The disposable VisuMax Femtosecond (FS) laser contact interface only touches the patient's cornea, eliminating the possibility of subconjunctival hemorrhage, which is commonly seen with interface suction rings on other FS laser systems that grab onto the conjunctiva. In addition, the curved applanation window reduces the pressure experienced by the patient. Image courtesy of Carl Zeiss Meditec. FS.

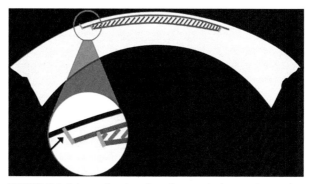

FIGURE 8-4 Schematic showing the posterior and anterior (cap) cuts, the lenticule side cut and the opening incision created by the VisuMax FS laser for SMILE. Image courtesy of Carl Zeiss Meditec.
FS; SMILE, small-incision lenticule extraction.

aspect of lenticule and cap zone). The cap cut proceeds from the center and spirals outward. The diameter of the cap is 7.5 mm in the United States or 7.0 mm if the optical zone is decreased to 6.0 mm in a sphere-only treatment. The depth of the cap is set at 120 microns in the United States. Finally, the opening incision is made superiorly, centered on the 12 o'clock meridian, at the peripheral aspect of the cap cut. This cut up to the corneal surface is typically 60° wide in the United States but can be increased to 90°.

If a suction break occurs during the posterior cut, the procedure should be converted to LASIK or PRK or postponed. If a suction break occurs during the cap cut, the eye can be re-docked using the same patient interface, and the procedure can be completed.

Lenticule Dissection and Removal

Once the patient interface is disengaged following laser treatment, the bed translates the patient under the operating microscope. During transit, the conjunctiva adjacent to the limbus where the surgeon will fixate the eye using forceps can be anesthetized with a cotton swab soaked in 4% lidocaine. A small dissector is used to open the surface incision and define the anterior and posterior planes of the lenticule. A spoon-shaped dissector is then used to separate the anterior plane of the lenticule from the cap. Finally, the dissector is used to separate the posterior plane of the lenticule from the posterior stroma, freeing up the lenticule, which is then removed from the interface. A sponge is used to smooth the anterior corneal surface and make sure there is no missing epithelium from the posterior edge of the surface incision. Antibiotic and anti-inflammatory drops are instilled, and the lid speculum is removed.

Key VisuMax Laser Settings

Choosing the appropriate VisuMax laser settings for SMILE is paramount in achieving an easy dissection and rapid recovery of vision following the procedure. There are two key parameters that can be adjusted: laser spot energy and spot spacing. The VisuMax laser fires 500,000 shots per second to perform the cutting of the lenticule. The higher the spot energy, the more overall energy deposition occurs. The closer the spot spacing, the more overall energy deposition occurs and the longer the procedure takes. If too much energy deposition occurs, opaque bubble layer (OBL) formation can occur. This can distort the tissues, block subsequent laser spots from having their full efficacy, and can lead to more challenging dissection with more tissue manipulation. This, in turn, can delay the visual recovery. Laser spot energy and spacing must be optimized for each individual laser installation. Once these parameters have been determined, the laser will typically perform in a consistent manner assuming temperature and humidity constraints are obeyed.

- *Minimum laser spot energy in the United States:* 125 nJ
- *Maximum laser spot spacing in the United States:* 4.5 microns

It is important to note that, prior to the FDA approval of myopic astigmatism in the United States, surgeon's were limited to a 3.0-micron spot spacing. This dramatically increased the energy deposition (high energy), creating more OBL and prolonging the visual recovery (see "SMILE vs. LASIK" section for more details). The goal is to choose the minimum spot energy with the widest spot spacing (low energy) that allows for easy dissection of the lenticule. Care must be taken to avoid choosing too low of an energy, which, if below the plasma threshold of the tissue, will result in no cutting action and a lenticule that cannot be dissected.

POSTOPERATIVE CARE/CO-MANAGEMENT (FOLLOW-UP SCHEDULE)

Key Postoperative Considerations

- Immediate postoperative period
- Postoperative drop regimen
- Postoperative limitations
- Treatments for dry eye symptoms
- Transient glare/halos
- Postoperative manifest refraction

Immediate Postoperative Period

For 3 to 4 hours following surgery, the eyes are light sensitive, scratchy, and tearing due to the reepithelialization that needs to occur at the small surface incision. This is typically a shorter duration than what occurs with LASIK as the incision is only 60° instead of 300° wide. Patients can be given acetominophen/diphenhydrmine (Tylenol PM) following surgery. This, together with the alprazolam administered prior to surgery, assists the patient to sleep through this healing period. When they wake up, the vision will be foggy, like "in a sauna." This will persist for 1 to 3 days typically and is determined primarily by how much OBL occurred during the laser application and how much force was required to dissect the lenticule. The more force is required, the more microtrauma occurs with the interface tissues. This can lead to edema that can take several days to resolve. The edema leads to backscatter of light, causing the foggy vision. In rare cases with significant OBL and difficult dissection, foggy vision can last for several weeks. Postoperative day 1 slit lamp appearance will show ground glass appearance of varying severity, which correlates with level of vision (Figure 8.5). Even best corrected vision can be reduced on postoperative day 1 due to backscatter.

Postoperative Drop Regimen

Prophylactic antibiotic drops (e.g., moxifloxacin) three to four times daily should be used for several days following surgery. Anti-inflammatory corticosteroid drops (e.g., prednisolone acetate 1%) should be used three to four times daily for at least one week following surgery. If significant OBL and/or challenging lenticule dissection occurs, a stronger steroid (e.g., difluprednate) and/or more frequent dosing should be implemented.

Postoperative Limitations

One of the most attractive aspects of the SMILE procedure for patients is the minimal need for lifestyle restrictions. Because there is no flap, there is no concern of a flap being shifted by rubbing the eye. Consequently, there is no need for the patient to wear goggles while sleeping for a week following surgery. There is also no need to limit the use of eye makeup beyond the first night after surgery. Also, for patients who are active, engaged in sports, which might involve taking a finger to the eye (e.g., basketball), there is no concern over a flap becoming dislodged. The small incision heals quickly, within a matter of hours. Thus, the risk of infection is minimal after the first 24 hours. Consequently, there is no need to limit activities such as swimming beyond a day or two.

Treatments for Dry Eye Symptoms

Dry eye symptoms include any combination of the following: transient blurred vision, particularly toward the end of the day and in patients who spend hours per

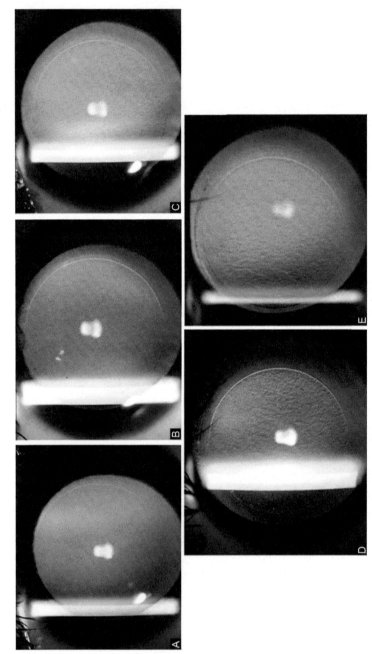

FIGURE 8-5 Retroillumination photographs after dilation showing the five templates of interface roughness grade. **A,** interface roughness grade—0 (clear), **B,** interface roughness grade—1 (mild interface roughness), **C,** interface roughness grade—2 (moderate interface roughness), **D,** interface roughness grade—3 (severe interface roughness), **E,** interface roughness grade—4 (severe interface roughness with Bowman's folds in the visual axis). Reproduced with permission from Sri Ganesh, MD, Department of Phacorefractive, Nethradhama Superspeciality Eye Hospital, Bengaluru, Karnataka, India.

day looking at monitors or cell phone, intermittent sandy, gritty feeling, mild conjunctival redness, and reflex tearing. Patients undergoing LASIK should expect to experience some or all of these symptoms for 6 to 12 months following surgery, decreasing in severity and frequency as time goes by. This time frame is shortened to one to three months for patients undergoing SMILE because many fewer sub-basal afferent corneal nerves are severed by the 60° small incision compared with the 310° LASIK side cut (Figure 8.6). Consequently, there are fewer nerves that need to regenerate which shortens the period of dry eye symptoms. Treatments include preservative-free artificial tears, punctal occlusion, topical cyclosporine 0.05% or 0.09%, topical lifitegrast 5%, or a short course of low-potency steroid (e.g., loteprednol 0.5%, fluorometholone 0.1%).

Transient Glare and Halos

Patients should understand that, with any refractive surgery, we are instantaneously changing the optics that their brain has become accustomed to. Much like the adaptation that occurs with a new pair of glasses, the patient will experience adaptation to their new optics following SMILE. Nighttime glare and halos may be noticed for several weeks to months following surgery, which will eventually subside as adaptation occurs. These halos are typically less than what is seen following LASIK for the same correction. This is due to slightly less induction of spherical aberration with SMILE compared to LASIK. See the "SMILE vs. LASIK" section for more details.

Postoperative Manifest Refraction

Accurate postoperative manifest refraction in SMILE patients is also very important, not just to confirm accuracy for individual patients, but also to record in a database to generate a surgeon nomogram. Nomograms for sphere and cylinder should be developed based on patient outcomes to improve consistency of refractive results for a given surgeon and laser installation. The accuracy of these nomograms relies on the accuracy of the manifest refraction. Postoperative manifest refraction data should be at least 45 days following surgery to be entered into a nomogram database. Once the surgeon has accumulated 40 to 50 eyes in the database, a nomogram equation can be generated. To use this, a desired sphere and cylinder correction is entered into the system. The nomogram inputs these entries as the "achieved" result and calculates, based on past results, what parameters should be entered into the laser to achieve the desired result. One such example of an outstanding nomogram system is the cloud-based "SurgiVision DataLink Zeiss Edition," which is made available to VisuMax-trained surgeon's.[7] Another option that resides on a local computer is "Datagraph-med."[8]

Removing tissue from deeper corneal layers results in less impact on the corneal surface and nerves.

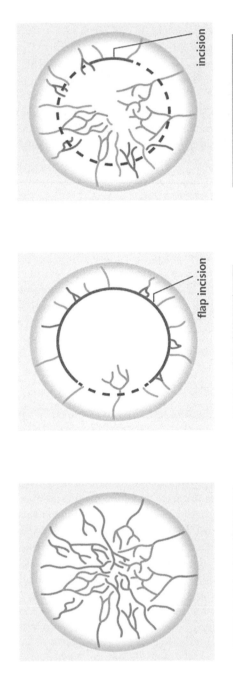

Normal nerve network   LASIK   SMILE

FIGURE 8-6 Schematic demonstrating the reduced severing of subbasal afferent corneal nerves with the small 60° SMILE opening incision compared with the 310° LASIK flap side cut. Image courtesy of Carl Zeiss Meditec. LASIK, laser in situ Keratomileusis; SMILE, small-incision lenticule extraction.

POTENTIAL COMPLICATIONS AND THEIR TREATMENT

Key Complications to Look for the Following:

- Overcorrection
- Undercorrection
- Epithelial ingrowth/implantation
- Retained lenticule fragment
- Decentration
- Diffuse lamellar keratitis
- Corneal ectasia
- Infectious keratitis

Overcorrection/Undercorrection

As with any refractive surgery technique, one can expect rare cases where the outcome differs from the intended target. Fortunately, for SMILE, the enhancement rate for patients appears to be roughly one third that of LASIK. In the author's experience, the enhancement rate is less than 1%. The reason for this low enhancement rate has to do with how the SMILE technique is fundamentally different than PRK or LASIK. Once the surgeon has passed the learning curve of the technique, the SMILE procedure is inherently less susceptible to variability in outcomes arising from amount of attempted correction or from differences in surgical technique. For example, the stromal bed is exposed to the air during the excimer ablation with both LASIK and PRK. The time of exposure is related both to the amount of correction and the technique of the surgeon. The differential tissue hydration that results from exposure to air can have an impact on the nomogram and outcomes. A higher correction with PRK/LASIK requires a longer ablation, more tissue drying, and potential overcorrection. In addition, certain excimer lasers correct sphere first followed by astigmatism. In higher myopic corrections, this may lead to variability in the astigmatic correction relative to lower myopic corrections. With SMILE, there is no exposure of the tissue being treated to air. In addition, the laser treatment time is identical regardless of the amount of sphere and cylinder correction is performed. Thus, the variability caused by tissue exposure is eliminated with SMILE. If clinically significant over- or undercorrection does occur, wait for three months for refractive stability and then enhancement can be done, either with thin flap (e.g., 90 micron) LASIK or surface ablation.

Epithelial Ingrowth/Implantation

The SMILE procedure requires a surface incision to allow for access and removal of the lenticule. The width of this incision is typically 60° in U.S. and smaller outside U.S. This is significantly smaller than the 310° side-cut incision used with a LASIK flap. While there is a theoretical risk of epithelial ingrowth occurring as a fistula of epithelium extending into the SMILE interface, that risk, as it relates to the width of the incision, is less than LASIK. With the advent of femtosecond laser flaps and the ability to create a 90° side-cut angle (vertical angle of perpendicular side-cut and lamellar flap plane), the incidence of epithelial ingrowth decreased dramatically relative to that seen with microkeratome flaps where the side-cut angle was flatter. The SMILE side-cut angle can also be programmed to 90°, thus minimizing the epithelial growth risk. SMILE differs from LASIK in that there is friction placed on the posterior edge of the surface incision during lenticular dissection. This friction is not present during the LASIK flap lift maneuver. Consequently, particularly in older patients with loosened epithelium from topical proparacaine, there is risk of introducing epithelial tags into the SMILE interface. This epithelial implantation can produce an island of epithelial cells that can proliferate, leading to distortion of the corneal surface shape, inducing irregular astigmatism, and decreasing vision (Figure 8.7). The risk of these epithelial islands proliferating is lower than with traditional LASIK epithelial ingrowth where there is a fistula track continuously delivering fresh epithelial cells from the corneal surface. Observation is appropriate in patients who are asymptomatic and show no sign of focal cap thinning, which can occur when the epithelial cells thicken in the interface. Interface irrigation and removal can be easily accomplished if the patient is symptomatic and/or there is evidence of cap thinning.

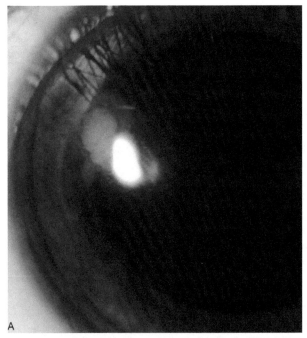

A

FIGURE 8-7 A, Front view of epithelial island resulting from epithelial implantation during SMILE lenticule dissection.

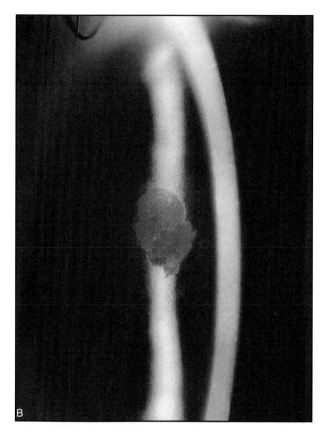

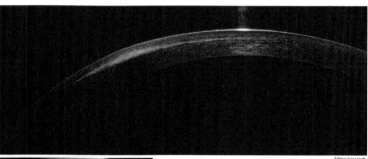

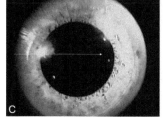

FIGURE 8-7 (*Continued*) **B,** Retroillumination view. **C,** Anterior segment OCT showing thickness and lateral extent of epithelial island.

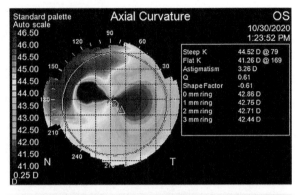

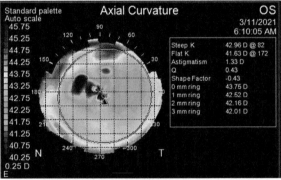

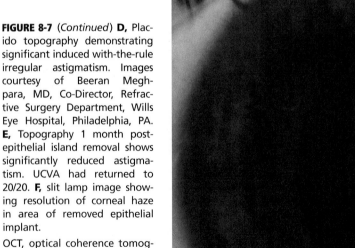

FIGURE 8-7 (*Continued*) **D,** Placido topography demonstrating significant induced with-the-rule irregular astigmatism. Images courtesy of Beeran Meghpara, MD, Co-Director, Refractive Surgery Department, Wills Eye Hospital, Philadelphia, PA. **E,** Topography 1 month post-epithelial island removal shows significantly reduced astigmatism. UCVA had returned to 20/20. **F,** slit lamp image showing resolution of corneal haze in area of removed epithelial implant.

OCT, optical coherence tomography; OS, left eye; SMILE, small-incision lenticule extraction.

Retained Lenticule Fragment

Lenticule laceration can occur during dissection, leading to retention of a lenticular fragment. This can be identified at the time of surgery by smoothing out the removed lenticule on the corneal surface to confirm it is 100% intact prior to discarding the tissue. If the lenticule is not inspected upon removal, it is possible that a lenticular fragment remains in the interface. The most likely portion of the lenticule to be retained is a peripheral crescent. In myopic corrections in the United States, the edge thickness of the lenticule is set at 15 microns. Consequently, a retained lenticule crescent is likely to be very thin and will often have no impact on the patient's vision. Conversely, if a patient demonstrates decreased UDVA or CDVA, a tomographic exam showing curvature and pachymetry or an anterior segment optical coherence tomography exam can be helpful in identifying the presence and location of a lenticular fragment. These can then be removed under the operating microscope using dissecting instrumentation and forceps.

Decentration

When creating a flap for LASIK using a femtosecond laser, the flap needs to be reasonably centered to allow the entire excimer ablation, the refractive correction, to fit within the flap. The centration of the treatment, therefore, occurs at the excimer laser, typically using pupil tracking, not at the femtosecond laser. With SMILE, the refractive correction is performed by the femtosecond laser, thus requiring more accurate centration than is required when creating the LASIK flap. Fortunately, the VisuMax docking design tends to auto-center the treatment on the visual axis. It is possible, however, to get a decentered treatment if the patient is not fixating appropriately on the target light as suction is applied or if the applanation cone is off center when suction is applied. The best way to confirm appropriate centration is to bring a photo into the laser room that shows the position of the visual axis relative to the pupil. This allows the surgeon a reference image to look at during the docking process, confirming that the fixation light (i.e. visual axis) is in the proper location relative to the pupil. Clinically significant decentration can manifest with a mild-to-moderate mixed astigmatic postoperative refraction, poor quality of vision, particularly at night, and a decentered treatment zone appearing on postoperative topography. If the tomography systems capture corneal wave front information, significant coma will be observed. A topography-guided PRK procedure can be performed (off-label use of excimer laser) to correct some of the aberrations resulting from the decentration.

Diffuse Lamellar Keratitis

Diffuse lamellar keratitis (DLK) is exceedingly rare these days as standardized sterilization techniques have been established to eliminate DLK arising from endotoxin residue on instruments. Epithelial defects or hemorrhage can lead to DLK but these are usually mild and successfully treated with topical corticosteroid drops. If Stage II or III DLK is observed (e.g., wave of white cells in the interface extending into the visual axis or clumping of white cells in the interface), interface washout should be done with BSS as well as injection of corticosteroid into the interface, together with topical steroid drops. Oral steroids can also be added in severe cases of DLK.

Corneal Ectasia

The surface incision with the SMILE procedure, typically 60°, is much smaller than the larger flap incision with LASIK, typically 310°. As a result, the anterior stromal biomechanical strength is relatively preserved, thus reducing the risk of ectasia development in topographically normal eyes. This hypothesis is supported by mathematical modeling.[9] As SMILE matures and long-term follow-up becomes available, studies are looking at the incidence of ectasia at 3 years and beyond.

There are a number of recent papers presenting SMILE treatment for myopia greater than –10.0D. Follow-up ranged from 15 months to 3 years, with no ectasia reported in any of these studies.[10–12] A particularly interesting recent report presents 3-year data for a series of 495 eyes of Egyptian patients with preoperative myopia exceeding –10.0 D in which no eyes developed ectasia over the course of the study, despite the high incidence of keratoconus in the Middle Eastern population.[13]

A review of the literature from 2011 to 2017 found seven cases of ectasia after SMILE in 4 patients after 750,000 cases of SMILE had been performed worldwide. Two of the patients had abnormal topographies in both eyes, whereas only one eye of one patient with normal topography developed ectasia.[14] It is very important to understand that even though the ectasia risk appears to be lower with SMILE than LASIK for an equivalent amount of correction on the same cornea, the identification of normal preoperative tomographic features is still requisite to avoiding the risk of ectasia with SMILE.

Infectious Keratitis

While exceedingly rare, infectious keratitis can occur, either with introduction of bacteria into the interface from contaminated instrumentation or migration of bacteria into the interface postoperatively prior to reepithelialization of the surface incision. Prophylactic antibiotics should be used just prior to surgery and should be continued for at least several days following surgery. Povidone-iodine prep should also be performed and eyelids should be draped prior to surgery.

VIDEO OF PROCEDURE

Video 8.1—This SMILE procedure uses a single femtosecond laser to create a lenticule in the anterior corneal stroma as well as an incision from the lenticule up to the corneal surface, through which the lenticule is extracted. The procedure begins with docking the laser to the patient's cornea. Care is taken to ensure proper centration over the patient's visual axis. The first cut performed by the laser is the posterior or "power" cut, proceeding from the corneal periphery toward the center. The depth of this cut is determined by the amount of nearsightedness and astigmatism being treated. The next cut, almost imperceptible, is the lenticule side cut. This cut is 15 microns in depth and occurs right at the edge of the power cut. The next cut is the anterior or "cap" cut, proceeding from the corneal center toward the periphery. This cut is currently fixed at 120 microns for lasers in the United States. Notice this cut extends peripheral to the power cut. This larger diameter facilitates the dissection of the lenticule. The final cut is the surface cut, always centered at the 12 o'clock meridian (at bottom of screen) and extends for 60°, allowing access for lenticule dissection. Following laser application, the patient bed translates to the operating microscope so that the surgeon can dissect and remove the lenticule. Lidocaine 4% is used to anesthetize the conjunctiva (swab to the right), allowing the surgeon to grasp the conjunctiva and Tenon's layer to fixate the globe. A dissector is then used to identify the anterior and posterior dissection planes. Following identification, the anterior lenticule plane is dissected first, followed by the posterior lenticule plane. Once the lenticule is freed up, the surgeon reaches in with microforceps and removes the lenticule in one piece. A circular merocel sponge is used to smooth out the cap. Antibiotic and anti-inflammatory drops are applied and the procedure concludes.

EFFICACY

SMILE versus LASIK

Refractive surgeon's have become accustomed to rapid, overnight visual recovery, excellent accuracy, and long-term stability with the LASIK procedure. Since SMILE requires the expense of a specific laser (VisuMax) and involves a surgical learning curve to become comfortable performing the procedure, barriers are in place for refractive surgeon's to adopt this newer technique. Yet, SMILE has advantages over LASIK regarding postoperative dry eye symptoms, corneal biomechanical properties, and attractiveness of the procedure (single laser, no sound, no smell, no flap). The first question that comes to mind when considering the new procedure is as follows: How do the results from SMILE compare with the stellar results achieved with LASIK? Will my patients still achieve that "WOW" factor I am used to with LASIK?

A study recently published by our group is the first to compare early postoperative SMILE results in eyes treated after the approval of myopic astigmatism correction and expanded energy settings (low energy) with those treated prior to the approval (high energy) and with results from wave front–optimized (WO) LASIK.[15]

The study comprises eyes from a single site in the United States treated by a single surgeon using SMILE and WO LASIK. Our group found that SMILE patients whose surgeries were performed with low energy had significantly better postoperative day 1 (POD1) vision (20/19.86) compared with high-energy patients (20/27.67) ($p < 0.001$). Moreover, the mean UDVA on POD1 for the low-energy SMILE group was equivalent to that of the WO LASIK group (20/19.50) ($p = 0.498$) (see Figure 8.2). Importantly, the percent of patients with UDVA 20/20 or better on POD1 was equivalent when comparing the low-energy SMILE group to the WO LASIK group (Figure 8.8). Furthermore,

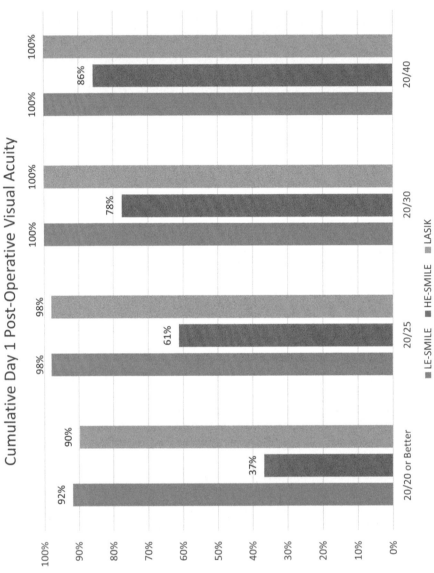

FIGURE 8-8 Cumulative postoperative day 1 uncorrected visual acuities (20/X): Comparison of LE SMILE, HE SMILE, and WO LASIK.
HE SMILE, high-energy small-incision lenticule extraction; LE SMILE, low-energy small-incision lenticule extraction; WO LASIK, wave front–optimized laser in situ keratomileusis.

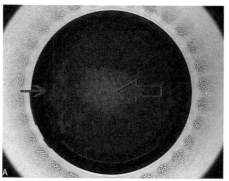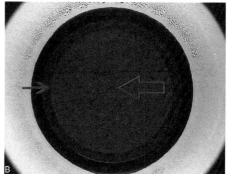

FIGURE 8-9 Comparison of bubble pattern for high-energy optimized treatments: **A,** Bubble pattern with high-energy, manifesting significant OBL in the visual axis and fluffy irregularity at the side cut; **B,** bubble pattern with optimized energy without OBL or black spots and a sharp lenticular border, suggestive of an easier dissection.
OBL, opaque bubble layer.

induced higher-order aberrations were equivalent between low-energy SMILE and WO LASIK at postoperative month 1 (POM1), with the exception of induced SA measured at a 6.0-mm optical zone (OZ), which was lower in the low-energy density SMILE group (0.136 μm) compared to WO LASIK (0.186 μm, p = 0.034).

These improved outcomes underscore the importance of energy optimization when performing SMILE, a concept that is new to refractive surgeon's, who are used to significant flexibility in femtosecond laser energy levels for LASIK flap formation. The bubble pattern appearance resulting from laser application during the SMILE procedure is useful to the surgeon both in anticipating the difficulty of dissection, but also to guide patient expectations for early postoperative visual acuity recovery (see Figure 8.9). By comparison, the bubble pattern appearance following LASIK flap creation using FS laser is much less important with regard to ease of flap dissection and typically has no impact on early postoperative visual acuity recovery.[13]

Long-Term Safety and Efficacy

Ten years after Sekundo et al.'s first published article on SMILE,[1] long-term data demonstrate excellent safety and efficacy of the procedure.

A study by Blum et al. presenting 10-year SMILE data for 56 eyes treated for myopia and myopic astigmatism found 64.3% were within ±0.50D of target, and 82.1% were within ±1.00D at 10 years. UDVA remained stable from one month through ten years with mid regression of 0.30D in manifest refraction spherical equivalent (MRSE).[16] Among the studied eyes, 29% gained at least 1 line of CDVA, 14% lost 1 line, and no eyes lost 2 or more lines, suggesting a favorable safety profile. No ectasia was observed within this cohort, and no patients required management of ocular surface disease after POM3.

The past 2 years have also seen several reports from Turkey and China presenting promising safety and stability data through 5 years.

In two 5-year Turkish studies of 54 and 24 SMILE eyes, respectively, 93% and 91% of patients remained within 0.5D of intended correction, with the majority of refractive error resulting from undercorrection of high myopia. Safety was also evaluated, with Agca et al. reporting 0 of 54 patients and Ayugin et al. reporting 1 eye in 24 (4%) losing a line of CDVA. In neither study, did any patient lose 2 or more lines of CDVA.[17,18]

Chinese studies by Han et al. and Li et al. followed SMILE eyes for 3 and 5 years, respectively. Han et al. found 80% to be within 0.5 D of attempted spherical equivalent at 3 years; whereas Li et al. observed 90% of eyes within 0.50 D of target at 5 years. These studies found 2% and 9% of SMILE eyes losing 1 line of CDVA, with no eyes losing 2 or more lines.[19,20]

CONCLUSION

SMILE represents a promising laser vision correction modality that addresses many of the fear issues that keep refractive surgery candidates on the sidelines: no sound or smell during the procedure, no flap, no pain, and minimal restrictions after surgery. As other ophthalmic surgical device companies develop their version of the technique and bring new equipment to market, further refinement of the technique is inevitable. With visual outcomes, safety, and predictability already comparable to LASIK, and with potential advantages in postoperative dry eye and biomechanical stability, expect SMILE to become a standard technique in the armamentarium of the refractive surgeon for the treatment of myopic astigmatism.

CODING/BILLING MODIFIERS

Myopia H52.1x
Regular Astigmatism H52.22x
Laser surgery is usually not covered by medical insurance. Some insurance companies will offer partial payments.

REFERENCES

1. Kezirian G, Fatnani L, Opoku E, et al. Forecast of laser refractive surgery in China 2013–2023. Lecture notes from Physician CEO program, Kellogg Northwestern School of Management, 12/2013.
2. Kobashi H, Kamiya K, Shimizu K. Dry eye after small incision lenticule extraction and femtosecond laser-assisted LASIK: Meta-analysis. *Cornea.* 2017 Jan;36(1):85–91.
3. Zhang Y, Shen Q, Jia Y, Zhou D, Zhou J. Clinical outcomes of SMILE and FS-LASIK used to treat myopia: A meta-analysis. *J Refract Surg.* 2016 Apr;32(4):256–265.

4. Ajazaj V Kacaniku G, Asani M, et al. Intraocular pressure after corneal refractive surgery. *Med Arch.* 2018 Oct;72(5):341–343.

5. Vetter JM, Faust M, Gericke A, Pfeiffer N, Weingartner WE, Sekundo W. Intraocular pressure measurements during flap preparation using 2 femtosecond lasers and 1 microkeratome in human donor eyes. *J Cataract Refract Surg.* 2012;38:2011–2018.

6. Vetter JM, Holzer MP, Teping C, et al. Intraocular pressure during corneal flap preparation: Comparison among four femtosecond lasers in porcine eyes. *J Refract Surg.* 2011;27:427–433.

7. SurgiVision Consultants Inc. SurgiVision DataLink Ophthalmic Applications. Available at: http://web.surgivision.net/Home/SVCHome.html

8. Datagraph med. Datagraph-med outcomes analysis software for cataract and refractive surgery. Available at: http://www.datagraph.eu/?menuid=1&getlang=en

9. Spiru B, Torres-Netto EA, Kling S, Lazaridis A, Hafezi F, Sekundo W. Biomechanical properties of human cornea tested by two-dimensional extensiometry ex vivo in fellow eyes: PRK versus SMILE. *J Refract Surg.* 2019;35(8):501–505.

10. Yang W, Liu S, Li M, Shen Y, Zhou X. Visual outcomes after small incision lenticule extraction and femtosecond laser-assisted LASIK for high myopia. *Ophthalmic Res.* 2020;63(4):427–433.

11. Qian Y, Chen X, Naidu RK, Zhou X. Comparison of efficacy and visual outcomes after SMILE and FS-LASIK for the correction of high myopia with the sum of myopia and astigmatism from –10.00 to –14.00 dioptres. *Acta Ophthalmologica.* 2020 Mar;98(2):e161-e172.

12. Zhou X, Shang J, Qin B, Zhao Y, Zhou X. Two-year observation of posterior corneal elevations after small incision lenticule extraction (SMILE) for myopia higher than –10 dioptres. *Br J Ophthalmol.* 2020;104:142–148.

13. Elmassry A, Ibrahim O, Osman I, et al. Long-term refractive outcome of small incision lenticule extraction in very high myopia. *Cornea.* 2020;Jun;39(6):669–673.

14. Moshirfar M, Albarracin JC, Desautels JD, Birdsong OC, Linn SH, Hoopes PC Sr. Ectasia following small-incision lenticule extraction (SMILE): A review of the literature. *Clin Ophthalmol.* 2017 Sep 15;11:1683–1688.

15. Hamilton DR, Chen AC, Khorrami R, Nutkiewicz M, Nejad M. Comparison of early visual outcomes following low-energy Small Incision Lenticule Extraction (SMILE), high-energy SMILE and LASIK for myopic astigmatism. *J Cataract Refractive Surg.* 2021 Jan 1;47(1):18–26.

16. Blum M, Lauer AS, Kunert KS, Sekundo W. 10-year results of small incision lenticule extraction. *J Refract Surg.* 2019;35(10):618–623.

17. Agca A, Tülü B, Yasa D, Yıldırım Y, Yıldız BK, Demirok A. Long-term (5 years) follow-up of small-incision lenticule extraction in mild-to-moderate myopia. *J Cataract Refract Surg.* 2019;45:421–426.

18. Aygün BT, Çankaya KI, Agca A, et al. Five-year outcomes of small-incision lenticule extraction vs femtosecond laser–assisted laser in situ keratomileusis: A contralateral eye study. *J Cataract Refract Surg.* 2020;46:403–409.

19. Li M, Li M, Chen Y, et al. Five-year results of small incision lenticule extraction (SMILE) and femtosecond laser LASIK (FS-LASIK) for myopia. *Acta Ophthalmol.* 2019;97:e373–e380.

20. Han T, Xu Y, Han X, et al. Three-year outcomes of small incision lenticule extraction (SMILE) and femtosecond laser-assisted laser in situ keratomileusis (FS-LASIK) for myopia and myopic astigmatism. *Br J Ophthalmol.* 2019;103:565–568.

9 Femtosecond Laser in Corneal Transplantation

Michael D. Greenwood • Nicholas C. Risbrudt

The femtosecond laser has played an integral role in laser vision correction as well as cataract surgery. In recent years, ophthalmology has been utilizing this technology in corneal transplantation with femtosecond laser–assisted keratoplasty (FLAK). Corneal disease ranks as the fifth leading cause of blindness in the world with the cornea being the most commonly transplanted human tissue worldwide.[1] Since the first successful full-thickness corneal transplant performed by Eduard Zirm in 1905,[2] corneal transplantation techniques have continued to evolve as improvements in medicine and technology advance.

Conventional corneal transplantation, in the procedure of penetrating keratoplasty (PKP), removes the diseased host corneal tissue and involves replacing it with the full-thickness donor tissue. Since the cornea is a multilayered structure, many pathologies only affect individual layers of the cornea, hence selective lamellar replacement of the diseased layers only while retaining the unaffected layers represents a new paradigm shift in the field.[3] For corneal pathologies in which the corneal endothelium is spared, Deep Anterior Lamellar Keratoplasty (DALK) may be the preferred approach. DALK is a partial-thickness corneal transplant where the host endothelial cell layer and Descemet's membrane (DM) complex are retained and the layers of the cornea anterior to that are replaced. Descemet's Membrane Endothelial Keratoplasty (DMEK) is a single-layer corneal transplant where the host endothelial layer and DM are replaced but all other corneal layers are retained. This is becoming the preferred approach for many surgeon's when dealing with pathologies affecting only the endothelium such as Fuchs corneal dystrophy. Descemet's stripping endothelial keratoplasty (DSEK) is similar to DMEK in that it is a partial-thickness corneal transplant. However, DSEK involves transplantation of donor endothelium, DM, and also some stromal tissue. Indications for DMEK and DSEK are similar, however, more surgeon's are preferring DMEK to approach pathologies isolated to the endothelial layer as it has shown to provide more rapid patient recovery.[4,5]

Advancements in surgical techniques and technology are allowing surgeon's to customize their approach while performing different forms of manual, microkeratome, and femtosecond laser–assisted corneal transplantation. The femtosecond laser has the ability to create accurate vertical, horizontal, and oblique incisions in the cornea with minimum collateral damage to adjacent corneal tissues and is now being used to do precise corneal trephination for donor and recipients.[6,7] FLAK can currently be used for PKP and DALK.

INDICATIONS

Key Indications

- Keratoconus
- Corneal scarring or opacification
- Previously failed PKP
- Pellucid marginal degeneration
- Corneal ectasia
- Various corneal dystrophies
- Chemical and mechanical trauma

The most common indication for PKP varies by region and is highly dependent on socioeconomic and geographical location. The leading etiologies of corneal blindness worldwide are primarily due to anterior corneal pathology with a normal endothelium, with the highest prevalence being in developing countries.[8]

Generally, indications for DALK can be considered for all corneal pathologies other than those affecting the corneal endothelium. The most common indication for DALK is likely keratoconus as these patients may benefit the most by retaining their own endothelium.[9] Thankfully, corneal collagen cross-linking has greatly limited the need for cornea transplantation due to keratoconus.

CONTRAINDICATIONS FOR PENETRATING KERATOPLASTY

Severe ocular surface disease with limbal stem cell deficiency is relative contraindications for a full-thickness corneal transplant as they may preclude to poor healing.[10] Examples include the following:

- Stevens–Johnson syndrome
- Advanced aniridia
- Ocular cicatricial pemphigoid
- Neurotrophic keratitis
- Chemical and thermal burns

The National Health Services Blood and Transplant Agency in the United Kingdom has the following absolute contraindications: transplant unlikely to restore corneal function or integrity or remove tissue that would otherwise have led to further damage to the eye.[11]

CONTRAINDICATIONS FOR DEEP ANTERIOR LAMELLAR KERATOPLASTY

Contraindications for DALK include all corneal pathologies in which the patient's corneal endothelium and/or DM are damaged or compromised. Bullous keratopathy is the major contraindication of DALK, which requires deeper corneal transplantation techniques.[10] Also, keratoconus patients with scars due to acute hydrops may not be good candidates for DALK since air may escape through the break in DM and prevent complete dissection.[8]

PREOPERATIVE PREPARATION FOR CORNEAL TRANSPLANT

A full ocular examination, complete with medical history, including current medication and allergies, is performed prior to the procedure. Since many of the patients undergoing corneal transplantation are older with other existing conditions, guidance should be given to them regarding their current medications before and following surgery. Health care providers may have protocols regarding different classes of medications and stopping/starting schedules for patients to follow.

Prior to corneal transplantation, more conservative treatments for vision rehabilitation should be exhausted, such as a change in glasses prescription, specialty contact lenses, and when indicated corneal cross-linking. The success rates for PKP and DALK are high compared to other organ transplants because of the low incidence of immunologic rejection.[7] Unfortunately, when rejection does occur, secondary procedures are inevitably less successful.[7] When comparing rejection rates of PKP and DALK, DALK has a lower rejection rate due to the host retaining the endothelial layer, which is a common site of rejection to occur.

Risks and benefits of the operation must be discussed in depth with each patient, as well as quality of life after surgery. Corneal transplantation requires lifelong follow-up appointments between the doctor and the patient, and success rates are highly dependent on the diligence of the patient to adhere to postoperative instructions given by the doctor.

If the indication for corneal transplantation is due to scarring from since fungi are microbes, could it be stated as bacterial, fungal, protozoan, or inflammatory etiologies time is needed to achieve a quiet eye prior to surgery. Often times, six months or up to a year may be needed to accomplish this. In patients with corneal neovascularization, time is also needed to quiet the eye as corneal vasculature drastically increases the levels of graft failure and rejection. If corneal transplantation is initiated too soon after suffering any of the etiologies stated previously, graft rejection and failure rates significantly increase. Often times, a long course of pharmaceutical therapies such as corticosteroids, antibiotics and immunomodulators are needed to prepare an eye for surgery.

It is of utmost importance to appropriately set patient expectations prior to corneal transplantation. Refractive error including astigmatism, myopia, and hyperopia following transplantation can at times be unpredictable as outcomes are dependent on individual patient healing. In the far majority of cases, after a successful corneal transplant, the patient will require vision correction in the form of glasses and/or specialty rigid contact lenses to achieve highest vision potential postoperatively.

PROCEDURE

The procedures for femtosecond laser PKP and DALK are similar except that the PKP is full thickness while the DALK spares the host DM and endothelium.

The first step for a PKP is preparing the donor graft with an artificial anterior chamber. Once that is completed, the donor cornea is placed underneath the femtosecond laser and the appropriate graft is cut (Figure 9.1). The donor graft is then dissected from the donor tissue and is set aside (Figure 9.2). If the procedure is a DALK, the donor endothelium is removed at this time. The host tissue is then cut by the femtosecond laser using a matching pattern (Figures 9.3 and 9.4). Some surgeon's may choose to have the donor tissue be 0.25 mm larger in diameter. The host tissue is then removed (Figures 9.5 and 9.6), and the donor tissue is put in its place (Figure 9.7). Sutures are then placed and the case is completed (Figures 9.8 and 9.9). The femtosecond laser allows the surgeon to create different trephination patterns in the host and donor corneal tissue. Traditionally, the most common pattern for manual PKP is a "top-hat." This pattern provides increased biomechanical stability and a strong resistance to leakage. With the femtosecond laser, more customizable trephination patterns can be achieved to create more surface area at the graft–host junction, thus, increasing the tensile strength and resulting in a faster recovery. Zigzag and Christmas tree shapes are examples of trephination patterns that allow for more surface area between the graft and the host, providing excellent safety, and may allow for earlier suture removal.

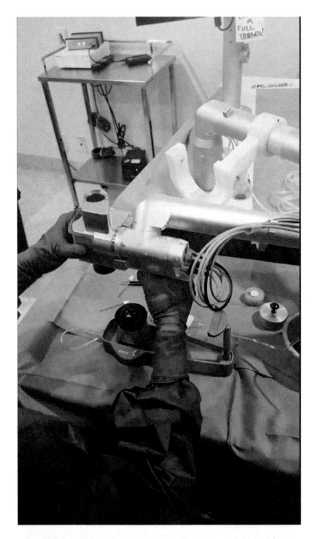

FIGURE 9-1 Preparing to place the femtosecond laser on the donor cornea in a DALK case. Image courtesy of Arturo S. Chayet and Denisse Pinkus.

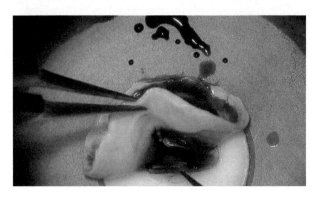

FIGURE 9-2 Dissection of the donor cornea. Image courtesy of Arturo S. Chayet and Denisse Pinkus.

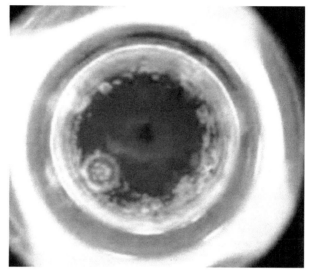

FIGURE 9-3 Host cornea under the femtosecond laser in a PKP case. Note the central "dot" for centration and the peripheral marks showing where the laser would cut. Image courtesy of Audrey Talley Rostov.
PKP, penetrating keratoplasty.

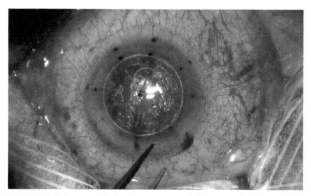

FIGURE 9-4 Image of the host cornea following the femtosecond laser procedure for a DALK. Image courtesy of Arturo S. Chayet and Denisse Pinkus.
DALK, Deep Anterior Lamellar Keratoplasty.

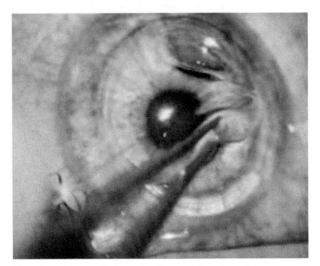

FIGURE 9-5 Removing the host cornea in a PKP. Image courtesy of Audrey Talley Rostov.
PKP, penetrating keratoplasty.

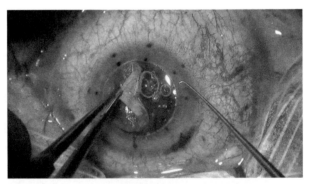

FIGURE 9-6 Dissection of the host cornea. Image courtesy of Arturo S. Chayet and Denisse Pinkus.

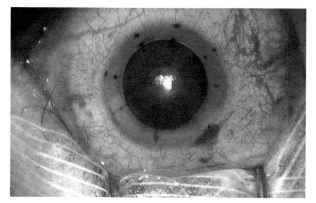

FIGURE 9-7 Image of the donor cornea on the host cornea. Note the precise match between the tissues. Image courtesy of Arturo S. Chayet and Denisse Pinkus.

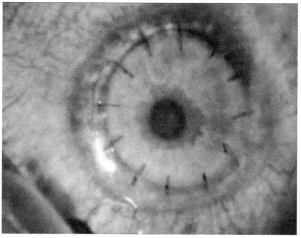

FIGURE 9-8 Completion of the full-thickness cornea transplant. Image courtesy of Audrey Talley Rostov.

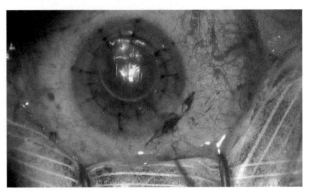

FIGURE 9-9 Completed femtosecond DALK procedure. Image courtesy of Arturo S. Chayet and Denisse Pinkus. DALK, Deep Anterior Lamellar Keratoplasty.

POSTOPERATIVE CARE/CO-MANAGEMENT (FOLLOW-UP SCHEDULE)

Postoperative care is extremely important and the most time-consuming part of the patient's journey through corneal transplant. Patients should be carefully followed for inflammation, infection, graft rejection, and suture-related complications. Postoperative follow-up schedules for PKP and DALK are very similar but may vary depending on surgeon's preference. Typically, the patient will be seen at one day, one week, and one-month postoperatively, and then every two to three months for up to a year.

Roughly 20% to 30% of patients with a full-thickness corneal transplant suffer a rejection episode within the first five years of the procedure, although the risk varies widely depending on the indication of the transplant. Urgent cases for a perforated ulcer are much more likely to have a rejection episode. Graft rejection occurs when the body's immune defenses recognize the donor tissue as foreign and attack it. Prophylactic treatment with topical corticosteroids is used to prevent graft rejection. For repeat transplants in which the previous donor graft was rejected or failed, or other high-risk cases, the surgeon may add oral corticosteroids temporarily in the postoperative regimen as well. Difluprednate ophthalmic emulsion 0.05% (Alcon) is the preferred steroid of many surgeon's as it is the most potent topical steroid available. Difluprednate 0.05% is dosed anywhere from four to eight times a day for two months with a slow taper depending on surgeon preference and individual patient case. Difluprednate 0.05% may also be switched to a less potent steroid during the course of the patient's follow-up appointments, such as prednisolone acetate 1% or loteprednol 0.5%. In some cases, the patient may be on low-dose steroid therapy indefinitely. The postoperative drops for DALK are identical, but the dosing regimen will vary patient to patient depending on the graft status.

It is well established that many patients are "steroid responders" in which intraocular pressure (IOP) can increase secondary to topical steroid therapy. It is imperative that the doctor or technician check the patient's IOP at every follow-up appointment after a corneal transplant to monitor for this. Should the patient get high IOP at any point in the course of their follow-up care, changing the topical steroid or initiating topical IOP-lowering medications can be used to combat this. Typically, IOP returns to normal as the steroid taper begins and/or the patient is switched over to a "soft" steroid.

Sutures are used in both PKP and DALK to hold the donor graft tissue in place postoperatively and to achieve a secure graft–host junction. Different suture techniques are used depending on surgeon's preference. The most common are monofilament nylon sutures. These sutures will be removed at the discretion of the surgeon once they feel the graft–host junction is secure. The sutures may be in place for up to a year prior to removal. The surgeon may utilize corneal topography to remove the sutures systematically, reducing corneal astigmatism. If the patient's vision is good, the sutures may remain permanently. The suture knots are usually buried within the incision, and the suture on the surface quickly heals over with epithelium, therefore the sutures do not cause discomfort or foreign body sensation. Loose or broken sutures can cause a foreign body sensation, inflammation, or an abscess, and so need to be monitored closely and if indicated, removed.

POTENTIAL COMPLICATIONS AND THEIR TREATMENT

Complications of Penetrating Keratoplasty

Graft rejection continues to be one of the most prevalent complications following a PKP. Rahman et al. performed a retrospective case study where they reviewed 203 manual PKPs from January 1, 2003 to December 31, 2003 at Manchester Royal Eye Hospital.[12] Graft rejection remained the most common complication of PKP at 21% (43 patients).[12] Other complications were graft failure 18% (36 patients), postkeratoplasty glaucoma (PKG) 18% (37 patients), and microbial keratitis 16% (8 patients).[12] Pramanik et al. in their retrospective, consecutive, noncomparative case series reported a graft failure rate of 6.3% at 20 years for manual PKP.[13]

The best management for graft rejection is to prevent it from occurring in the first place. Irreversible graft rejection is the main cause of graft failure in the intermediate and late postoperative period. Early detection of graft rejection is key in saving the transplanted cornea. Corticosteroid therapy, both topical and systemic, is the mainstay of management.[14] Difluprednate 0.05% is preferred due to its potency, but prednisolone acetate 1% is an alternative. Topical corticosteroids are dosed every 1 to 2 hours until improvement is seen. The corticosteroid dosing schedule is then reduced appropriately. After a rejection episode, topical corticosteroids are rarely discontinued altogether. Vigilant attention to IOP is needed following a corneal transplant as it is well known that topical corticosteroids can cause an IOP spike. Often times, the patient is switched to less potent or "soft" corticosteroids throughout their course of recovery to reduce the risk of IOP spikes. Insufficient control of IOP after a PKP is a significant cause of graft failure.[15]

PKG has been reported to be one of the most serious complications following PKP and the second leading cause of graft failure after graft rejection.[16,17] Diagnosis and management of PKG is more difficult to treat compared to a non-PKP glaucomatous eye.[18] First-line therapy for a post-PKP IOP spike is topical glaucoma drops as they are the least invasive. If topical therapy fails to control IOP, glaucoma surgery should be considered. Minimally invasive glaucoma surgeries may be indicated in less complex cases. Tube shunt and trabeculectomy may be required in complex eyes with difficult to control PKG.

Microbial infections are treated with topical antibiotics. Cultures may be taken to determine the infectious organism. Treatment should be initiated immediately with a broad-spectrum antibiotic. Newer generation fluoroquinolones are often preferred. Intracameral antibiotic injections may also be required. Corticosteroids may be added to reduce scarring if there is no or minimal epithelial defect present.

Complications of Deep Anterior Lamellar Keratoplasty

The most frequent complication of DALK that is performed manually or with femtosecond laser is perforation of DM and entering the anterior chamber from the stroma.[19] Tears or perforations of DM during DALK have been reported to occur in 10% to 30% of cases.[20] Noble et al.[21] found an incidence of DM perforation of 13.8% in their study during manual DALK (M-DALK). Other authors have reported variable rates of DM perforation. Gadhvi et al.[22] compared complications of M-DALK and femtosecond DALK (F-DALK). They found that perforation of DM during surgery occurred in 15/58 (25.9%) of F-DALK cases compared with 148/326 (45.4%) of M-DALK cases.[22] Repair of a tear or perforation of DM during surgery depends on the size of the tear. Most DM detachments can be managed by injecting air or an air–gas mixture (sulfur hexafluoride + air) into the anterior chamber which creates a tamponade to seal the defect in DM.[23,24] However, some patients may still require to be converted to PKP if repair efforts fail.

Graft rejection is significantly less common in DALK compared to PKP since with DALK the patient retains their own endothelium. However, since rejection can occur at any layer of the donor corneal graft, it is still a real concern. Graft rejection with DALK has been reported at rates as low as 5% to 8%.[25] Graft rejection in DALK is treated in the same manner as graft rejection in PKP (with topical and/or oral corticosteroids).

VIDEOS OF PROCEDURE

Video 9.1—This video shows the host cornea undergoing the femtosecond laser procedure followed by the removal of the host cornea and placement of the donor cornea. The donor cornea was also cut by the femtosecond laser. Note the host cornea has a center "dot" to ensure centration. Viscoelastic is placed in the anterior chamber and the host cornea is removed, and the new donor cornea is placed. Sixteen interrupted sutures are placed to secure the donor tissue. Video courtesy of Audrey Talley Rostov.

Video 9.2—This video shows the preparation and procedure of an F-DALK in a patient with previous radial keratotomy (RK) surgery. Video courtesy of Arturo S. Chayet and Denisse Pinkus.

EFFICACY—STUDY DATA

Femtosecond Laser–Assisted Deep Anterior Lamellar Keratoplasty

Using a femtosecond laser over current manual trephination techniques has many advantages in corneal transplantation. Both PKP and DALK can be performed using femtosecond laser.[26] Femtosecond laser has the capabilities of performing accurate and precise tissue ablation in the form of different patterns in both the recipient and donor corneal tissue. More accurate alignment of the graft–host junction reduces postoperative astigmatism and allows better healing. Creating a pattern trephination with the femtosecond laser increases graft–host interface surface area, therefore increasing the strength of the graft–host junction and decreasing the risk for graft dehiscence.[27] While microkeratome-assisted lamellar keratoplasty helps in dissection of predetermined depth, FLAK, when combined with intraoperative optical coherence tomography, allows for a more accurate consideration of the depth of opacity and preparation of corneal grafts.[28]

Gadhvi et al.[22] compared the outcomes of 58 eyes that underwent F-DALK for keratoconus to 326 eyes that underwent M-DALK at Moorfields Eye Hospital London. The F-DALK cases were performed from August 1, 2015 to September 1, 2018, and big-bubble M-DALK from September 1, 2012 to September 31, 2016. Perforation of DM during surgery occurred in 15/58 (25.9%) of F-DALK cases compared with 148/326 (45.4%) of M-DALK cases. Conversion to PKP intraoperatively was carried out in 2/58 (3.4%) of F-DALK cases compared with 80/326 (24.5%) of M-DALK cases. In the F-DALK group, 86.5% of eyes had a best-corrected visual acuity (BCVA) of 20/40 or more (15 ± 7.3 months after surgery) compared with 83.7% of M-DALK eyes (24.9 ± 10.6 months after surgery). The investigators concluded that laser automation of some steps in DALK for keratoconus may reduce the rate of intraoperative DM perforation and conversion to PKP, in a multi-surgeon setting.

Yoo et al. performed F-DALK in 12 eyes with anterior stromal scarring. They found that femtosecond laser–assisted sutureless anterior lamellar keratoplasty could improve uncorrected visual acuity (UCVA) and BCVA in patients with anterior corneal pathology. Also, of important note, is that there were no intraoperative complications. UCVA was improved in 7 eyes (58%) compared with preoperative visual acuity. The mean difference between preoperative and postoperative UCVA was a gain of 2.5 lines (range, unchanged–7 lines). BCVA was unchanged or improved in all eyes compared with preoperative levels. The mean difference between preoperative and postoperative BCVAs was a gain of 3.8 lines (range, unchanged–8 lines). In 2 eyes, additional surgical procedures were performed (one treated with phototherapeutic keratectomy and the other with photorefractive keratectomy).

Femtosecond Laser–Assisted Penetrating Keratoplasty

Farid et al.[29] compared 49 eyes of 43 patients that underwent femtosecond laser zigzag incision pattern PKP versus 17 eyes of 14 patients that underwent conventional Barron suction trephination PKP. They measured topographically determined astigmatism, best-corrected spectacle visual acuity (BCSVA), and recovery of full visual potential. They found a significant difference in astigmatism between the two groups and postoperative months 1 and 3. By month 3, the average astigmatism was 3 diopters in the zigzag group compared to 4.46 diopters in the conventional group. In patients with normal macular and optic nerve function, they found a significant difference in BCSVA at one month and three months. Eighty-one percent of the of zigzag group achieved BCSVA of 20/40 or more by three months compared to 45% of the conventional group. This study shows that the femtosecond laser generated zigzag-shaped incision resulted in faster recovery postoperatively while inducing less corneal astigmatism compared to the conventional blade trephination PKP group.

Chamberlain et al.[30] performed a similar retrospective, comparative surgical series study. Fifty patients were designated to the FLAK group receiving full-thickness corneal transplant with the femtosecond laser, and 50 patients were in the conventional PKP group. Outcome measures involved looking at topographic astigmatism, BCSVA, UCVA, pinhole visual acuity, and timing of selective suture removal, or adjustment over follow-up during a period of two years. They found that the FLAK group had significant improvement in astigmatism before but not after the six-month postoperative follow-up period. Earlier suture removal was seen in the FLAK group. No significant improvement in BCSVA was noted at any time point. There were no complications or difficulties with trephination in the FLAK procedure across a wide range of corneal pathologies.

While both manual and femtosecond techniques are used at this time, femtosecond laser may become the preferred method for corneal transplantation in the future. More research will be needed for surgeon's to fully adopt this technology in treating their patients. However, the femtosecond laser is allowing more customized transplantation techniques, which may ultimately lead to better postoperative visual outcomes for patients undergoing corneal transplantation.

CODING/BILLING MODIFIERS

A major barrier to FLAK is the cost of the femtosecond laser. The laser is expensive to acquire, and there are ongoing costs with maintenance and click fees for each cut the laser makes. For keratoplasty, you need to make a cut on the donor and also the host. As of today, insurance does not cover the use of a laser for keratoplasty.

REFERENCES

1. Flaxman SR, Bourne RRA, Resnikoff S, et al. Vision loss expert group of the global burden of disease study. Global causes of blindness and distance vision impairment 1990–2020: A systematic review and meta-analysis. *Lancet Glob Health.* 2017 Dec;5(12):e1221–e1234.

2. Crawford AZ, Patel DV, McGhee CNj. A brief history of corneal transplantation: From ancient to modern. *Oman J Ophthalmol.* 2013;6(Suppl 1):S12–S17. doi: 10.4103/0974-620X.122289.

3. Steinert RF, Ignacio TS, Sarayba MA. "Top hat"-shaped penetrating keratoplasty using the femtosecond laser. *Am J Ophthalmol.* 2007;143:689–691.

4. Lin SR, Prapaipanich P, Yu F, et al. Comparison of endothelial keratoplasty techniques in patients with prior glaucoma surgery: A case-matched study. *Am J Ophthalmol.* 2019;206:94–101. doi: 10.1016/j.ajo.2019.03.020.

5. Li S, Liu L, Wang W, et al. Efficacy and safety of Descemet's membrane endothelial keratoplasty versus Descemet's stripping endothelial keratoplasty: A systematic review and meta-analysis. *PLoS One.* December 18, 2017;12(12):e0182275. doi: 10.1371/journal.pone.0182275.

6. Mehta JS, Parthasarthy A, Por YM, Cajucom-Uy H, Beuerman RW, Tan D. Femtosecond laser-assisted endothelial keratoplasty: A laboratory model. *Cornea.* 2008;27:706.

7. Tan DT, Anshu A, Mehta JS. Paradigm shifts in corneal transplantation. *Ann Acad Med Singapore.* 2009;38(4):332–338.

8. Mathews PM, Lindsley K, Aldave AJ, Akpek EK. Etiology of global corneal blindness and current practices of corneal transplantation: A focused review. *Cornea.* 2018;37(9):1198–1203. doi: 10.1097/ICO.0000000000001666.

9. Shimmura S. Component surgery of the cornea. *Cornea.* 2004;23(8 Suppl):S31–S35. doi: 10.1097/01.ico.0000136669.05036.d8.

10. Nassiri N, Djalilian AR. Keratoplasty: Moving to the front. *J Ophthalmic Vis Res.* 2009;4(1):5–7.

11. Maghsoudlou P, Sood G, Akhondi H. Cornea transplantation. [Updated 2020 Jul 7]. In: StatPearls [Internet]. Treasure Island, FL: StatPearls Publishing; 2020 Jan. Available at: https://www.ncbi.nlm.nih.gov/books/NBK539690/

12. Rahman I, Carley F, Hillarby C, Brahma A, Tullo AB. Penetrating keratoplasty: Indications, outcomes, and complications. *Eye.* 2009;23:1288–1294.

13. Pramanik S, Musch DC, Sutphin JE, Farjo AA. Extended long-term outcomes of penetrating keratoplasty for keratoconus. *Ophthalmology.* 2006;113(9):1633–1638. doi: 10.1016/j.ophtha.2006.02.058.

14. Panda A, Vanathi M, Kumar A, Dash Y, Priya S. Corneal graft rejection. *Surv Ophthalmol.* 2007;52(4):375–396. doi: 10.1016/j.survophthal.2007.04.008.

15. Schanzlin DJ, Robin JB, Gomez DS. Results of penetrating keratoplasty for aphakic and pseudophakic bullous keratopathy. *Am J Ophthalmol.* 1984;98(3):302–312.

16. Ing JJ, Ing HH, Nelson LR, Hodge DO, Bourne WM. Ten-year postoperative results of penetrating keratoplasty. *Ophthalmology.* 1998;105(10):1855–1865.

17. Thompson RW Jr, Price MO, Bowers PJ, Price FW Jr. Long-term graft survival after penetrating keratoplasty. *Ophthalmology.* 2003;110(7):1396–1402. doi: 10.1016/S0161-6420(03)00463-9.

18. Karadag O, Kugu S, Erdogan G, Kandemir B, Eraslan Ozdil S, Dogan OK. Incidence of and risk factors for increased intraocular pressure after penetrating keratoplasty. *Cornea.* 2010;29(3):278–282.

19. Vishak J, Goins KM, Afshari NA. Deep anterior lamellar keratoplasty. *EyeNet Magazine.* September 2007. Retrieved from https://www.aao.org/eyenet/article/deep-anterior-lamellar-keratoplasty.

20. Trimarchi F, Poppi E, Klersy C, Piacentini C. et al. Deep anterior lamellar keratoplasty. *Ophthalmologica.* 2001;215:389–393.

21. Noble BA, Agrawal A, Collins C, Saldana M, Brogden PR, Zuberbuhler B. Deep Anterior Lamellar Keratoplasty (DALK): Visual outcome and complications for a heterogeneous group of corneal pathologies. *Cornea.* 2007;26(1):59–64.

22. Gadhvi KA, Romano V, Fernández-Vega Cueto L, et al. Femtosecond laser assisted deep anterior lamellar keratoplasty for keratoconus: Multi-surgeon results. *Am J Ophthalmol.* July 21, 2020;220:191–202.

23. Anwar M, Teichmann KD. Deep lamellar keratoplasty: Surgical techniques for anterior lamellar keratoplasty with and without baring of Descemet's membrane. *Cornea.* 2002; 21(4):374–383. doi: 10.1097/00003226-200205000-00009. PMID: 11973386.

24. Shimmura S, Tsubota K. Deep anterior lamellar keratoplasty. *Curr Opin Ophthalmol.* 2006; 17:349–355.
25. Watson SL, Ramsay A, Dart JK, Bunce C, Craig E. Comparison of deep lamellar keratoplasty and penetrating keratoplasty in patients with keratoconus. *Ophthalmology.* 2004;111(9):1676–1682.
26. Farid M, Steinert RF. Deep anterior lamellar keratoplasty performed with the femtosecond laser zigzag incision for the treatment of stromal corneal pathology and ectatic disease. *J Cataract Refract Surg.* 2009;35(5):809–813.
27. Yoo SH, Kymionis GD, Koreishi A, et al. Femtosecond laser-assisted sutureless anterior lamellar keratoplasty. *Ophthalmology.* 2008;115(8):1303–1307, 1307.e1.
28. Wirbelauer C, Winkler J, Bastian GO, Häberle H, Pham DT. Histopathological correlation of corneal diseases with optical coherence tomography. *Graefes Arch Clin Exp Ophthalmol.* 2002;240(9):727–734.
29. Farid M, Steinert RF, Gaster RN, Chamberlain W, Lin A. Comparison of penetrating keratoplasty performed with a femtosecond laser zig-zag incision versus conventional blade trephination. *Ophthalmology.* 2009;116(9):1638–1643. doi: 10.1016/j.ophtha.2009.05.003.
30. Chamberlain WD, Rush SW, Mathers WD, Cabezas M, Fraunfelder FW. Comparison of femtosecond laser–assisted keratoplasty versus conventional penetrating keratoplasty. *Ophthalmology.* 2011;118(3):486–491. doi: 10.1016/j.ophtha.2010.08.002.

SUPPLEMENTAL READINGS

van Dijk et al.[A] used the femtosecond laser to transplant isolated Bowman's layer to reduce and stabilize the cornea in patients with progressive advanced keratoconus. In their prospective, nonrandomized cohort study, 22 eyes of 19 patients that were not eligible for corneal collagen cross-linking underwent Bowman's layer corneal transplantation. The study showed that with isolated Bowman layer transplantation, they achieved reduction and stabilization of corneal ectasia in eyes with progressive, advanced keratoconus with a low incidence of complications.

Parker et al.[B] also demonstrated Bowman's layer corneal transplantation as an alternative treatment for reversing corneal ectasia in eyes with advanced keratoconus. This surgical technique may allow patients to get back to wearing their contact lenses with improved comfort and delaying or avoiding PKP or DALK.

REFERENCES FOR SUPPLEMENTAL READINGS

A. van Dijk K, Liarakos VS, Parker J, et al. Bowman layer transplantation to reduce and stabilize progressive, advanced keratoconus. *Ophthalmology.* 2015;122:909–917 doi:10.1016/j.ophtha.2014.12.005.
B. Parker JS, van Dijk K, Melles GR. Treatment options for advanced keratoconus: A review. *Surv Ophthalmol.* 2015;60:459–480. doi: 10.1016/j.survophthal.2015.02.004. Epub 2015 Mar 5. PMID: 26077628.

Corneal Cross-Linking

Y. Ralph Chu • Jessica Heckman

Corneal ectasia is the progressive steepening and thinning of the cornea that can occur naturally or be induced surgically. A patient with corneal ectasia will often experience an increase in ocular aberrations and decreased best corrected visual acuity (BCVA). Due to these aberrations and loss of BCVA, these patients report varying degrees of visual symptoms including glare, halo, multiple images, and ghosting. A patient with corneal ectasia may need to wear gas permeable or other specialty contact lenses to obtain their best visual acuity due to the corneal irregularity. Often glasses are not able to fully correct a patient with corneal ectasia.

Various forms of ectasia exist including keratoconus, pellucid marginal degeneration, wound ectasia after penetrating keratoplasty (PK), and keratoglobus. The reported incidence and prevalence rates reported for keratoconus tend to vary widely from an incidence as high as 1 in 400, to a long-term study in the United States reporting 54.5 per 100,000.[1,2] It has been generally considered to occur equally in men and women; however, more recent studies have shown an increased risk of development of keratoconus in men, African-Americans, and Latinos and lower risk in women, Asian-Americans, and people with diabetes.[1] Keratoconus can begin before puberty and may continue to progress even after the age of 40. The weakening and degradation of the corneal collagen results in the progressive thinning and steepening observed in eyes with keratoconus.[3]

Corneal ectasia can also occur after laser-assisted keratomileusis (LASIK), small incision lenticule extraction, and photorefractive keratectomy. Risk factors for corneal ectasia include high preoperative myopia, thin residual stromal bed, high total percentage of tissue altered, and forme fruste keratoconus on preoperative topography.[4] Corneal ectasia can develop in a normal appearing cornea preoperatively.[5] Similar to keratoconus, in corneal ectasia following corneal refractive surgery, there is a suspected weakening and degradation of the corneal collagen resulting in biomechanical instability of the cornea in the residual stromal bed.[6,7]

In April 2016, the Food and Drug Administration (FDA)-approved corneal cross-linking for progressive keratoconus and corneal ectasia following refractive surgery. Corneal cross-linking is performed to slow or halt the progression of keratoconus and corneal ectasia by increasing the biomechanical rigidity of the cornea. It is thought to achieve this by replicating the age-related cross-linking that occurs in the cornea naturally with time.[8] The procedure is performed using ultraviolet-A (UV-A) light

165

and topical riboflavin as a photosensitizing agent to result in local photopolymerization.[9] Different from other corneal ectasia surgical treatments (intrastromal corneal ring segments and PK), this procedure can be performed in earlier stages of disease progression to prevent further vision loss from progressive corneal ectasia.

INDICATIONS

Key Indications

- Progressive keratoconus
- Corneal ectasia following refractive surgery

Corneal cross-linking is indicated for progressive keratoconus and corneal ectasia following refractive surgery. The definition of progression is at the discretion of the physician. There are many factors that have been evaluated as progressive determinants for keratoconus and ectasia following refractive surgery including topometric, pachymetry, and refractive changes.[10] Topometric changes indicative for progression include an increasing maximum keratometry and/or steepening of the anterior or posterior corneal surface.[11,12] Thinning pachymetry, as well as an increase in the rate of corneal thickness change from the periphery to the thinnest point of the cornea are also considerations for progression.[11,12] Insurance carriers often require documentation of specific criteria.[13,14]

These criteria may include the following:

- An increase of greater than or equal to 1 diopter of steepest keratometry value within 24 months
- An increase of greater than or equal to 1 diopter of cylinder in subjective refraction within 24 months
- A decrease of greater than or equal to 0.1 mm in back optical zone radius (base curve) in rigid gas permeable contact lens wearer within 24 months
- Progressive deterioration of best spectacle corrected visual acuity.

CONTRAINDICATIONS

Key Contraindications

- Pregnant and nursing mothers
- Age consideration
- History of herpes simplex keratitis
- Thin cornea

The safety and efficacy of corneal cross-linking has not been evaluated during pregnancy or in nursing mothers. There is no contraindication to operation of the device by pregnant operators.

While there is no specific age range in the indication statement for corneal cross-linking, the United States clinical trials that led to FDA approval included only patients aged 14–65.[15,16] If the procedure is being submitted to a patient's insurance, this may play a role in coverage determination for the patient if outside this age range.

Exposure to UV light may cause reactivation of herpes simplex virus keratitis.[17] Due to this, caution should be exercised in patients with history of prior herpes simplex virus keratitis.

To prevent endothelial cell damage, the last contraindication to corneal cross-linking is corneal stromal thickness below 400 microns at the time of UV light exposure. Hypotonic riboflavin may be used to thicken a cornea to or above the 400-micron threshold at the time of the procedure.[15,16]

The last relative contraindication is a patient's ability to tolerate the procedure and comply with procedure instructions. The patient does need to maintain fixation underneath the UV light for 30 minutes. A patient who is unable to remain in the proper position for this duration of time, or if there are concerns regarding a patient's ability to follow and comply with procedure or postoperative instructions, may not be an ideal candidate for this procedure.

INFORMED CONSENT CONSIDERATIONS

Key Informed Consent Adverse Events Listed

- Blurred vision
- Eye pain
- Dry eye
- Corneal opacity (haze)
- Corneal edema
- Slowly healing cornea/persistent epithelial defect
- Light sensitivity/photophobia
- Corneal infection/infectious keratitis
- Ineffectiveness of the procedure

Informed consent should include a description of the procedure in plain language, for example, "The very superficial layer of the cornea will be temporarily removed, and eye drops along with UV light will be used over the course of one hour to strengthen the cornea."

Potential alternative treatments, such as continuing to wear eyeglasses and/or contact lenses, monitoring, other corneal surgeries including corneal transplant penetrating keratoplasty (PKP), Intacs, among others, should be listed. Risks and complications, inherent to the procedure, include but are not limited to blurred vision, eye pain, dry eye, corneal haze or edema, a slowly healing cornea following the procedure, light sensitivity, and corneal infection, as well as ineffectiveness of the procedure.

The patient should sign and date the consent to indicate their understanding of the procedure and acceptance of risks.

PREOPERATIVE CARE

Key Preoperative Considerations

- Full corneal assessment
- Management of ocular surface disease
- Patient education

A full examination of ocular and specifically corneal health including but not limited to topography, pachymetry, and ocular surface assessment is done on the preoperative exam evaluating for any potential contraindications as well as assessing for signs of progressive corneal disease.[17] It is often beneficial, if appropriate for the patient situation, to obtain corneal measurements out of contact lenses. If the patient is new to the physician and is determined to have keratoconus or corneal ectasia, it may be necessary to obtain old examination records to assist in determination of progression.

Dry eye, epithelial defects, and punctate keratitis are known potential postoperative complications of the corneal cross-linking procedure.[15,16] Secondary to this, careful evaluation of the ocular surface preoperatively is important as well as consideration of the need for any ocular surface treatment prior to undergoing the corneal cross-linking procedure.

Lastly, proper patient education regarding expectations of the procedure, postoperative healing, and goals of the procedure is important for these patients. Often other anterior segment procedures, such as laser vision correction, cataract surgery, etc., result in relatively quick visual recovery and significant improvement in visual function. An emphasis with patient education is stabilization of the existing disease versus resolution of visual blur.

SETTINGS AND PROCEDURE

Medications and Devices for the Procedure

- Topical anesthetic
- PHOTREXA VISCOUS (riboflavin 5′-phosphate in 20% dextran ophthalmic solution) 0.146% for topical ophthalmic use
- PHOTREXA (riboflavin 5′-phosphate ophthalmic solution) 0.146% for topical ophthalmic use

- KXL system (Figures 10.1 and 10.2)
- Ultrasound pachymetry

The FDA-approved (Dresden protocol) corneal cross-linking procedure is a 60-minute monocular treatment.

Topical anesthetic is used to anesthetize the cornea of the procedure eye. After the patient is anesthetized, the epithelium is debrided using standard aseptic technique. Once the epithelium is removed, one drop of PHOTREXA VISCOUS is instilled topically on the eye every 2 minutes for 30 minutes (Figure 10.3). After 30 minutes, it is important the eye is examined with a slit lamp to confirm the presence of a yellow

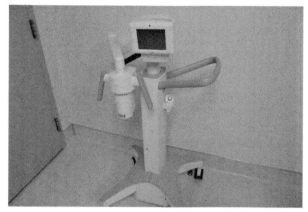

FIGURE 10-1 The KXL system has a touch screen for planning patient treatment, a moveable arm for aligning the UV irradiation, and handheld surgeon control.

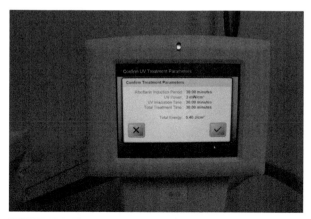

FIGURE 10-2 The KXL system touch screen shows treatment parameters of UV power, irradiation time, and total energy. UV, ultraviolet.

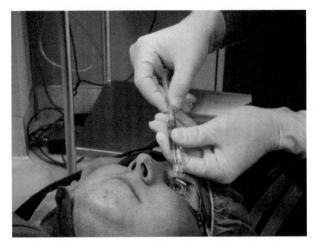

FIGURE 10-3 PHOTREXA VISCOUS (riboflavin 5′-phosphate in 20% dextran ophthalmic solution) 0.146% for topical ophthalmic use is instilled in the patient's eye at a rate of one drop every 2 minutes for 30 minutes prior to and during ultraviolet irradiation.

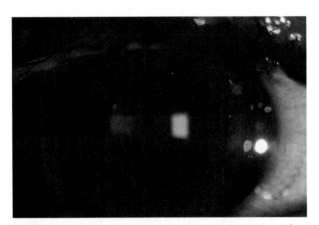

FIGURE 10-4 The eye is examined with a slit lamp to confirm the presence of yellow flare in the anterior chamber. Photo courtesy of Clark Y. Chang, OD, MS, FAAO.

flare in the anterior chamber (Figure 10.4). If flare is not present, PHOTREXA VISCOUS should be instilled at a rate of 1 drop every 2 minutes for an additional 2 to 3 drops. After these additional drops, the eye is again examined with a slit lamp to confirm the presence of yellow flare. This process can be repeated as necessary until yellow flare is confirmed in the anterior chamber.

Ultrasound pachymetry is performed once yellow flare is observed in the anterior chamber to confirm the corneal thickness is at a minimum of 400 microns

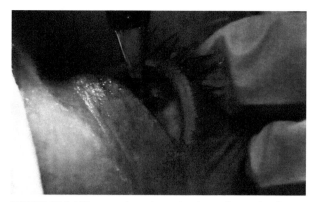

FIGURE 10-5 Ultrasound pachymetry is performed prior to irradiation to confirm 400-micron corneal thickness.

(Figure 10.5). If the corneal thickness is less than 400 microns, 2 drops of PHO-TREXA should be instilled every 5 to 10 seconds until the corneal thickness increases to at least 400 microns. It is a contraindication to irradiate the cornea unless this 400-micron threshold thickness is met and yellow flare is seen.

Once each yellow flare is visualized and the corneal stromal thickness has met the threshold of 400-micron thickness, the eye is irradiated using the KXL system. The KXL system delivers a metered dose of 365 nm UV-A light, exposure at 3 mW/cm^2 irradiance (Figure 10.6). During the irradiation, the instillation of PHOTREXA VISCOUS is continued at a rate of one drop every 2 minutes for the 30-minute irradiation period. This treatment results in a total treatment dose of 5.4 J/cm^2.

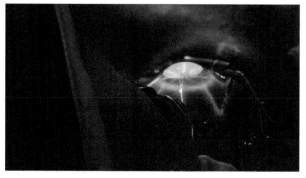

FIGURE 10-6 Corneal irradiation is performed for 30 minutes after the presence of yellow flare is confirmed in the anterior chamber and the cornea is a minimum of 400-microns thick.

A bandage contact lens (BCL) is placed on the eye for patient comfort at the end of the procedure.

Performing corneal cross-linking without removing the epithelium (epithelium-on procedure) is not currently FDA approved, thus considered an off-label use of the technology. Several studies have shown good safety with this technique and variable efficacy.[18,19,20]

POSTOPERATIVE CARE/CO-MANAGEMENT (FOLLOW-UP SCHEDULE)

Key Postoperative Considerations

- Postoperative drops: antibiotic, steroid, nonsteroidal anti-inflammatory.
- Return to contact lenses at one month.
- Monitor corneal topography.

Postoperatively, a topical antibiotic and steroid taper are prescribed. Often a nonsteroidal anti-inflammatory is prescribed for the first few days after the procedure to help with pain control. Preservative-free artificial tears are often encouraged for use to assist with comfort.

A typical postoperative follow-up schedule entails an exam at postoperative day 1, day 4 to 7, 1 month, 3 months, and 6 to 12 months. At the postoperative day-1 exam, it is expected for the patient to experience blurred vision and discomfort. At this exam, the eye is evaluated for signs of normal healing, and the bandage contact lens is assessed to ensure it is present and well positioned. At postoperative day 4 to 7, the corneal epithelium is monitored for closure. The BCL is removed once the epithelium is closed.

At the 1-month postoperative exam, visual acuity and refraction are able to be assessed more accurately. Slit lamp examination is done to confirm the healing process. Corneal haze and/or a demarcation line may be expected at this time point[15,16] (Figure 10.7). Corneal topography may appear to look worse relative to baseline. At this point, the patient may return to contact lens wear.

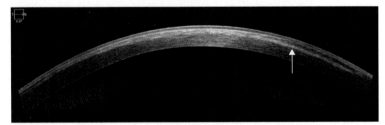

FIGURE 10-7 A demarcation line is often visible at the 1-month postoperative examination. OCT can be used to image and measure treatment depth. OCT, optical coherence tomography.

Corneal haze is often resolved or near resolution at the three-month postoperative exam. Visual acuity and refraction are assessed. A patient may need a contact lens refit if significant change to corneal topography and/or refraction is seen.

Corneal topography is used to monitor these patients every 6 to 12 months for stability.

POTENTIAL COMPLICATIONS AND THEIR TREATMENT

Key Potential Complications

- Corneal opacity (haze)
- Punctate keratitis
- Corneal striae
- Persistent epithelial defect
- Eye pain
- Dry eye
- Reduced visual acuity
- Photophobia
- Infectious keratitis
- Corneal edema

The most common ocular adverse reactions occurring in patients who underwent corneal cross-linking for progressive keratoconus in the phase III clinical trial were corneal opacity (haze), punctate keratitis, corneal striae, corneal epithelial defect, eye pain, reduced visual acuity, and blurred vision.[15] The most common ocular adverse reactions occurring in patients who underwent corneal cross-linking for corneal ectasia in the phase III clinical trial were corneal opacity (haze), corneal epithelial defect, corneal striae, dry eye, eye pain, punctate keratitis, reduced visual acuity, and blurred vision.[16] In these clinical trials, most of the reported adverse events resolved within the first month. However, persistent epithelial defects, corneal striae, punctate keratitis, photophobia, dry eye, eye pain, and decreased visual acuity took up to six months to resolve in some instances. There are no contraindicated ocular surface treatments after corneal cross-linking. The patient may be managed with the appropriate ocular surface treatment for the clinical presentation. Corneal opacity or haze took up to 12 months to resolve with non-resolution in some patients at the conclusion of the studies. It has been suggested that many of these complications are the result of the removal of or damage to the epithelium of the cornea.[21,22] A patient with preexisting ocular surface disease may benefit from treatment of the ocular surface prior to proceeding with corneal cross-linking. Corneal edema is likely caused by endothelial cell damage, and the risk of this complication is minimized by ensuring 400-micron minimum corneal thickness at the time of the procedure. Typically, corneal edema will resolve with a postoperative course of topical corticosteroid if sufficient endothelial cell function exists.

VIDEO OF PROCEDURE

Video 10.1—This corneal cross-linking procedure is performed following the FDA-approved Dresden protocol with the Avedro KXL system. This treatment begins with the removal of the epithelium. Then PHOTREXA VISCOUS is instilled at a rate of one drop every 2 minutes for 30 minutes. After a confirmed pachymetry of 400 microns, the cornea is irradiated for 30 minutes along with continued PHOTREXA VISCOUS instillation at the same rate of 1 drop every 2 minutes for the duration of the irradiation. A bandage contact lens is placed after completion of the procedure for patient comfort.

EFFICACY

The goal of corneal cross-linking is to stabilize the progression of keratoconus and corneal ectasia. The data that supported the FDA approval from the phase III clinical trials of corneal cross-linking for progressive keratoconus and ectasia showed this to be an effective treatment.

The phase III study of corneal collagen cross-linking for progressive keratoconus included 205 participants in multiple centers across the United States. Patients were placed into a treatment group or sham treatment group. The maximum keratometry value in the treatment group decreased by 1.6 diopters from baseline at the 1-year postoperative time. Eyes with keratoconus in the control group continued to progress. Additionally, in 31.4% of patients receiving the cross-linking treatment, the maximum keratometry decreased by 2.0 diopters or more and 24% of patients in the treatment group gained 2 lines or more of best corrected distance visual acuity.[14]

The phase III clinical trial for corneal collagen cross-linking for corneal ectasia included 179 participants across multiple centers in the United States. Similar to the progressive keratoconus phase III clinical trial, patients who received the corneal cross-linking treatment showed a decrease of the maximum keratometry value over the course of a year. On average, the maximum keratometry value decreased by 0.7 diopter in the treatment group while there was continued progression of the control group. Most patients in the treatment group also gained best corrected distance visual acuity.[17]

Additionally, since the introduction of corneal cross-linking, the number of penetrating keratoplasties for keratoconus has reduced.[23,24] This further supports the effectiveness of corneal cross-linking as well as advances in contact lens technology.[20,21]

CODING/BILLING AND MODIFIERS

Since FDA approval of corneal cross-linking in April of 2016, the procedure has been billed with a Category III code 0402T: collagen cross-linking of cornea (including removal of the corneal epithelium and intraoperative pachymetry when performed).

As of January 2019, the appropriate Healthcare Common Procedure Coding System (HCPCS) code is J2787 Riboflavin 5′-Phosphate, ophthalmic solution, up to 3 mL. Since the procedure requires the use of 6 mL of solution, 2 units are submitted. The National Drug Code (NDC) number and description for the PHOTREXA cross-linking kit are NDC 25357-025-03 PHOTREXA cross-linking kit. For payers that require an 11-digit NDC, a zero is added to the NDC: 25357-0025-03. There is no global period for corneal cross-linking, so a provider may bill each postoperative examination. Generally, insurance does not cover non-FDA–approved procedures and many insurance policies have detail regarding epithelium-off corneal cross-linking as the only FDA-approved treatment for progressive keratoconus.[13]

REFERENCES

1. Woodward MA, Blachley TS, Stein JD. The association between sociodemographic factors, common systemic diseases, and keratoconus: An analysis of a nationwide health care claims database. *Ophthalmology*. 2016;123:457–465. http://www.ncbi.nlm.nih.gov/pubmed/26707415.
2. Kennedy RH, Bourne WM, Dyer JA. A 48-year clinical and epidemiologic study of keratoconus. *Am J Ophthalmol*. 1986;101:267–273.
3. Gefen A, Shalom R, Elad D, Mandel Y. Biomechanical analysis of the keratoconic cornea. *J Mech Behav Biomed Mater*. 2009;2:224–236.
4. Randleman JB, Russell B, Ward MA, et al. Risk factors and prognosis for cornea ectasia after LASIK. *Ophthalmology*. 2003;110:267–275.
5. Klein SR, Epstein RJ, Randleman JB, Stulting RD. Corneal ectasia after laser in situ keratomileusis in patients without apparent preoperative risk factors. *Cornea*. 2006;25:388–403.
6. Meek KM, Tuft SJ, Huang Y, et al. Changes in collagen orientation and distribution in keratoconus corneas. *Invest Ophthalmol Vis Sci*. 2005;46:1948–1956.
7. Dawson DG, Randleman JB, Grossniklaus HE, et al. Corneal ectasia after excimer laser keratorefractive surgery: Histopathology, ultrastructure, and pathophysiology. *Ophthalmology*. 2008;115:2181–2191.
8. Cartwright NEK, Tyrer JR, Marshall J. Age-related differences in the elasticity of the human cornea. *Invest Ophthalmol Vis Sci*. 2011;52:4324–4329.
9. Klyce SD. UVA-riboflavin collagen cross-linking: A misnomer perhaps, but it works! *Invest Ophthalmol Vis Sci*. 2013;54(3):1635.
10. Gomes JA, Tan D, Rapuano CJ, et al. Global consensus on keratoconus and ecstatic diseases. *Cornea*. 2015;34(4):359–369.
11. Belin MW, Meyer JJ, Duncan JK, Gelman R, Borgstrom M, Ambrosio R. Assessing progression of keratoconus & crosslinking efficacy: The Belin ABCD progression display. *Int J Kerat Ect Cor Dis*. 2017;6(1):1–10.
12. Duncan JK, Belin MW, Borgstrom M. Assessing progression of keratoconus: Novel tomographic determinants. *Eye Vis*. 2016;3:6.
13. Is Cross-Linking Covered by Insurance? 2020. Retrieved September 6, 2020, from https://www.livingwithkeratoconus.com/is-cross-linking-right-for-me/is-cross-linking-covered-by-insurance/.
14. Fact Sheet for Coding Corneal Collagen Cross-Linking. January 24, 2019. Retrieved September 6, 2020, from https://www.aao.org/practice-management/news-detail/fact-sheet-coding-corneal-collagen-cross-linking/.
15. Hersh PS, Stulting RD, Muller D, Durrie DS, Rajpal RK, United States Crosslinking Study G. United States multicenter clinical trial of corneal collagen crosslinking for keratoconus treatment. *Ophthalmology*. 2017;124(9):1259–1270.
16. Hersh PS, Stulting RD, Muller D, Durrie DS, Rajpal RK, Group USCS. U.S. multicenter clinical trial of corneal collagen crosslinking for treatment of corneal ectasia after refractive surgery. *Ophthalmology*. 2017;124(10):1475–1484.

17. Garcia-Ferrer FJ, Akpek EK, Amescua G, et al. November 13, 2018. Corneal Ectasia PPP – 2018. Retrieved September 6, 2020, from https://www.aao.org/preferred-practice-pattern/corneal-ectasia-ppp-2018/.
18. Lombardo M, Serrao S, Raffa P, Rosati M, Lombardo G. Novel technique of transepithelial corneal cross-linking using iontophoresis in progressive keratoconus. *J Ophthalmol.* 2016;2016:7472542. doi: 10.1155/2016/7472542.
19. Khairy HA, Marey HM, Ellakwa AF. Epithelium-on corneal cross-linking treatment of progressive keratoconus: A prospective, consecutive study. *Clin Ophthalmol.* 2014;8:819–823. Published April 29, 2014. doi: 10.2147/OPTH.S60453.
20. Salah Y, Omar K, Sherif A, Azzam S. Study of demarcation line depth in transepithelial versus epithelium-off Accelerated Cross-Linking (AXL) in Keratoconus. *J Ophthalmol.* 2019;2019:3904565. Published September 26, 2019. doi: 10.1155/2019/3904565.
21. Stulting RD. Corneal collagen cross-linking. *Am J Ophthalmol.* 2012;154(3):423–424.
22. Hovakimyan M, Guthoff RF, Sachs O. Collagen cross-linking: Current status and future directions. *J Ophthalmol.* 2012;2012:Article ID 406850.
23. Sandvik GF, Thorsrud A, Raen M, Ostern AE, Saethre M, Drolsum L. Does corneal collagen cross-linking reduce the need for keratoplasties in patients with keratoconus? *Cornea.* 2015;34(9):991–995.
24. Godefrooij DA, Gans R, Imhof SM, Wisse RP. Nationwide reduction in the number of corneal transplantations for keratoconus following the implementation of cross-linking. *Acta Ophthalmol.* 2016;94(7):675–678.

SECTION 3

Glaucoma Procedures

11 Argon Laser Trabeculoplasty

Myranda R. Partin • Steven R. Sarkisian, Jr.

Argon laser trabeculoplasty (ALT) was introduced by Wise and Witter in 1979.[2] Many attempts using different lasers were tried earlier but these lasers were either unstable or their parameters caused too many side effects. ALT dominated the market until the FDA approval of selective laser trabeculoplasty (SLT) for the treatment of open-angle glaucoma in 2002.[3] Argon laser trabeculoplasty remained the standard-of-care method of laser therapy to the trabecular meshwork (TM) for open-angle glaucoma until 2005.[4] The Glaucoma Laser Trial performed over two decades ago had demonstrated equivalency between ALT and medical treatment as initial treatment modalities in patients with glaucoma. This was revolutionary for its time as there were very few hypotensive eye drops available and other glaucoma surgical alternatives were invasive.

ALT uses thermal energy to achieve an IOP decrease. The melanin absorbs the laser light energy and converts it into heat, which in turn creates thermal damage with subsequent coagulative necrosis.[5] The amount of damage is not limited to the treatment area but extends beyond the trabecular cells that contain melanin.[6] The surrounding tissue also obtains considerable damage. According to Hollo, following ALT, the uveoscleral meshwork is severely destroyed around the area of the laser spots, and the surrounding collagen fibers are heat damaged.[7] A membrane is formed by migrating endothelial cells, which covers the meshwork between the laser spots and is responsible for the late pressure rise and treatment failure after ALT. This endothelial membrane and thermal damage were not seen after 532-nm SLT.[7] According to the mechanical theory, ALT causes coagulative damage to the TM, which results in collagen shrinkage and subsequent scarring of the TM (Figure 11.1). This tightens the meshwork around the area of each burn and reopens the adjacent, untreated intertrabecular spaces.[6] The cellular theory proposes that in response to coagulative necrosis induced by the laser there is a migration of macrophages, which phagocytose debris and thus clear the TM (Figure 11.1).[2]

179

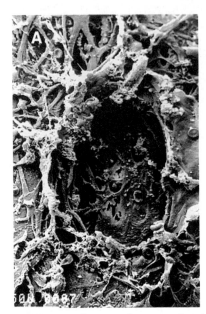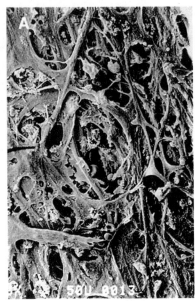

FIGURE 11-1 Electron microscopy showing TM modification seen by argon laser trabeculoplasty on the left and selective laser trabeculoplasty on the right. The argon laser trabeculoplasty laser burns and leaves a definite scar behind.[8] (Reprinted with permission from Pham H, Mansberger S, Brandt JD. I. Argon laser trabeculoplasty. The gold standard: Argon laser trabeculoplasty versus selective laser trabeculoplasty. *Surv Ophthalmol.* 2008;53(6):641–646.)

INDICATIONS

Key Indications

- Primary open-angle glaucoma (POAG)
- Ocular hypertension
- Pigment dispersion syndrome (PDS) or pigmentary glaucoma
- Pseudoexfoliation syndrome (PXE) or pseudoexfoliative glaucoma
- Normal tension glaucoma (NTG) also known as low-tension glaucoma
- Primary angle closure (PAC) or PAC glaucoma (PACG) after successful angle-closure treatment.

Gonioscopy should always be performed before initiating any laser trabeculoplasty to ensure an open angle and to document any angle abnormalities or previous surgical changes. POAG, pseudoexfoliative glaucoma, and pigmentary glaucoma respond best to ALT. In POAG and PXE, patient's ALT success rate ranges from 80% to 97%.[1,2,9] Pigmentary glaucoma patients still have great success at 44% to 80% at one year.[10]

A study done to evaluate the effectiveness of SLT versus ALT in PXE and pseudoexfoliative glaucoma showed an equivalent efficacy between the two lasers. Laser trabeculoplasty has been thought to be of great success due to hyperpigmentation in the TM from the accumulation of proteinaceous material in PXE patients.

Patients with NTG in one study showed a 4.9-mm Hg decrease in IOP at 12 months with a gradual tapering of the pressure-lowering effect over the course of a 21.6-month follow-up.[11] As with all types of glaucoma, the pressure-lowering effect diminishes over time with ALT. There are not many other studies conducted studying ALT in NTG. However, one other study with SLT also concluded laser trabeculoplasty as a successful treatment option for NTG.[12]

As with SLT and most other glaucoma treatments, a lower preoperative IOP such as in low-tension glaucoma is likely thought to be a negative predictor of success. The treating clinician should factor that in when gauging expectations of IOP reduction following any laser trabeculoplasty, including ALT, in low-tension glaucoma.

ALT can be very effective after the opening of the angle from peripheral iridotomy in PACG patients. A study conducted with 19 Japanese patients, after peripheral iridotomy, had a 66% probability of success at the end of three years after ALT.[13]

CONTRAINDICATIONS

Key Contraindications

- PAC or PACG
- A relatively high preoperative IOP (>30 mm Hg) in conjunction with advanced optic nerve damage, in which cases a possible postoperative transient IOP elevation is thought to pose a significant risk for the patient's vision
- Glaucoma associated with uveitis, trauma, ischemia/neovascularization, juvenile open-angle glaucoma, or angle dysgenesis
- A history of previous ALT failure in the same or fellow eye
- Little or no trabecular pigmentation (negative predictor for success)
- Aphakic or pseudophakic glaucoma (relative contraindication)
- Young age (relative contraindication)

ALT will likely be unsuccessful if a majority of the angle is not seen. The exact amount of visible TM needed is unknown but speculated to be at least half.

Patients with previous or active uveitis are poor responders to laser trabeculoplasty due to inflammatory debris in the angle or angle structure modification. ALT could possibly cause further damage by reactivating inflammation or further damaging the angle.[10,14]

An IOP spike in a patient who has advanced glaucoma or an impending central visual field defect may be at too high of a risk to consider ALT. Without prophylactic hypotensive eye drops such as brimonidine or apraclonidine, about one third of patients have a rise in IOP over 5 mm Hg, and 12% to 50% will have spiked over 10 mm Hg 1 hour after treatment. Thankfully these prophylactic hypotensive eye drops can effectively prevent a rise in IOP in all but about 3% to 5% of cases.[1,15]

Repeating ALT is typically contraindicated if the patient has previously had 360° of treatment. Around 30% of cases can respond with an adequate drop in IOP.[1,16] This drop in IOP can be short lived due to the rapid loss of effectivity in two thirds of those cases at one year.[1,16] SLT can be utilized successfully over previous ALT burns or in eyes who had failed with ALT.[17]

Patients with aphakia typically have a poor response to ALT; however, an IOP-lowering effect of around 6 mm Hg has been reported.[1] However, if there is any vitreous in the anterior chamber, ALT has a high failure rate. It is still unknown the mechanism behind ALT failure along with glaucoma secondary to complicated cataract surgery.[18]

Patients who are younger than 40 years of age or those with congenital or juvenile-onset glaucoma respond poorly to ALT.[19] In one study, glaucoma-filtering surgery was needed in 60% of cases in only two years.[1,19]

INFORMED CONSENT CONSIDERATIONS

Key Informed Consent Adverse Events Listed as Follows

- IOP spike
- Inflammation
- Transient blurring of vision
- Bleeding/hyphema
- Lack of efficacy
- Loss of efficacy over time

Informed consent is important not only for liability purposes but also to help the patient understand more about the procedure. A brief summary in laymen terms should include how the laser works on the pigmented region of the drain in their eye. The mechanism by which this occurs is twofold: mechanically pulling open the TM by creating small burn spots and cellular from their immune cells cleaning out the drain. The combination of these two mechanisms is likely what lowers the eye pressure, which is the only modality of treatment. Although laser trabeculoplasty is considered a minor procedure, it still needs to be taken seriously.

Key informed consent adverse events include but are not limited to an IOP spike, postoperative inflammation, discomfort during or after the procedure, transient blurring of vision, ineffectiveness of the procedure, bleeding, or corneal edema. It should be documented that the patient was counseled on alternative options, informed of risks of the procedure including that the procedure may not work, and future alternative methods of treatment could be required. Such alternatives include hypotensive eye drops, monitoring, or more invasive glaucoma surgery.

A note from the counseling physician should be included and phrased similar to, "I have counseled this patient as to the nature of the proposed procedure, the attendant risks involved, and the expected results." The patient's and doctor's names should be printed and signed with the date as well as a witness signature.

PREOPERATIVE CARE

Key Preoperative Considerations

- Pre-laser measurement of IOP
- Gonioscopy assessing for openness of the angle, amount of pigment in the TM, indications and contraindications
- Fluorescein rinsed from the eye
- Preoperative drops: Alpha-agonist such as brimonidine or apraclonidine, proparacaine, and pilocarpine

Pretreatment IOP influences the overall outcome. Studies have shown that patients with higher starting IOPs receive the greatest effect from the laser.[20]

Gonioscopy should always be performed before recommending laser trabeculoplasty. Documentation must include which angles were viewed along with the amount of openness, pigmentation, and any obstructing factors such as peripheral anterior synechiae, stents, or tubes.

Argon laser energy may be absorbed by fluorescein and can cause corneal opacities. Therefore, excess fluorescein should be irrigated from the conjunctival sac prior to treatment.[1]

Patients may be pretreated 30 minutes before the procedure with a drop of pilocarpine (1%–2%) to stretch and momentarily cause paralysis to the iris, creating more space and therefore preventing inadvertent laser-induced peripheral anterior synechiae formation. Secondarily, a drop of apraclonidine 0.5% or brimonidine 0.1% to 0.2% is added to decrease the incidence and the severity of a possible postoperative transient IOP elevation.

SETTINGS AND PROCEDURE

Key ALT Settings

- Power
  - 600–800 mW (standard grade 1–2 meshwork pigmentation)
  - 800–1200 mW (light meshwork pigmentation)
  - 300–600 mW (heavy meshwork pigmentation)
- Spot size
  - 50 μm
- Pulse duration
  - 0.1 second

The appropriate laser settings are a spot size of 50 μm, a duration of 0.1 sec, and a power of 300 to 1200 mW, dependent on the level of TM pigmentation. In general, the more pigmented the TM, the less power required. Due to the laser being absorbed by pigment, the power level is titrated to produce minimal depigmentation during the procedure. This can vary angle to angle as pigment often accumulates more heavily inferiorly or in eyes that have PDS or PXE. The spot size of the ALT is usually 50 μm and the pulse duration of ALT is usually 0.1 second compared to SLT's 3 nanoseconds.[21] Both the spot size and pulse duration settings can be altered in ALT, which is in contrast to the SLT where both settings are fixed and therefore non-alterable.

Key Procedural Points

- Magnification—medium
- Illumination tower variable to wherever produces the best view
- Laser lens mirror placement
  - Ritch trabeculoplasty lens
  - Goldmann gonioscopy lens
- Approximately 100 nonoverlapping laser pulses for 360° of treatment, and 50 laser pulses for 180° of treatment
- 180–360° of treatment

The magnification setting should be comfortable for the treating physician to view the angle's structures but not too high as to cause a loss of focus. The illumination tower should be angled out approximately 30° to get an unobstructed view without causing glare or losing the light beam. Placing the lens does not have to be specific but it should be consistent. Using a mirrored lens such as the Goldmann gonioscopy lens or the Ritch trabeculoplasty lens (Figure 11.2), start at the 9 or 3 o'clock position to work one hemisphere at a time. 360° of the angle can be done during treatment, but often 180° is preferable for safety and repeatability reasons. If choosing to do only 180°, the inferior half is usually chosen first due to it often containing greater pigment and a wider angle.[22,23]

The lens is placed on the cornea following proparacaine installation, and adequate visualization of the angle structures is ensured. The spot size needs to stay round while focusing on the TM. If not, the treating clinician most likely is tipping the prism to view the angle over the iris surface. The laser beam is aimed at the junction of pigmented and nonpigmented TM (Figures 11.3 and 11.4), and the laser power is adjusted until a mild blanching effect is observed. Vapor bubble formation is a sign of excessive power and should be avoided. To ensure maximal delivery of the power, the aiming beam should be kept in the center of the Goldmann mirror. Around 50 laser spots are delivered equally spaced to 180°, similar to the SLT. Some studies show treating all 360° is typically more effective, with better long-term success with ALT correlated with applying 100 or more burns to the

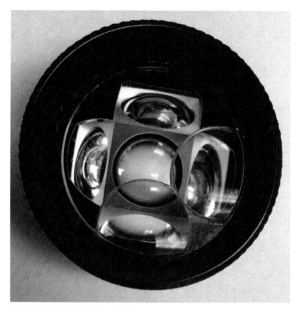

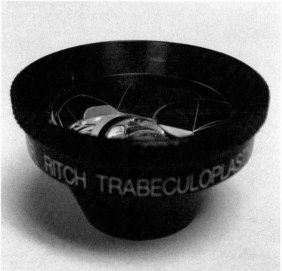

FIGURE 11-2 Laser lenses that can be used during argon laser trabeculoplasty.[23,24]

entire angle.[22,23] A typical ALT treatment protocol would involve approximately 100 spots delivered over 360° of the TM. If the treating clinician is unsure about treating 360° all at once or is concerned for a clinically significant pressure spike or inflammatory response, it is also permissible, and often recommended, to treat 180° per session.

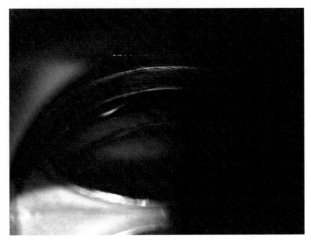

FIGURE 11-3 View of the superior mirror (inferior angle) during an argon laser trabeculoplasty procedure. Notice the small spot size (50 microns) and its placement right in the middle of the trabecular meshwork.

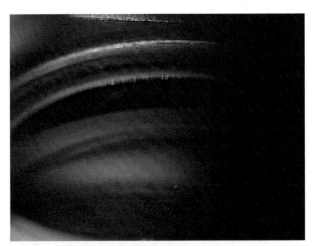

FIGURE 11-4 More magnified view of the superior mirror (inferior angle) during an argon laser trabeculoplasty procedure. Notice the proper placement of the aiming beam right in the middle of the trabecular meshwork.

The routine use of brimonidine or apraclonidine post-laser has diminished acute IOP spikes to 5%, even following 360° of treatment.[1] After four to six weeks, the pressure is reassessed and the second 180° can be treated or saved until necessary, if a positive response was achieved. If there was a negative response, then an alternative solution to treat the patient's glaucoma can be utilized if needed.

POSTOPERATIVE CARE/CO-MANAGEMENT (FOLLOW-UP SCHEDULE)

Key Postoperative Considerations

- Postoperative drops: Alpha-agonist in-office and anti-inflammatory prescribed
- IOP check 30 to 60 minutes post-procedure
- IOP check and anterior chamber assessment one to two weeks post-procedure
- Final IOP check to assess the full effectiveness of the procedure 6 to eight weeks post-procedure

The number of laser shots, power per shot, and total amount of power used should be recorded in the patient's chart. Information on how the patient tolerated the procedure should also be recorded. Immediately after the procedure has finished, another 1 to 2 drops of brimonidine or apraclonidine should be instilled into the operative eye. After 30 to 60 minutes, the pressure should be checked and determined if there is a significant rise in IOP.

Patients are instructed to use a topical corticosteroid eye drop such as prednisolone acetate 1%, 4 times daily for 5 to 7 days after the procedure, along with all their previous glaucoma medications.[9,25] The anticipated IOP-lowering response can be delayed up to six weeks after the procedure. Glaucoma hypotensive drops should not be stopped immediately but tapered accordingly at postoperative visits.

POTENTIAL COMPLICATIONS AND THEIR TREATMENT

Key Potential Complications to Look for the Following

- IOP spike
- Inflammation
- Redness, pain, photophobia
- Peripheral anterior synechiae
- Corneal edema/haze

A transient IOP elevation may occur. The incidence and severity of IOP elevations are significantly reduced if patients are pretreated with brimonidine 0.1%–0.2% or apraclonidine 0.5%. Most of the IOP spikes manifest within 1 to 5 hours after the procedure. Therefore, checking the IOP approximately 1 hour after ALT is recommended to determine if additional actions are necessary. The incidence of IOP elevation has been reported as high as 12% (>10 mm Hg) on the first postoperative days.[6]

A mild iritis is not unusual after ALT and peaks the second day after the procedure, causing occasional pain and photophobia. Treating the patient with a short course of topical corticosteroids for 5 to 7 days after the procedure is recommended.

One complication found with ALT, but much less likely with SLT or micropulse laser trabeculoplasty (MLT), is the formation of peripheral anterior synechiae. The rate of PAS may reach 12% to 47% after ALT but in SLT as low as 0% to 2.86%.[17,23] This difference speaks to the thermal nature of ALT compared with SLT and MLT. These may form if the laser energy is directed too posterior toward the iris, a higher power is used, and are more common in narrow angles. In most cases, peripheral anterior synechiae are small and not clinically significant.[1]

Disruption of endothelial cells with polymorphism and an increase in cell size has also been reported.[23] Transient epithelial burns can be also observed and are more likely with high power settings.[23] Finally, an increase in the incidence of bleb encapsulation after trabeculectomy, which may represent the next step in the treatment of medically uncontrolled glaucoma, has been reported.[26]

VIDEOS OF PROCEDURE

Video 11.1—This is a simulation of an ALT procedure on an actual eye showing proper aiming beam placement and spacing during the procedure. Laser burns would be spaced out approximately 2 to 3 spot sizes in between each ALT laser burn. Mild blanching of the TM along with possible small champagne bubble formation is the desired tissue endpoint for each laser burn. Video courtesy of Nate Lighthizer.

Video 11.2—Treatment is applied to the junction between the nonpigmented and pigmented trabecular meshwork. Laser Settings: laser power 800 mW and adjusted to achieve slight blanching or small bubble formation. Laser duration 0.1 seconds, spot size 50 μm in equally spaced and nonoverlapping applications while maintaining a round spot size. Lens: three-mirror Goldmann lens with anti-reflective coating features. Video courtesy of Leonid Skorin, Jr.

EFFICACY—RELEVANT ARGON LASER TRABECULOPLASTY STUDY DATA

ALT after Maximal Medical Therapy and as a First-Line Treatment

The Advanced Glaucoma Intervention Study (AGIS) compared the effectiveness of ALT to trabeculectomy in patients who were on maximal medical therapy and were continuing to progress with vision loss. ALT was favorable in African patients, despite higher IOPs, compared to those who received trabeculectomy.[27] Caucasian patients however managed better with a trabeculectomy over ALT.[27] The Glaucoma Laser Trial, a multicenter, randomized clinical trial involving 271 patients, was designed to assess the efficacy and safety of ALT as an alternative treatment to topical medication for controlling IOP in patients with newly diagnosed, previously untreated POAG.[28] Each patient had one eye randomly assigned to ALT (the laser first eye) and the other eye assigned to timolol maleate 0.5% (the medication first eye). The medication was initiated or changed for either eye according to the same stepped regimen if the IOP was not controlled. Throughout the two-year follow-up, laser first eyes had lower mean IOPs than medication first eyes (1–2 mm Hg), and fewer laser first eyes than medication first eyes required simultaneous prescription of two or more medications to control IOP.[28]

Long-Term Efficacy

Unfortunately, the IOP-lowering effects of ALT diminish with time. The five-year success rate with ALT is reported to be 50%, with a decrease of 6% to 10% per year.[1,26] However, ALT still showed success in up to 32% of patients after ten years.[1]

Previous Trabeculectomy

ALT can be successful in eyes with prior trabeculectomy in up to 70% of patients.[10,14,25] The AGIS appeared to confirm this, although it still found that the IOP decrease was greatest with filtration surgery.[27]

Repeat ALT

ALT is effective, but its most significant problem is that its effectiveness decreases with retreatment because the tissue it targets is changed by the laser, rendering repeat treatments less effective.[6] One of the most important potential clinical advantages of SLT over ALT is based on the premise that it causes less damage to the tissue it targets.[4] Only around 35% of repeat ALTs are successful, and of the ones that are classified as successful, two thirds will fail by one year.[5] There is also an associated risk of an IOP spike of 10 to 37 mm Hg in 12% to 17%, which can cause progressive optic nerve damage and visual field loss.[1,14] SLT retreatment can produce a clinically useful decrease in IOP at one year, similar to that obtained by ALT, in patients who have had prior argon laser treatment. SLT may be a useful adjunctive therapy when 360° of ALT has already been performed.[29]

Effect of Race and Age on Efficacy

Race does not seem to affect ALT response rate. Age however does. Patients who are 40 years of age and younger fail more often and 60% of them will go on to need more invasive surgery within two years.[19,25]

Anterior versus Posterior Placement of Laser Burns

Initially, it was thought a posterior placement of each laser burn would provide a better outcome due to heavier pigmentation; however, this ended up causing more inflammation and pain. The side effects were diminished by straddling each burn on the junction of the pigmented and nonpigmented region of the TM.[20]

180- versus 360-Degree Treatment

Treating all 360° is typically more effective.[21] In addition, better long-term success with ALT has been correlated with applying 100 or more burns to the entire angle.[22] A typical ALT treatment protocol would involve approximately 100 laser spots delivered over 360° in the middle of the TM. By treating all 360° at once, it potentially saves the patient an extra expense and the inconvenience of two treatments. However, many treating clinicians prefer the safety of treating 180° per session. If the treating physician is unsure about treating 360° all at once or is concerned for a clinically significant pressure spike or inflammatory response, it is permissible, and often recommended, to treat 180° increments. After four to six weeks, the pressure is reassessed, and the second 180° can be treated or saved until necessary, if a positive response was achieved.

Argon laser trabeculoplasty is an effective means for reducing IOP in many open-angle glaucoma patients followed for an extended time. However, up to one-half of eyes within five years of ALT and two thirds of eyes within ten years may require additional laser or surgical intervention for glaucoma control. Laser trabeculoplasty is attractive as a therapeutic option because it can complement or supplant topical medical therapy. One laser treatment session can reduce the IOP for years, thus eliminating the side effects or poor compliance associated with medication use.

CODING/BILLING

The CPT code 65855, *Trabeculoplasty by laser surgery*, is used for all trabeculoplasty procedures. Medicare assigns a 10-day postoperative period to laser trabeculoplasty, which makes laser trabeculoplasty a minor procedure according to Medicare. If both eyes are done in the same session, use modifier-50 after the CPT code. Typically, it is recommended to perform one eye at a time unless patient factors necessitate bilateral same-day treatment. When treating the fellow eye during the global period of the first procedure, use modifier-79 after the CPT code.

Common ICD-10 codes that support this procedure include the following:

H40.1111 to H40.1134 (primary open-angle glaucoma)
H40.011 to H40.029 (open angle with borderline findings)
H40.1310 to H40.1394 (pigmentary glaucoma)
H40.051 to H40.53 (ocular hypertension)
H40.1211 to H40.1294 (low-tension glaucoma)
H40.1411 to H40.1494 (capsular glaucoma with pseudoexfoliation of lens)
H40.2210 to H40.2294 (chronic angle-closure glaucoma)

REFERENCES

1. Morrison JC, Pollack IP, eds. *Glaucoma: Science and Practice*. 1st edition. New York: Thieme; 2011.

2. Wise JB, Witter SL. Argon laser therapy for open-angle glaucoma. A pilot study. *Arch Ophthalmol*. 1979 Feb;97(2):319–322. doi:10.1001/archopht.1979.01020010165017. PMID: 575877.

3. Alon S. Selective laser trabeculoplasty: a clinical review [Internet]. *Journal of Current Glaucoma Practice*. Jaypee Brothers Medical Publishers (P) Ltd; 2013 [cited 2020 Dec 22]. 7:58–65. Available from: https://pubmed.ncbi.nlm.nih.gov/26997784/

4. Latina MA, Park C. Selective targeting of trabecular meshwork cells: in vitro studies of pulsed and CW laser interactions. *Exp Eye Res* [Internet]. 1995 [cited 2020 Dec 22];60(4):359–371. Available from: https://pubmed.ncbi.nlm.nih.gov/7789416/

5. Shingleton BJ, Richter CU, Dharma SK, Tong L, Bellows AR, Hutchinson BT, et al. Long-term efficacy of argon laser trabeculoplasty: a 10-year follow-up study. *Ophthalmology* [Internet]. 1993 [cited 2020 Dec 22];100(9):1324–1329. Available from: https://pubmed.ncbi.nlm.nih.gov/8371919/

6. Kramer TR, Noecker RJ. Comparison of the morphologic changes after selective laser trabeculoplasty and argon laser trabeculoplasty in human eye bank eyes. *Ophthalmology* [Internet]. 2001 [cited 2020 Dec 22];108(4):773–779. Available from: https://pubmed.ncbi.nlm.nih.gov/11297496/

7. Holló G. Argon and low energy, pulsed Nd: YAG laser trabeculoplasty. A prospective, comparative clinical and morphological study. *Acta Ophthalmol Scand* [Internet]. 1996 [cited 2020 Dec 22];74(2):126–131. Available from: https://pubmed.ncbi.nlm.nih.gov/8739675/

8. Ophthalmology management—ALT vs. SLT: is one better than the other? [Internet]. [cited 2020 Dec 25]. Available from: https://www.ophthalmologymanagement.com/issues/2013/february-2013/alt-vs-slt-is-one-better-than-the-other

9. Schwartz AL, Whitten ME, Bleiman B, Martin D. Argon laser trabecular surgery in uncontrolled phakic open angle glaucoma. *Ophthalmology*. 1981 Mar;88(3):203–212. doi:10.1016/s0161-6420(81)35048-9. PMID: 7231908.

10. Robin AL, Pollack IP. Argon laser trabeculoplasty in secondary forms of open-angle glaucoma. *Arch Ophthalmol*. 1983 Mar;101(3):382–384. doi:10.1001/archopht.1983.01040010382005. PMID: 6830487.

11. Schwartz AL, Perman KI, Whitten M. Argon laser trabeculoplasty in progressive low-tension glaucoma. *Ann Ophthalmol* [Internet]. 1984 Jun 1 [cited 2020 Dec 27];16(6):560–566. Available from: https://europepmc.org/article/med/6742697

12. Lee JW, Ho WL, Chan JC, Lai JS. Efficacy of selective laser trabeculoplasty for normal tension glaucoma: 1 year results. *BMC Ophthalmol* [Internet]. 2015 Dec 12 [cited 2020 Dec 14];15(1):1–6. Available from: https://link.springer.com/articles/10.1186/1471-2415-15-1

13. Shirakashi M, Iwata K, Nakayama T. Argon laser trabeculoplasty for chronic angle-closure glaucoma uncontrolled by iridotomy. *Acta Ophthalmol* [Internet]. 1989 [cited 2020 Dec 27];67(3):265–270. Available from: https://pubmed.ncbi.nlm.nih.gov/2763814/

14. Fellman RL, Starita RJ, Spaeth GL, Poryzees EM. ALT: argon laser trabeculoplasty following failed trabeculectomy. *J Ophthalmic Nurs Technol*. 1986 Mar-Apr;5(2):65–68. PMID: 3634021.

15. Robin A. Argon laser trabeculoplasty medical therapy to prevent the intraocular pressure rise associated with argon laser trabeculoplasty—PubMed [Internet]. *Ophthalmic Surgery*. 1991 [cited 2020 Dec 28]. p. 7. Available from: https://pubmed.ncbi.nlm.nih.gov/2014108/

16. Richter CU, Shingleton BJ, Bellows AR, Hutchinson BT, Jacobson LP. Retreatment with argon laser trabeculoplasty. *Ophthalmology* [Internet]. 1987 [cited 2020 Dec 28];94(9):1085–1089. Available from: https://pubmed.ncbi.nlm.nih.gov/3684226/

17. Damji KF, Shah KC, Rock WJ, Bains HS, Hodge WG. Selective laser trabeculoplasty v argon laser trabeculoplasty: a prospective randomised clinical trial. *Br J Ophthalmol* [Internet]. 1999 [cited 2020 Dec 28];83(6):718–722. Available from: https://pubmed.ncbi.nlm.nih.gov/10340983/

18. Wise JB, Witter SL. Argon laser therapy for open-angle glaucoma: a pilot study. *Arch Ophthalmol* [Internet]. 1979 Feb 1 [cited 2020 Dec 22];97(2):319–322. Available from: https://jamanetwork.com/journals/jamaophthalmology/fullarticle/632881

19. Safran MJ, Robin AL, Pollack IP. Argon laser trabeculoplasty in younger patients with primary open-angle glaucoma. *Am J Ophthalmol* [Internet]. 1984 [cited 2020 Dec 23];97(3):292–295. Available from: https://pubmed.ncbi.nlm.nih.gov/6702966/

20. Schwartz LW, Spaeth GL, Traverso C, Greenidge KC. Variation of techniques on the results of argon laser trabeculoplasty. *Ophthalmology*. 1983 Jul;90(7):781–784. doi:10.1016/s0161-6420(83)34488-2. PMID: 6622016.

21. Lustgarten J, Podos SM, Ritch R, Fischer R, Stetz D, Zborowski L, et al. Laser trabeculoplasty: a prospective study of treatment variables. *Arch Ophthalmol* [Internet]. 1984 Apr 1 [cited 2020 Dec 23];102(4):517–519. Available from: https://jamanetwork.com/journals/jamaophthalmology/fullarticle/635005

22. Wise JB. Ten year results of laser trabeculoplasty does the laser avoid glaucoma surgery or merely defer it? *Eye* [Internet]. 1987 [cited 2020 Dec 23];1(1):45–50. Available from: https://pubmed.ncbi.nlm.nih.gov/3556659/

23. Fillippopoulos TM. Argon laser trabeculoplasty: overview, indications, contraindications [Internet]. *Medscape*. 2016 [cited 2020 Dec 25]. Available at: https://emedicine.medscape.com/article/1844064-overview#a5

24. Ritch Trabeculoplasty [Internet]. [cited 2020 Dec 18]. Available at: https://www.eyecareandcure.com/ECC-Products/SLT-Iridectomy-Capsulotomy/Ritch-Trabeculoplasty

25. Thomas JV, Simmons RJ, Belcher CD 3rd. Argon laser trabeculoplasty in the presurgical glaucoma patient. *Ophthalmology*. 1982 Mar;89(3):187–97. doi: 10.1016/s0161-6420(82)34807-1. PMID: 7088501.

26. Herndon LW, Moore DB. Take-home messages from the advanced glaucoma intervention study—glaucoma today. [cited 2020 Dec 22]; Available at: https://glaucomatoday.com/articles/2013-may-june/take-home-messages-from-the-advanced-glaucoma-intervention-study

27. AGIS Investigators. The advanced glaucoma intervention study (AGIS): 9. Comparison of glaucoma outcomes in black and white patients within treatment groups. *Am J Ophthalmol*. 2001;132(3):311–320. https://doi.org/10.1016/S0002-9394(01)01028-5

28. Krug J, Chiavelli M, Borawski G, Devaney M, Epstein D, Berson F, et al. The Glaucoma Laser Trial (GLT) and glaucoma laser trial follow-up study: 7. Results. *Am J Ophthalmol* [Internet]. 1995 [cited 2020 Dec 22];120(6):718–731. Available from: https://pubmed.ncbi.nlm.nih.gov/8540545/

29. Birt CM. Selective laser trabeculoplasty retreatment after prior argon laser trabeculoplasty: 1-Year results. *Can J Ophthalmol* [Internet]. 2007 [cited 2020 Dec 22];42(5):715–719. Available from: https://pubmed.ncbi.nlm.nih.gov/17891199/

12 Selective Laser Trabeculoplasty

Nate Lighthizer

Selective laser trabeculoplasty (SLT), introduced by Latina and Park in the mid-1990s and FDA approved in 2001, has been a mainstay of glaucoma therapy for nearly two decades. SLT uses a 532-nm Q-switched, frequency-doubled Nd:YAG laser with a short-pulse duration of 3 ns. The quick-pulse duration allows SLT to achieve selective photothermolysis, which is the process by which energy can be selectively absorbed by a pigmented cell population within a tissue to cause only localized damage and permit target selectivity, thereby reducing collateral damage.[1] Selective photothermolysis is achieved due to the fact that the 3-ns pulse duration of SLT is quicker than the thermal relaxation time of melanin, which is approximately 1 μs. Therefore, SLT laser energy, which is selectively absorbed by melanin within the trabecular meshwork (TM), is not spread collaterally as a photocoagulation or thermal burn within the TM. The effect is "biologic" or "inflammatory" in effect or better described as selective photothermolysis.

The mechanism by which SLT lowers intraocular pressure (IOP) is not completely understood and is likely multifactorial.[2] Numerous studies have shown that SLT increases aqueous outflow through the TM.[3] Since limited structural damage occurs to the TM, the mechanical and structural theories, which have been suggested to explain the mechanism of action of argon laser trabeculoplasty (ALT), do not fully apply to SLT. Moreover, SLT has been demonstrated to induce biological changes that modulate increased aqueous outflow through the TM, including changes in gene expression, cytokine secretion, matrix metalloproteinase induction, and TM remodeling.[1,4]

Recent studies described light microscopy, scanning electron microscopy (SEM), and transmission electron microscopy findings from cadaver eye sections that were treated with either ALT or SLT using power ranging from 0.4 to 2.0 mJ. Eyes treated with ALT demonstrated significant disruption of TM architecture. Eyes treated with SLT showed normal TM architecture on light microscopy, but transmission electron microscopy did show some disruption of TM cells with cracked extracellular pigment granules even at low power settings. On SEM, TM treated with high power (2.0 mJ) showed more obvious tissue destruction. This suggests that treatment with SLT does have the potential to cause structural damage to the TM and that dose titration remains important.[2,5]

INDICATIONS

Key Indications (in order)

- Primary open-angle glaucoma (POAG)
- Ocular hypertension (OHT)
- Normal-tension glaucoma (NTG)
- Pigment dispersion syndrome or pigmentary glaucoma
- Pseudoexfoliation syndrome or pseudoexfoliative glaucoma
- Primary angle closure (PAC) or PAC glaucoma (PACG) after successful angle-closure treatment

When considering a laser procedure into the anterior chamber angle, it is critical to ensure that the patient has an open angle. POAG and OHT are the two strongest indications to consider SLT due to the fact that studies show positive predictors for success include the following:

- Pre-laser IOP with higher IOPs being more predictive of greater IOP lowering.[6,7]
- Fewer number of medications the patient is on at the time of the SLT. As with eye drops, typically SLT earlier in the course of therapy leads to more robust lowering of IOP.
- Some research indicates that lack of prostaglandin analogue drop use at the time of SLT may increase chances of robust IOP lowering.[8]

Despite higher pre-laser IOPs being likely the most predictive factor of SLT success, there still is an indication for NTG. The IOP-lowering effect is more modest in NTG compared to POAG, with studies showing a 12% to 15% IOP reduction with 27% to 41% fewer medications one to two years postoperatively.[9,10] Additionally, SLT also has a positive effect on diurnal IOP fluctuations, which may be an additional benefit in NTG patients.[11,12]

Pigmentation in the TM has been shown in some studies to be another predictive factor for SLT success with heavier pigmentation being more predictive of greater IOP lowering.[7] Patients with pigmentary glaucoma have similar success rates with SLT as patients with other types of open-angle glaucoma.[2,13,14] However, caution must be taken when considering SLT in pigmentary glaucoma, as the high levels of pigmentation can cause an overproduction of the biologic or inflammatory SLT effect. Studies have suggested there may be an increased complication rate, including eye pain, inflammation, IOP spikes, and a greater need for surgical intervention, after SLT in patients with highly pigmented TM.[2,14] In a case series of four patients with post-SLT IOP spikes lasting four days to three months, three patients had pigmentary glaucoma and the other had a heavily pigmented angle. Three of these patients eventually required trabeculectomy. Lowering power settings and treating 180° or less may be necessary in patients with heavily pigmented angles.[2,15]

Patients with pseudoexfoliative glaucoma seem to have similar IOP-lowering efficacy, failure rate, and adverse event rate compared with patients with other open-angle glaucomas. The presence of pseudoexfoliation does not seem to be a risk factor for IOP spikes or complications after SLT.[2,16]

Many patients with PAC or PACG will require additional therapy beyond the angle-closure treatment to maintain IOP control.[2,17] One study examined subjects with at least 180° of open angle after peripheral iridotomy and found a 17% IOP reduction with SLT.[18] Consequently, even though it is counterintuitive, SLT may be an additional IOP-lowering option in patients with PAC or PACG whose anterior chamber angles have been opened with angle-closure therapy and the TM remains healthy without synechiae.[2,18]

CONTRAINDICATIONS

Key Contraindications

- Narrow angles or angle closure where adequate TM is not visible
- Inflammatory glaucoma
- Neovascular glaucoma
- Angle recession glaucoma
- Juvenile glaucoma
- Prior SLT that failed
- Significant corneal endothelial disease

The presence of less than 90° to 180° of visible posterior pigmented TM on gonioscopy likely is a contraindication for performing SLT. Numerous secondary glaucomas, including inflammatory, neovascular, angle recession, and juvenile, are either absolutely or relatively contraindicated due to the potential for worsening the condition (inflammatory glaucoma), needing other therapy (neovascular glaucoma), or likely noneffectiveness of treatment (angle recession and juvenile glaucoma).

The effect of SLT on the corneal endothelium may be transient, and long-term effects are probably negligible in normal corneas. However, in compromised corneas and corneas with pigment deposits on the endothelium, there may be a risk of corneal endothelial compromise, especially after repeated SLT.[19] Therefore, it may be wise to limit the number of shots and energy when considering SLT in a patient with a compromised corneal endothelium.

INFORMED CONSENT CONSIDERATIONS

Key Informed Consent Adverse Events Listed as Follows

- IOP spike
- Inflammation
- Pain/discomfort during and/or after the procedure
- Transient blurring of vision
- Ineffectiveness of the procedure
- Corneal haze/edema (rare)
- Bleeding/hyphema (rare)
- Macular edema (rare)
- Hyperopic or myopic shift (rare)[20]

Informed consent should include a description of the procedure in plain language. For example, "A laser will be used to place gentle laser pulses in the drainage area of the eye. The laser energy will work on the pigmented area of the drain which in turn will recruit the body's own natural immune cells to travel up to the area and clean out the debris in the drain. This will help lower the eye pressure which is the main known modifiable risk factor in glaucoma."

Potential alternative treatments, such as eye drops, monitoring, minimally invasive glaucoma surgery, or invasive surgery, should be listed. Risks and complications inherent to any laser procedure, including SLT, include but are not limited to increased eye pressure; eye inflammation; irritation or pain during or after the procedure; temporary blurring of vision, swelling of the cornea, hyphema or micro-hyphema; as well as ineffectiveness of the procedure.

A note from the counseling clinician should be included and phrased similar to "I have counseled this patient as to the nature of the proposed procedure, the attendant risks involved, and the expected results." The patient's and doctor's names should be printed and signed with the date as well as a witness signature (typically a staff member).

PREOPERATIVE CARE

Key Preoperative Considerations

- Gonioscopy assessing for openness of the angle, amount of pigment in the TM, indications, and contraindications
- Preoperative drops: Alpha-agonist, proparacaine, and pilocarpine (rare)

If not already performed, angles should be viewed via gonioscopy to assess visible structures, amount of pigmentation in the TM and any pathology such as peripheral anterior synechiae.

The amount of pigmentation in the TM will affect starting energy level with lighter pigmented meshworks requiring higher energy levels and heavier pigmented meshworks requiring lower energy levels.

Approximately 15 to 30 minutes prior to the procedure, one or two drops of an alpha-agonist such as brimonidine (0.1%–0.2%) or apraclonidine 1% should be instilled into the selected eye to blunt any potential IOP spike. Pilocarpine 1% may also be used to help move the iris out of the angle and visualize more of the TM and angle structures. Immediately before the procedure, proparacaine should be instilled into both eyes; instillation in the fellow eye will help control blinking during the procedure.

SETTINGS AND PROCEDURE

Key SLT Settings

- Energy
    - 0.8 to 1.0 mJ (standard grade 1–2 meshwork pigmentation)
    - 1.1 to 1.4 mJ (light meshwork pigmentation)
    - 0.4 to 0.7 mJ (heavy meshwork pigmentation)
- Spot size
    - 400 microns (fixed/not adjustable)
- Pulse duration
    - 3 ns (fixed/not adjustable)

A laser lens (Latina lens or Rapid SLT lens) is required. The procedure has been studied and theoretically can be performed without a laser lens by applying trans-scleral laser pulses near the perilimbal scleral area over the area of the TM.[21] This technique however is experimental and has not reached widespread clinical practice. The use of a lens has several advantages: (1) it helps stabilize the eye and minimize eye movements and prevents the upper lid from blocking the doctor's view; (2) it helps to focus and concentrate the laser energy; and (3) it provides an easy and inconspicuous method of staunching a rare angle bleed and potential hyphema. The most effective way to stop bleeding is to apply gentle pressure with the laser lens for 30 to 60 seconds.

A small amount of cushioning agent should be instilled into the lens well. While 1% carboxymethylcellulose (Celluvisc) drops can be used, a gel formulation such as Genteal or Systane gel (both hypromellose 0.3%) has the advantage of better contact with the SLT lens and less potential for air bubbles thus providing a better view through the lens. After applying the laser lens to the patient's anesthetized eye, the initial treatment mirror should be placed in the initial treatment position.

SLT Settings

Due to the laser spot size and pulse duration being internally fixed and not adjustable for the doctor, there are less laser settings to dial in for an SLT compared to other laser procedures. Typical starting energy setting is between 0.8 and 1.0 mJ and is adjusted based on TM pigmentation. Angles with heavy pigmentation (grade 3 or 4) may require titrating the energy down to 0.4 to 0.7 mJ depending on the patient and tissue reaction during the procedure. Angles with light pigmentation (trace pigmentation or less) may require titrating the energy up to 1.1 to 1.4 mJ or more.

As with every laser procedure, the laser shot counter should be reset or "zeroed" before starting, with the last thing done before beginning the procedure is turning the laser on.

The Procedure

Key Procedural Points

- Magnification—12.5 to 20x (medium mag)
- Illumination tower variable to wherever produces the best view
- Laser lens mirror placement:
  - Latina lens 1 mirror placed at 9:00 (for clockwise rotation) or 3:00 (for counterclockwise rotation) if desiring to treat the inferior 180° first which is typical
  - Rapid SLT lens 4 mirrors placed at 12:00, 3:00, 6:00, and 9:00
- Approximately 100 nonoverlapping laser pulses for 360° treatment, and 50 laser pulses for 180° treatment
- Desired tissue reaction = lowest laser energy, which produces champagne bubbles approximately 50% to 75% of the time
- 360° treatment for POAG, OHT, NTG
- 180° treatment for pigmentary or pseudoexfoliative glaucoma

Many of the same skills and slit lamp settings necessary for gonioscopy are utilized in SLT. Magnification is usually high enough to visualize angle structures such as the TM but not too high as to cause the treating clinician to lose orientation. The illumination tower should be positioned in a manner that gives the best view possible with minimal glare and reflections. Clinically speaking, it has been the author's experience that the illumination tower on the opposite side of the mirror (e.g., working in the right mirror with the illumination tower slightly to the left) generally gives the brightest, clearest view while minimizing reflections and glare.

Laser lens placement on the eye depends on which laser lens is being used. Traditionally, the inferior 180° is the first half of the eye treated as it is the most open half of the angle and usually contains the most pigment in the TM. With the 1-mirror Latina lens (Figures 12.1 and 12.2), the mirror should initially be placed at 9:00 (if moving clockwise) or 3:00 (if moving counterclockwise). The single-aiming beam should be placed to cover the entire width of the TM, and 8 to 12 nonoverlapping laser pulses are usually placed in the mirror followed by rotating the mirror to the next location. The Latina lens typically requires 8 to 12 mirror rotations during a 360° treatment session. With the 4-mirror Rapid SLT lens (Figures 12.3 and 12.4), the mirrors should be placed at 12:00, 3:00, 6:00, and 9:00. It is recommended to start in the 12:00 mirror since it provides a direct view of the inferior TM and continue to the 3:00 mirror, 6:00 mirror, and then 9:00 mirror. The aiming beam should again be placed to cover the entire width of the TM (Figure 12.5), and 10 to 15 nonoverlapping laser pulses should be placed in each mirror, giving approximately 50 shots after completing the 4 mirrors. If treating 360°, the Rapid SLT lens should then be rotated 45° one time to place the 4 mirrors in the oblique locations, and treatment continues with the 10:30, 1:30, 4:30, and finally 7:30 mirror locations. Approximately 90 to 110 laser pulses are typically placed for a 360° SLT treatment session, with 45 to 55 laser pulses for a 180° SLT treatment session.

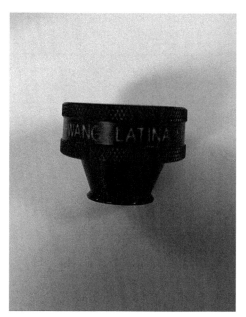

FIGURE 12-1 Latina selective laser trabeculo-plasty lens.

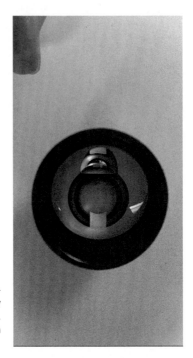

FIGURE 12-2 Latina selective laser trabeculoplasty lens (doctor perspective). Note the 1 mirror shown at the 12:00 position.

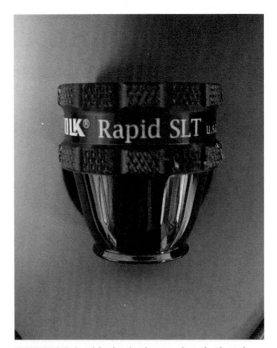

FIGURE 12-3 Rapid selective laser trabeculoplasty lens.

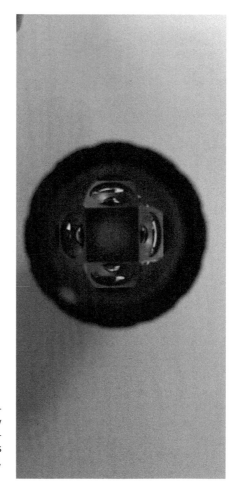

FIGURE 12-4 Rapid selective laser trabeculoplasty lens (doctor perspective). Note the 4 mirrors shown at the 12:00, 3:00, 6:00, and 9:00 positions.

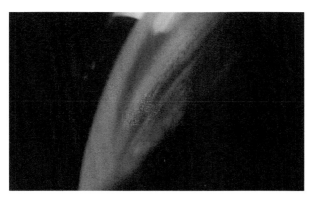

FIGURE 12-5 Aiming beam correctly placed with the width of the beam covering the entire TM.

With the mechanism of action of SLT being photothermolysis/biologic/inflammatory, minimal tissue reaction will be seen while performing an SLT. The desired tissue reaction is the appearance of small cavitation or champagne bubbles after the majority of laser pulses (Figure 12.6). If champagne bubbles are present for the first four to five laser pulses, the energy should then be titrated down to 0.1 mJ to determine if champagne bubbles are present at the lower energy level. If no champagne bubbles are seen with the first four to five laser pulses, the energy should be titrated up until champagne bubble formation is seen. The lowest energy setting that produces champagne bubbles approximately 50% to 75% of the time is currently considered the most appropriate laser energy setting for SLT.[14,22–25]

How many degrees of the angle to treat depends on clinician preference and the type of glaucoma being treated. The early days of SLT generally recommended 180° of treatment consistent with prior ALT treatment protocols. Due to the mechanism of action, minimal structural damage in the angle, lower side effect profile, and repeatability, it has become generally accepted to perform 360° of SLT treatment for POAG, OHT, and NTG.[2,23,24,26–29] Conversely, some studies indicate that fewer degrees of treatment may be as effective as a full 360° treatment while reducing the incidence and magnitude of postoperative IOP elevation.[2,22–24,30,31] Heavier amounts of pigment in the angle can potentially cause an overproduction of inflammation leading to higher rates of potential adverse events. Therefore, the general consensus is to perform 180° or less in patients with heavy pigmentation in the TM, pigmentary glaucoma, or pseudoexfoliative glaucoma.[2,14]

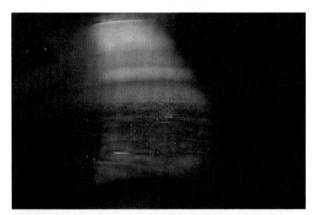

FIGURE 12-6 Selective laser trabeculoplasty procedure being performed in the inferior quadrant (mirror is currently at the 12:00 position). Notice the correct placement of the aiming beam covering the trabecular meshwork, and the appearance of multiple champagne or cavitation bubbles. Also note no difference in appearance of the trabecular meshwork that has not been treated yet (to the right of the aiming beam) compared to already treated trabecular meshwork (to the left of the aiming beam).

POSTOPERATIVE CARE/CO-MANAGEMENT (FOLLOW-UP SCHEDULE)

Key Postoperative Considerations

- Postoperative drops: Alpha-agonist in-office and anti-inflammatory prescribed
- IOP check 30 to 60 minutes post-procedure
- IOP check and anterior chamber assessment one week post-procedure
- Final IOP check to assess full effectiveness of the procedure six to eight weeks post-procedure

Immediately after completing the procedure and removing the SLT laser lens, another 1 to 2 drops of brimonidine or apraclonidine should be instilled into the postoperative eye. After 30 to 60 minutes, IOP should be assessed and treated if a significant rise in IOP is noted.

The number of shots, energy per shot, and total amount of energy used should be recorded in the chart. A notation similar to "The patient tolerated the procedure well and left in no apparent distress" should be added to the chart.

Traditionally, a topical non-steroidal anti-inflammatory drug (NSAID) as needed or no anti-inflammatory eye drops have been used post-operatively as to not overly suppress the inflammation needed to necessitate SLT effectiveness. Numerous studies have concluded anti-inflammatory drops after SLT do not cause a significant reduction in inflammation or altered IOP-lowering efficacy.[1,32,33] More recently studies have shown that a topical steroid or topical NSAID for three to five days post-SLT may lead to a better 12-week SLT IOP reduction than no drops used post-procedure.[34] Prednisolone acetate four times a day, Durezol (difluprednate) twice a day, a topical NSAID as directed, or no anti-inflammatory drops postoperatively are all acceptable options for the postoperative eye for three to five days. A follow-up visit for one week is scheduled with instructions to the patient to return if any increased redness, increased pain, or decreased vision is noted. Specific patient education is given regarding ocular soreness for the two to three days following the SLT due to the nature of the procedure.

At the one-week follow-up, the doctor should inspect the anterior chamber for degree of inflammation, and IOP should be measured. Patient education should discuss the importance of continuing any current glaucoma drop therapy until the six- to eight-week follow-up visit when the full effect of the SLT procedure is better known.

At the six- to eight-week follow-up, the doctor should again inspect the anterior chamber for degree of inflammation, and IOP should be measured. Studies indicate it takes anywhere from 4 to 12 weeks to see the full IOP-lowering effect following SLT, with the general consensus being approximately six to eight weeks.[1,35,36]

Decisions regarding any possible glaucoma drop discontinuation or addition are generally made once the full effect of SLT is known.

POTENTIAL COMPLICATIONS AND THEIR TREATMENT

Key Potential Complications to Look for:

- IOP spike
- Inflammation
- Redness, pain, and/or blurred vision
- Peripheral anterior synechiae (rare)
- Bleeding/hyphema (rare)
- Macular edema (rare)
- Corneal edema/haze (rare)
- Hyperopic or myopic refractive shifts (rare)

Complications due to SLT are infrequent and their effects are rarely permanent. A transient IOP increase of 5 mm Hg or more has been reported in 0% to 28% of eyes.[2] More specifically, a study[20,37] reported transient elevated IOP after SLT of 4.5%, which seems consistent with clinical experience. A systematic review found that prophylactic in-office treatment with IOP-lowering medication reduced the incidence of transient IOP elevation.[38] Heavily pigmented TMs may lead to potentially higher rates of IOP spike, with one study[15] reporting a series of four cases of severe IOP spike in patients with highly pigmented angle structures; thus, caution should be exercised in these patients. Most IOP spikes are initially detected at the 1-hour IOP check and often dissipate within 24 hours either on their own or with topical hypotensive therapy such as brimonidine.

Postoperative inflammation following SLT usually occurs one to three days following the procedure. It has been seen in 83% of eyes undergoing SLT, and the inflammation is usually transient and resolves in five days or less.[20] Conversely, one study[39] looked at 64 patients treated with 360° SLT and did not observe any anterior chamber cell or flare or vitreous haze at 24 hours or 14 days after treatment. It is important to remember that due to the mechanism of action of SLT, a certain degree of inflammation is expected, and potentially good, in the hours to days following the procedure. Risk factors for an excessive inflammatory response, possibly leading to IOP elevation, include a heavily pigmented TM or a history of prior ALT treatment.[20] Topical steroids or topical NSAIDS for three to five days post-SLT should be considered to ensure the inflammatory response is not excessive.

Other possible side effects, such as redness, pain/ocular soreness, and blurred vision, have also been described as transient and without sequelae in all studies.[15]

Peripheral anterior synechiae have been described but occur rarely after SLT. In a systematic review of 12 studies, PAS were observed in 2 eyes in 2 separate studies (1.1% and 2.85% of eyes), whereas none were observed in the other 10 studies.[2,38]

Bleeding/hyphema has been reported as a rare complication during SLT.[40,41] If bleeding occurs during an SLT, gentle pressure should be applied with the laser lens to the eye to stop bleeding. All reported cases of hyphema in the literature have resolved without sequela.

Macular edema has been reported in multiple case reports and studies as a rare complication of SLT.[42–44] Preexisting macular or retinal pathology, such as diabetic retinopathy, retinal vein occlusion, or post-cataract surgery cystoid macular edema (CME), has often been present. Management consists of the typical CME treatment options, including topical steroids and/or NSAIDs.

Multiple corneal changes have been reported following SLT including corneal edema, corneal haze, white spots on the endothelium, decreased endothelial cell count, and SLT-induced keratitis with a hyperopic shift. These changes are usually transient without long-term sequalae. The incidence of corneal edema after SLT is 0.8%.[20]

VIDEOS OF PROCEDURE

Video 12.1—This is an SLT procedure being done 360° with the Latina lens starting in the 9:00 position and rotating clockwise. The procedure is being done at 0.8 mJ. Notice the abundance of champagne bubbles particularly in the inferior quadrant (superior mirror). The single-aiming beam is being aimed to cover the entire width of the TM with crisp focus on the pigmented TM. IOP preoperatively was 22 mm Hg, and IOP six weeks after the procedure was 13 mm Hg.

Video 12.2—This is an SLT procedure being done 360° with the Rapid SLT lens starting in the 12:00 mirror (inferior angle) and continuing to the 3:00 mirror, followed by the 6:00 mirror, and then 9:00 mirror. A single 45° lens rotation is performed to orientate the mirrors in the oblique positions, and treatment continues in the 10:30, 1:30, 4:30, and finally 7:30 mirrors (last 3 mirrors not shown in the video). Notice the small champagne bubbles that are present during some, but not all, laser pulses. Approximately 100 laser pulses were placed for this entire SLT procedure.

Video 12.3—This is an SLT procedure being done 360° with the Rapid SLT lens. Only the oblique mirrors are shown in this video. Notice the small champagne bubbles that are present during some, but not all, laser pulses. Also note the dark appearance of the third mirror (7:30 position), and how the situation is corrected by repositioning the illumination tower. Approximately 100 laser pulses were placed for this entire SLT procedure.

Videos courtesy of Nate Lighthizer.

EFFICACY—RELEVANT SELECTIVE LASER TRABECULOPLASTY STUDY DATA

Efficacy as Primary/Initial Therapy

Generally speaking, the literature indicates that the practitioner can expect 20% to 35% IOP lowering for patients where SLT is used as primary therapy. The initial study by Latina et al.[35] demonstrated a mean IOP reduction of 23.8% at 26 weeks after a single treatment. The SLT: Med study showed the percentage of IOP reduction 9 to 12 months after treatment was 26.4% for the SLT group and 27.8% in the medical/prostaglandin arm with the two treatment arms being statistically equivalent.[28]

Overall success depends on how it is defined, with one study[29] showing 74.2% of patients being drop free three years after primary SLT treatment. The author educates patients that SLT is effective in 80% to 90% of patients with the effect tending to wane with time. SLT has repeatedly been shown to be equivalent to prostaglandins for first-line therapy,[28,29,45] with one study concluding SLT should be offered as a first-line treatment for open-angle glaucoma and OHT, supporting a change in clinical practice.[29]

Efficacy as Secondary/Adjunctive Therapy

SLT has also been investigated as an adjunct treatment for patients on concurrent topical therapy as a means of further IOP reduction. Weinand et al.[46] reported clinical outcomes of 52 POAG eyes that received adjunct SLT while on topical medical treatment. Average IOP reduction from baseline was 24.3% at one year, 27.8% at two years, 24.5% at three years, and 29.3% at four years. Similar to medications, the effect of SLT as adjunctive therapy is likely not as robust as primary therapy with the average IOP reduction being approximately 10% to 25% depending on number of medications the patient is on and the baseline IOP prior to the laser.

Use with Topical Glaucoma Medications

When used as adjunctive therapy, SLT pairs well with most all medications. A retrospective review found no difference between specific classes of antiglaucoma medications in regard to SLT success.[47] These findings confirm a role for SLT as an adjunct to antiglaucoma medications, including prostaglandin analogs, which have been suggested to possibly impair the effectiveness of SLT by competing for a common pathway to lower pressure.[8]

Efficacy in Different Patient Populations

SLT has been shown to have positive, but varying effects in different ethnicities. Analyzing different ethnic groups, one study[48] found a reduction of IOP of at least 20% at one year in 90% of African patients compared with 54% in the Indian subgroup and 83% in the Caucasian subgroup. At one year, African patients showed a reduction in their mean IOP of 52% from baseline compared with a reduction of 30% in the Indian group. Another study[49] showed a 20% reduction in IOP was sustained at 12 months in 90% of African eyes but in only 50% of Indian eyes. This supports the theory that SLT directly targets melanocytes in the TM, leading to the conclusion that while SLT works well for nearly all, darker pigmented angles tend to have the most robust results.

Predictive Factors for Success

While SLT works well for most, it does not work for all, and selecting patients based on factors that most likely lead to success of the SLT is critical. Several studies have shown that the strongest predictor of SLT success is higher preoperative IOP.[2,13,47]

Intuitively, the number of medications a patient is on likely affects the percentage of IOP reduction after SLT, with the more preoperative medications likely leading to a lower percentage of IOP reduction, and vice versa. Lee et al.[50] described results after analysis of 111 eyes treated with 360° SLT, finding that the use of 3 topical IOP-lowering medications was associated with SLT failure. Conversely, Woo et al.[30] described the five-year success rates of SLT and found no significant difference in success rate on the basis of the number of preoperative glaucoma eye drops patients were using. There was, however, an increased likelihood of patients requiring a second procedure (SLT or trabeculectomy) during the five-year follow-up period in those who were taking 2 or more preoperative IOP-lowering drops.

Increased angle pigmentation may correlate with SLT efficacy.[2] In a study by Wasyluk et al.,[51] patients were subdivided into three groups on the basis of angle pigmentation. Mean IOP fell by 2.06, 2.46, and 4.75 mm Hg in subgroups with low-, marked-, and high-angle pigmentation, respectively. Conversely, other studies have shown that angle pigmentation is not predictive of SLT success.[24] Considering the mechanism of action of SLT, pigmentation in the angle is an important variable to consider; however, angles with low pigmentation likely will still show clinically significant IOP-lowering effects provided treatment protocols are adjusted properly (increasing treatment energy).

Multiple other factors have been investigated yet were not found to be significant predictors of success including age, sex, previous ALT, angle grade, lens status, and central corneal thickness.[47]

How Long Does the Effect of Selective Laser Trabeculoplasty Last?

SLT treatment efficacy is known to diminish with time. Survival analysis indicates that the time for 50% of eyes to fail after SLT treatment is approximately two years.[46,52] The more recent LIGHT trial showed 74.2% of patients being drop free three years after primary SLT treatment.[29] It is recommended that patients be educated that the likely effectiveness of the procedure is somewhere between one and five years, with the option available to repeat the SLT when the IOP elevates or progression is shown.

Repeatability of Selective Laser Trabeculoplasty

As SLT causes minimal structural damage to the TM, retreatment is a viable option in patients that need further IOP reduction. Although this benefit of SLT was theoretical for many years, the body of evidence now supports the efficacy of repeat SLT.[53] It achieves a similar absolute level of IOP control with mean percent IOP reduction following repeat SLT perhaps slightly lower than the initial treatment. This is possibly related to the retreatment being done at an overall lower level of IOP. For example, an initial SLT was done at a baseline IOP of 24 mm Hg with a 30% IOP reduction to achieve a post-SLT treatment IOP of 17 mm Hg. The IOP elevated in the years following the initial SLT to 22 mm Hg. Repeat SLT achieved a 25% IOP reduction taking the IOP back to 17 mm Hg. The repeat SLT achieved the same IOP endpoint with a slightly lower percentage of IOP reduction.

One study demonstrated that repeat SLT can maintain IOP at or below target IOP in medication naive POAG and OHT eyes requiring retreatment with at least an equivalent duration of effect to the initial laser.[54]

Repeat treatments are not usually performed in the first six months after initial treatment, as the need for repeat treatment that early would indicate initial SLT failure.

Overall, repeat SLT appears to be comparable to initial SLT in regard to efficacy, duration of effect, and rate of complications.

Efficacy after Prior Argon Laser Trabeculoplasty

Just as repeat SLT after initial SLT has been shown to be comparable to the initial treatment, SLT after prior ALT has shown similar findings. SLT can be performed after prior ALT.

Diurnal Control Benefits of Selective Laser Trabeculoplasty

IOP fluctuation has been shown to be an independent risk factor for glaucomatous progression.[55] The ability to decrease IOP fluctuations is a significant benefit of SLT treatment, with the blunting of IOP fluctuations possibly being more evident at night.[12] The diurnal control with SLT likely is better with 360° treatment compared to 180°,[26] although even the 360° treatment may not offer as much diurnal control as prostaglandin therapy.[56]

CODING/BILLING AND MODIFIERS

For an SLT, CPT code 65855 is used: "Trabeculoplasty by laser surgery." This code has a 10-day postoperative global period. If both eyes are done in the same session, use modifier-50 after the CPT code. Typically, it is recommended to perform one eye in a treatment session, unless it is a repeat SLT without incident or complication on prior sessions or if patient factors necessitate bilateral same day treatment. When treating the fellow eye during the global period of the first procedure, use modifier-79 after the CPT code.

Common ICD-10 codes that support this procedure include the following:

H40.1110 to H40.1194 (primary open-angle glaucoma)
H40.011 to H40.029 (open angle with borderline findings)
H40.051 to H40.059 (ocular hypertension)
H40.1210 to H40.1294 (low-tension glaucoma)
H40.1310 to H40.1394 (pigmentary glaucoma)
H40.1410 to H40.1494 (capsular glaucoma with pseudoexfoliation of lens)
H40.2210 to H40.2294 (chronic angle-closure glaucoma)

REFERENCES

1. Garb A, Gazzard G. SLT past, present and future 2018. *Eye (Lond)*. 2018 May;32(5):863–876.
2. Kennedy J, SooHoo J, Kahook M, Seibold L. Selective laser trabeculoplasty: an update. *Asia Pac J Ophthalmol*. 2016;5:63–69.
3. Gulati V, Fan S, Gardner BJ, et al. Mechanism of action of selective laser trabeculoplasty and predictors of response. *Invest Ophthalmol Vis Sci*. 2017;58(3):1462–1468.
4. Kagan DB, Gorfinkel NS, Hutnik CM. Mechanisms of selective laser trabeculoplasty: a review. *Clin Exp Ophthalmol*. 2014;42(7):675–681.
5. SooHoo JR, Seibold LK, Ammar DA, et al. Ultrastructural changes in human trabecular meshwork tissue after laser trabeculoplasty. *J Ophthalmol*. 2015;2015:476138.
6. Bruen R, Lesk MR, Harasymowycz P. Baseline factors predictive of SLT response: a prospective study. *J Ophthalmol*. 2012;2012:642869.
7. Kuley B, Zheng C, Ed Zhang Q, et al. Predictors of success in selective laser trabeculoplasty. *Ophthalmol Glaucoma*. 2020;3(2):97–102.
8. Alvarado J, Iguchi R, Juster R, et al. From the bedside to the bench and back again: predicting and improving the outcomes of SLT glaucoma therapy. *Trans Am Ophthalmol Soc*. 2009 Dec;107:167–181.
9. Lee J, Shum J, Chan J, Lai J. Two-year clinical results after selective laser trabeculoplasty for normal tension glaucoma. *Medicine*. 2015 June;94(24):e984.
10. Lee J, Ho WL, Chan J, Lai J. Efficacy of selective laser trabeculoplasty for normal tension glaucoma: 1 year results. *BMC Ophthalmol*. 2015 Jan 8;15:1. doi:10.1186/1471-2415-15-1
11. Kiddee W, Atthavuttisilp S. The effects of selective laser trabeculoplasty and travoprost on circadian intraocular pressure fluctuations: a randomized clinical trial. *Medicine (Baltimore)*. 2017 Feb; 96(6):e6047.
12. Tojo N, Oka M, Miyakoshi A, et al. Comparison of fluctuations of intraocular pressure before and after selective laser trabeculoplasty in normal-tension glaucoma patients. *J Glaucoma*. 2014;23:e138–e143.
13. Hodge WG, Damji KF, Rock W, et al. Baseline IOP predicts selective laser trabeculoplasty success at 1 year post-treatment: results from a randomised clinical trial. *Br J Ophthalmol*. 2005;89:1157–1160.
14. Koucheki B, Hashemi H. Selective laser trabeculoplasty in the treatment of open-angle glaucoma. *J Glaucoma*. 2012;21:65–70.
15. Harasymowycz PJ, Papamatheakis DG, Latina M, et al. Selective laser trabeculoplasty (SLT) complicated by intraocular pressure elevation in eyes with heavily pigmented trabecular meshworks. *Am J Ophthalmol*. 2005;139:1110–1113.

16. Ayala M, Chen E. Comparison of selective laser trabeculoplasty (SLT) in primary open angle glaucoma and pseudoexfoliation glaucoma. *Clin Ophthalmol.* 2011;5:1469–1473.

17. Alsagoff Z, Aung T, Ang LP, et al. Long-term clinical course of primary angle-closure glaucoma in an Asian population. *Ophthalmology.* 2000;107:2300–2304.

18. Narayanaswamy A, Leung CK, Istiantoro DV, et al. Efficacy of selective laser trabeculoplasty in primary angle-closure glaucoma: a randomized clinical trial. *JAMA Ophthalmol.* 2015;133:206–212.

19. Ong K, Ong L, Franzco L. Corneal endothelial changes after selective laser trabeculoplasty. *Clin Exp Ophthalmol.* 2013;41:537–540. doi:10.1111/ceo.12068

20. Song J. Complications of selective laser trabeculoplasty: a review. *Clin Ophthalmol.* 2016;10:137–143.

21. Geffen N, Ofir S, Belkin A, et al. Transscleral selective laser trabeculoplasty without a gonioscopy lens. *J Glaucoma.* 2017;26:201–207.

22. American Academy of Ophthalmology. Primary Open Angle Glaucoma: Preferred Practice Pattern. 2015. https://www.aao.org/preferred-practice-pattern/primary-open-angle-glaucoma-ppp (accessed April 29, 2020).

23. Nagar M, Ogunyomade A, O'Brart DP, Howes F, Marshall J. A randomised, prospective study comparing selective laser trabeculoplasty with latanoprost for the control of intraocular pressure in ocular hypertension and open angle glaucoma. *Br J Ophthalmol.* 2005;89(11):1413–1417.

24. Alon S. Selective laser trabeculoplasty: a clinical review. *J Current Glau Prac.* 2013;7(2):58–65.

25. Leahy K, White A. Selective laser trabeculoplasty: current perspectives. *Clin Ophthalmol.* 2015;9; 833–841.

26. Prasad N, Murthy S, Dagianis JJ, et al. A comparison of the intervisit intraocular pressure fluctuation after 180 and 360 degrees of selective laser trabeculoplasty (SLT) as a primary therapy in primary open angle glaucoma and ocular hypertension. *J Glaucoma.* 2009;18:157–160.

27. Shibata M, Sugiyama T, Ishida O, et al. Clinical results of selective laser trabeculoplasty in open-angle glaucoma in Japanese eyes: comparison of 180 degree with 360 degree SLT. *J Glaucoma.* 2012;21:17–21.

28. Katz LJ, Steinmann WC, Kabir A, et al. Selective laser trabeculoplasty versus medical therapy as initial treatment of glaucoma: a prospective, randomized trial. *J Glaucoma.* 2012;21:460–468.

29. Gazzard G, Konstantakopoulou E, Garway-Heath D, et al. Selective laser trabeculoplasty versus eye drops for first-line treatment of ocular hypertension and glaucoma (LiGHT): a multicentre randomised controlled trial. *Lancet.* 2019;393:1505–1516.

30. Woo DM, Healey PR, Graham SL, et al. Intraocular pressure-lowering medications and long-term outcomes of selective laser trabeculoplasty. *Clin Exp Ophthalmol.* 2015;43:320–327.

31. McAlinden C. Selective laser trabeculoplasty (SLT) vs other treatment modalities for glaucoma: systematic review. *Eye (Lond).* 2014;28:249–258.

32. Realini T, Charlton J, Hettlinger M. The impact of anti-inflammatory therapy on intraocular pressure reduction following selective laser trabeculoplasty. *Ophthalmic Surg Lasers Imaging.* 2010;41(1):100–103.

33. Jinapriya D, D'Souza M, Hollands H, et al. Anti-inflammatory therapy after selective laser trabeculoplasty: a randomized, double-masked, placebo-controlled clinical trial. *Ophthalmology.* 2014;121(12):2356–2361.

34. Groth S, Albeiruti E, Nunez M, et al. SALT trial: Steroids after laser trabeculoplasty: impact of short-term anti-inflammatory treatment on selective laser trabeculoplasty efficacy *Ophthalmology.* 2019 Nov;126(11):1511–1516.

35. Latina M, Sibayan S, Shin D, et al. Q-switched 532-nm Nd:YAG laser trabeculoplasty (selective laser trabeculoplasty) a multicenter, pilot, clinical study. *Ophthalmology.* 1998;105:2082–2090.

36. Johnson PB, Katz LJ, Rhee DJ. Selective laser trabeculoplasty: predictive value of early intraocular pressure measurements for success at 3 months. *Br J Ophthalmol.* 2006 Jun;90(6):741–743.

37. Damji K, Shah K, Rock W, Bains H, Hodge W. Selective laser trabeculoplasty vs argon laser trabeculoplasty: a prospective randomized clinical trial. *Br J Ophthalmol.* 1999;83(6):718–722.

38. Wong MO, Lee JW, Choy BN, et al. Systematic review and meta-analysis on the efficacy of selective laser trabeculoplasty in open-angle glaucoma. *Surv Ophthalmol.* 2015;60:36–50.

39. Klamann MK, Maier AK, Gonnermann J, et al. Adverse effects and short-term results after selective laser trabeculoplasty. *J Glaucoma*. 2014;23:105–108.

40. Shihadeh W, Ritch R, Liebman J. Hyphema occurring during selective laser trabeculoplasty. *Ophthalmic Surg Laser Imaging*. 2006;37: 432–433.

41. Rhee DJ, Krad O, Pasquale LR. Hyphema following selective laser trabeculoplasty. *Ophthalmic Surg Lasers Imaging*. 2009;40:493–494.

42. Wechsler DZ, Wechsler IB. Cystoid macular oedema after selective laser trabeculoplasty. *Eye (Lond)*. 2010;24(6):1113.

43. Ha JH, Bowling B, Chen SD. Cystoid macular oedema following selective laser trabeculoplasty in a diabetic patient. *Clin Exp Ophthalmol*. 2014;24(2):200–201.

44. Wu ZQ, Huang J, Sadda S. Selective laser trabeculoplasty complicated by cystoid macular edema: report of two cases. *Eye Sci*. 2012;27: 193–197.

45. Waisbourd M, Katz LJ. Selective laser trabeculoplasty as a first-line therapy: a review. *Can J Ophthalmol*. 2014;49:519–522.

46. Weinand FS, Althen F. Long-term clinical results of selective laser trabeculoplasty in the treatment of primary open angle glaucoma. *Eur J Ophthalmol*. 2006;16(1):100–104.

47. Martow E, Hutnik CM, Mao A. SLT and adjunctive medical therapy: a prediction rule analysis. *J Glaucoma*. 2011;20(4):266–270.

48. Goosen E, Visser L, Sartorius B. Selective laser trabeculoplasty in primary open-angle glaucoma: primary versus secondary treatment outcomes. *African Vision and Eye Health*. 2016;71(1):a338.

49. Goosen E, Coleman K, Visser L, Sponsel WE. Racial differences in selective laser trabeculoplasty efficacy. *J Curr Glaucoma Pract*. 2017;11(1):22–27.

50. Lee JW, Liu CC, Chan JC, et al. Predictors of success in selective laser trabeculoplasty for Chinese open-angle glaucoma. *J Glaucoma*. 2014;23:321–325.

51. Wasyluk JT, Piekarniak-Wozniak A, Grabska-Liberek I, et al. The hypotensive effect of selective laser trabeculoplasty depending on iridocorneal angle pigmentation in primary open angle glaucoma patients. *Arch Med Sci*. 2014;10:306–308.

52. Bovell AM, Damji KF, Hodge WG, et al. Long term effects on the lowering of intraocular pressure: selective laser or argon laser trabeculoplasty? *Can J Ophthalmol*. 2011;46:408–413.

53. Guo Y, Ioannidou A, Jute P. Selective laser trabeculoplasty: a review of repeatability. *Ann Eye Sci*. 2019;4:20.

54. Garg A, Vickerstaff V, Nathwani N, et al. Efficacy of repeat selective laser trabeculoplasty in medication-naive open-angle glaucoma and ocular hypertension during the LiGHT trial. *Ophthalmology*. 2020;127:467–476.

55. Asrani S, Zeimer R, Wilensky J, et al. Large diurnal fluctuations in intraocular pressure are an independent risk factor in patients with glaucoma. *J Glaucoma*. 2000;9:134–142.

56. Nagar M, Luhishi E, Shah N. Intraocular pressure control and fluctuation: the effect of treatment with selective laser trabeculoplasty. *Br J Ophthalmol*. 2009;93(4):497–501.

13 MicroPulse Laser Trabeculoplasty

Myranda R. Partin • Steven R. Sarkisian, Jr.

The clinical management of glaucoma continuously evolves with more efficacious topical medications, less invasive surgeries, and safer laser procedures. Topical anti-glaucoma medications are commonly used as first-line treatments before surgery. In the past, argon laser trabeculoplasty (ALT) and selective laser trabeculoplasty (SLT) have demonstrated safe alternatives to eye drops. Recently, MicroPulse laser trabeculoplasty (MLT) offers another safe, effective alternative to pharmacotherapy in treating glaucoma patients. The procedure is performed with the Iridex IQ laser which is offered in various wavelengths of 532, 577, and 810 nm (Iridex Corporation, Mountain View, CA).[1] The platform has many other applications for ophthalmology, including transscleral cyclophotocoagulation, panretinal photocoagulation, iridotomy, and laser suture lysis.[2,3] The multifaceted Iridex IQ 577 nm is reserved for treatment zones within the macula. There is very little absorption within the macular xanthophyll and higher transmission through dense ocular media, while still targeting melanin in retinal pigment epithelium (RPE).[4] Singh has demonstrated efficacy using the IQ 577 nm continuous wave mode in conjunction with anti-VEGF injections for diabetic macular edema, panretinal photocoagulation, and retinopexy procedures.[5] Moreover, he has shown that pretreating patients with darker colored irides prior to Nd:YAG laser peripheral iridotomy may help decrease patient discomfort. The IQ 577 nm can be switched to MicroPulse mode for laser trabeculoplasty; however, the IQ 532 nm is the standard mode for laser trabeculoplasty because it is the equivalent to the SLT.[6] The 810 nm is reserved for laser cyclophotocoagulation using the MicroPulse P3 glaucoma device powered by Cyclo G6 Glaucoma Laser System.[5]

MicroPulse Technology is an advanced laser technology that breaks up a continuous-wave laser beam into very small, repetitive micropulses, which allow energy to be delivered with intermittent periods. The cooling periods in between the micropulses reduce thermal buildup and tissue damage while inducing beneficial biological effects. MLT is at work 15% of the time while the laser is at rest 85% of the time, effectively eliminating burn complications.[7,8] Each application delivers a 300-ms envelope of 150 2-ms micropulses. Each micropulse consists of 0.3 ms of laser on time (pulse width) and 1.7 ms of laser off time (pulse interval).[2] The permeability of the trabecular meshwork (TM) is increased after the laser due to the release of inflammatory cytokines, similar to how the SLT works but without the thermal damage.[9]

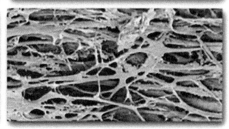

Trabecular meshwork after ALT
CW laser exposures can cause high thermal rise resulting in tissue damage.

MLT
Meshwork remains intact without the signs of tissue damage while still as effective as ALT*.

FIGURE 13-1 Electron microscopy showing how MLT thermally effects but does not destroy pigmented trabecular meshwork cells.[1] (From Gawęcki M. Micropulse laser treatment of retinal diseases. *J Clin Med.* 2019;8(2):242. Published 2019 Feb 13. doi: 10.3390/jcm8020242) ALT, argon laser trabeculoplasty; continuous-wave; MLT, MicroPulse laser trabeculoplasty.

Where MLT differs from SLT is that MLT thermally affects, not destroys, pigmented trabecular meshwork cells without thermal or collateral damage. Cycling the application on and off minimizes the rise in temperature; therefore, the tissue has time to cool off. Microscopic photos have proven that MLT generates enough thermal energy to injure but not alter the trabecular meshwork cells compared to the SLT and ALT lasers.[7] As with any trabeculoplasty, there appears to be an immediate release of cytokines followed by monocytic recruitment that facilitates greater permeability. The principle of laser trabeculoplasty may be explained by several mechanisms, including the mechanical pulling open of the uveoscleral trabecular meshwork and Schlemm's canal, cellular mechanisms that stimulate cell division, and biochemical mechanisms that alter cytokines and stimulate the macrophage-like capacity of trabecular-lining cells (Fig. 13.1).[7]

INDICATIONS

Key Indications

- Primary open-angle glaucoma (POAG)
- Ocular hypertension
- Normal-tension glaucoma (NTG)
- Pigment dispersion syndrome (PDS) or pigmentary glaucoma
- Pseudoexfoliation syndrome (PXE) or pseudoexfoliative glaucoma
- Primary angle closure (PAC) or primary angle closure glaucoma (PACG) after successful angle-closure treatment.

Laser treatments for glaucoma have been gaining popularity as first-line treatments because hypotensive drops cause disruption to the ocular surface, are costly to patients, and often are associated with poor compliance. Hyperemia and lash growth due to topical medications are generally considered minor cosmetic problems. However, hyperemia can be a burden for patients who are still working or have an active social life. Surgery may achieve lower intraocular pressure (IOP), but it is associated with greater risks and complications not seen with laser therapies. The concept behind pulsed laser delivery is to minimize thermal energy and physiological damage to ocular tissue. MLT offers advantages over other forms of trabeculoplasty and can be a great tool for any glaucoma practice.

The similarities between SLT and MLT are beneficial due to the significant research already done with the SLT laser. Ocular hypertension and POAG are well known to have the best response to laser therapy compared to other types of glaucoma. Several studies have shown MLT to reduce IOP of POAG patients by 12.2% to 21.3%.[10–12] In the past, success rates with SLT have been correlated with higher starting levels in IOP; however, NTG has also seen beneficial outcomes with laser therapies.[13,14] It would be reasonable to believe that MLT would also have similar outcomes although further research is still needed.

Laser trabeculoplasty, such as ALT and SLT, has been a successful option in the past for pigmentary and pseudoexfoliation glaucoma patients who need adjunctive therapy or wish to lessen their need for drops. The biochemical theory in which MLT mimics SLT would conjecture that it also would be a fair option; however, to this date, the authors know of no studies having been performed. Similar to SLT, the MLT laser settings likely should be titrated down for pigmentary glaucoma or those with heavier pigmented TM. Studies have shown a higher occurrence rate for post-laser IOP spikes in those with darker pigmented angles.[14,15] However, in patients with PXE, the success and adverse event rate compare similarly with POAG, and the presence of pseudoexfoliation does not increase the rate of a post-laser IOP spike.[14,16]

Even though SLT, ALT, and MLT need an open angle to be performed, those with PAC or PACG can still benefit from the IOP-lowering effects once their anterior chambers have been modified through angle opening therapies and a healthy TM remains.[13,14]

CONTRAINDICATIONS

Key Contraindications

- Any type of angle-closure glaucoma or angle closure where adequate TM is not visible
- A relatively high preoperative IOP (>30 mm Hg) in conjunction with advanced optic nerve damage, in which case a possible postoperative transient IOP elevation is thought to pose a significant risk for the patient's vision

- Glaucoma associated with uveitis, trauma, ischemia/neovascularization, juvenile open-angle glaucoma, or angle dysgenesis
- A history of previous MLT failure in the same or fellow eye
- Congenital glaucoma
- Significant corneal endothelial disease

Glaucoma associated with inflammatory conditions or neovascularization is contraindicated due to the potential of the laser worsening the condition. Numerous studies have been done on the ALT and SLT laser for such conditions but not yet the MLT. However, one can assume the outcome would be similar. One study done on uveitic patients with glaucoma who underwent SLT showed only 8% of quiet eyes (no inflammation for at least 90 days) had flare compared with 13% of controlled eyes (inflammation within 90 days but quiet on the day of the procedure). It was concluded that SLT was still considered a viable treatment modality.[17]

Those without any corneal endothelial disease have shown in previous studies an incidence of corneal edema post-SLT as approximately 0.8%.[18] At one-week postoperatively, thinning was documented and thought to be contributed by the laser heat dissipation causing stromal contractions. Normal corneal thickness readings were again found by one-month post-laser and postulated to be from keratocyte migration and stromal remodeling.[19] In compromised corneas, the effects of SLT may be transient but they have a higher long-term risk, especially after repeated SLT.[20] MLT likely follows a similar contraindication profile as SLT.

INFORMED CONSENT CONSIDERATIONS

Key Informed Consent Adverse Events Listed as Follows:

- IOP spike
- Inflammation
- Pain/discomfort during and/or after the procedure
- Macular edema
- Corneal haze/edema
- Transient blurring of vision
- Bleeding/hyphema
- Lack of efficacy
- Loss of efficacy over time

Informed consent is important not only for liability purposes but also to help the patient understand more about the procedure. A brief summary in laymen terms should include how the laser works on the pigmented region of the "drain" in their eye and that their body uses immune cells to help clean out the drain. In return, this lowers the eye pressure which is currently the only modality of treatment. Although laser trabeculoplasty is considered a minor procedure, it still needs to be taken seriously. While the incidence of an adverse event is low, the patient needs to be well educated by the attending physician.

Key informed consent adverse events include but are not limited to an IOP spike, postoperative inflammation, discomfort during or after the procedure, transient blurring of vision, ineffectiveness of the procedure, bleeding, or corneal edema. It should be documented that the patient was counseled on alternative options, informed of risks, including that the procedure may not work, and future alternative methods of treatment could be required. Such alternatives include hypotensive eye drops, minor invasive glaucoma surgeries, monitoring, or more invasive surgery.

A note from the counseling physician should be included and phrased similar to, "I have counseled this patient as to the nature of the proposed procedure, the attendant risks involved, and the expected results." The patient's and doctor's names should be printed and signed with the date as well as a witness signature.

PREOPERATIVE CARE

Key Preoperative Considerations

- Pre-laser measurement of IOP
- Gonioscopy assessing for openness of the angle, amount of pigment in the TM, indications, and contraindications.
- Preoperative drops: Alpha-agonist, proparacaine, and pilocarpine (rare)

Gonioscopy should always be performed before recommending laser trabeculoplasty. Documentation must include which angles were viewed along with the amount of openness, pigmentation, and any obstructing factors such as peripheral anterior synechiae, stents, or tubes.

A drop of apraclonidine 0.5% or brimonidine 0.1% to 0.2% should be instilled into the operative eye 15 to 30 minutes before the procedure to help control a postoperative IOP spike. Pilocarpine 1% to 2% can be utilized if more of the angle structures and TM need to be viewed to perform the procedure. A Goldmann 3-mirror lens is used to visualize the angle structures and direct the laser energy toward the TM. A coupling agent such as 2% or 2.5% hydroxypropyl methylcellulose (Gonak, Goniosoft, or Goniosol) is necessary since the radius of curvature of the Goldmann

3-mirror lens is smaller than that of the cornea. Immediately before the procedure, proparacaine should be instilled into both eyes; installation in the fellow eye will help control blinking during the procedure.

SETTINGS AND PROCEDURE

Key MLT Settings

- Energy
  - 1,000 mW[8]
- Spot size
  - 300 µm
- Pulse duration
  - 300 ms (0.3 s) with a 15% duty cycle (laser on time)
- Wavelength
  - 532 nm
- Magnification
  - 12.5 to 16× (medium range)

A power setting of 1,000 mW has been demonstrated to generate the greatest reduction of IOP at one and four months.[8] 360° of application is preferred but can be titrated based on the physician's clinical judgment. The spot size is 300 µm, compared to the SLT's 400 µm size, which may allow MLT to be more useful for more narrow angles.[1] The difference in spot size influences how much irradiance or energy per square area is applied to the TM. The MLT laser has multiple wavelength settings, with the trabeculoplasty setting being 532 nm, just like the SLT. It also has an additional wavelength setting of 577 nm (yellow), which is typically utilized more in retinal cases.

The patient must be seated comfortably in the chair and have their chin and forehead rested appropriately on the slit lamp. The laser procedure can then begin with patient education that they may see a flash of light or hear a click during the procedure, but not to pull back from the laser until the procedure is complete. MLT does not result in any visible tissue reaction (champagne bubbles or blanching of the tissue) during treatment, creating a more difficult challenge titrating energy levels compared to SLT and ALT. Although SLT energy is titrated based on visible microbubbles, typically requiring less energy in heavily pigmented TMs, it is not customary to deviate from the manufacturer's recommended energy setting (1,000 mW power, 300 µm spot size, 300 ms duration with a 15% duty cycle, 360° treatment) during MLT. Various methods were attempted in clinical trials of altering the power setting to 700, 800, and 1,000 mW. Clinical benefits were seen with each setting, with the 1,000-mW setting having the most robust IOP-lowering effects without any further complications. The 300-μm spot size is a factory setting and was intentionally chosen to help with smaller angles.[8] The pulse duration as discussed earlier is 300 ms; however, with the micropulse technology each 300 ms (0.3 s), laser pulse is broken down into 150 2-ms pulses, which represents a duty cycle of 15% work and 85% rest.

Key Procedural Points

- Magnification—medium
- Illumination tower variable to wherever produces the best view
- Laser lens mirror placement
  - Ritch trabeculoplasty lens
  - MLT laser lens
- Approximately 100 to 200 nonoverlapping laser pulses for 360° treatment, and 50 to 100 laser pulses for 180° treatment
- 360° treatment is typically recommended

The magnification setting should be comfortable for the treating physician to view the angle's structures but not too high as to cause a loss of focus. The illumination tower should be angled out approximately 30° to get an unobstructed view without causing glare or losing the light beam. Placing the lens does not have to be specific but it should be consistent. Using a one-mirrored lens such as the MLT lens, start at the 9 or 3 o'clock position to work one hemisphere at a time. 360° of the

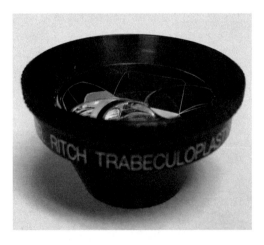

FIGURE 13-2 The Ritch trabeculoplasty laser lens is designed with two 59° and two 64° mirrors. A 1.4x magnifying button is placed over one of the 59° and 64° mirrors. The magnifying button reduces the laser spot size by 30% and increases the laser power by 2x. (From Alward W, Longmuir R. Principles of gonioscopy [Internet]. American Academy of Ophthalmology. 2017 [cited 2020 Dec 18]. Available from: https://www.aao.org/disease-review/principles-of-gonioscopy; Ritch Trabeculoplasty [Internet]. [cited 2020 Dec 18]. Available from: https://www.eyecareandcure.com/ECC-Products/SLT-Iridectomy-Capsulotomy/Ritch-Trabeculoplasty)

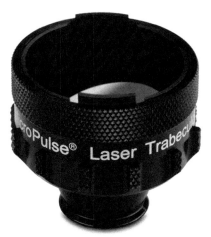 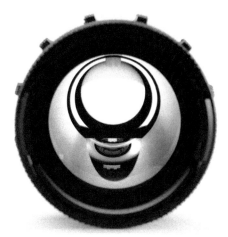

FIGURE 13-3 The MicroPulse laser trabeculoplasty laser lens has an integrated reference guide to assist the placement of subthreshold laser spots during MicroPulse laser trabeculoplasty. The reference guide allows 10 consecutive, 300 μm spots to be placed before the need to rotate. Twelve mirror rotations or "clicking rotations" of the mirror will cover 360°, and therefore a complete rotation of the lens (12 mirror rotations) allows for approximately 120 laser spots.[1] Note that one mirror is located in the 6:00 position (doctor's perspective).

angle is recommended during treatment but if choosing to do only 180°, the inferior half is usually chosen first due to it often containing greater pigment and a wider angle. Looking in the mirror, the single-aiming beam should be placed upon the TM starting near one side of the mirror, and then 10 nonoverlapping laser pulses are consecutively placed moving either clockwise or counterclockwise. The lens is then rotated and the next mirror treated with another approximate 10 nonoverlapping laser pulses. This sequence is then repeated until 360°, or the desired treatment zone, has been covered (Figs. 13.2 and 13.3).

POSTOPERATIVE CARE/CO-MANAGEMENT (FOLLOW-UP SCHEDULE)

Key Postoperative Considerations

- Postoperative drops: alpha-agonist in-office and anti-inflammatory prescribed
- IOP check 30 to 60 minutes post procedure
- IOP check one to two weeks post procedure
- Final IOP check to assess the full effectiveness of the procedure six to eight weeks post procedure

The number of shots, energy per shot, and total amount of energy used should be recorded in the patient's chart. Information on how the patient tolerated the procedure should also be recorded. Immediately after the procedure has finished, another 1 to 2 drops of brimonidine or apraclonidine should be instilled into the operative eye. After 30 to 60 minutes, the pressure should be checked and determined if there is a significant rise in IOP. In one study comparing MLT to SLT, none of the patients who received MLT had any significant rise in IOP, whereas 10% (5/50) of patients who received SLT experienced 1-hour postoperative IOP spikes of ≥5 mm Hg.[4]

It is debated whether or not a steroid should be indicated postoperatively. According to the Steroids after Laser Trabeculoplasty (SALT) trial for the SLT laser, postoperative steroids are beneficial. However, since the study did not include the MLT laser, it is left to the treating physician's discretion. For an IOP spike greater than 10 mm Hg, supplementary IOP-lowering medications may be indicated. A one-week follow-up is scheduled to monitor for a pressure spike, inflammation, ocular irritation, and patient reassurance and education. A minimum of six weeks is allowed after MLT has been performed before discussing repeat laser, considering other procedures, or changing medication, as six weeks is the approximate timeframe to determine the full effect of the procedure.[23,24]

POTENTIAL COMPLICATIONS AND THEIR TREATMENT

Key Potential Complications to Look for the Following

- IOP spike
- Inflammation
- Redness, pain, and/or blurred vision
- Peripheral anterior synechiae
- Corneal haze

In one study published in the journal *Medicine*, 7.5% of MLT patients had a mild, self-limiting anterior uveitis post-laser, which was found to be clinically significant.[9] In another study, only one patient with PDS had flare detected with the Kowa FM 500 flare.[12] In a third study, none of the patients reported side effects nor were there any cell or flare documented.[25] Conclusively, it is known that MLT has very mild if any side effects. The list of side effects mentioned earlier and the ones included in the laser consent form section are historically based on SLT post-laser complications.[26]

VIDEOS OF PROCEDURE

Video 13.1—Video showing a portion of an MLT procedure. Notice minimal to no reaction of the tissue is seen. Video courtesy of Dr. Ike K. Ahmed and Iridex.

Video 13.2—Sixteen-minute video giving a great tutorial and overview of MLT from world-renowned leading glaucoma expert Dr. Ike K. Ahmed. Video courtesy of Dr. Ike K. Ahmed and Iridex.

EFFICACY—RELEVANT MICROPULSE LASER TRABECULOPLASTY STUDY DATA

How Does MicroPulse Laser Trabeculoplasty Compare to Selective Laser Trabeculoplasty?

Coombs and Radcliff compared the effectiveness of SLT versus MLT. The study had 12 eyes that underwent MLT and 14 that underwent SLT. Eyes in both the MLT and SLT groups had significantly lower IOP after laser trabeculoplasty, with MLT mean IOP reduction equal to 3.9 mm Hg and SLT mean IOP reduction equal to 2.6 mm Hg. MLT eyes were on fewer drops following treatment, with mean pretreatment drops equal to 1.9 compared to mean posttreatment drops of 1.4. MLT eyes also had a greater decrease in the number of drops used compared to SLT eyes. The study concluded MLT appears comparable to SLT in lowering IOP and reducing the need for topical medication.[27]

How Much Does the MicroPulse Laser Trabeculoplasty Lower Intraocular Pressure?

Investigators in Hong Kong showed that MLT had a mean percentage IOP reduction of 24% and the success rate was 73%.[9] Ahmed and co-investigators showed a 30% decrease in overall IOP in their own clinical studies.[8] Just as with SLT, the percentage of IOP reduction is likely dependent upon multiple variables, including pre-laser IOP and the number of pre-laser IOP-lowering medications the patient is on. Overall, MLT is likely going to achieve a similar percentage of IOP reduction as SLT.

Efficacy in Different Patient Populations

Most of the MLT studies have been conducted in China and the United States.[28,29] A majority of these studies have looked at MLT in open-angle glaucoma or ocular hypertension. Currently, to the author's knowledge, there is no great literature studying MLT in normal tension or angle closure following successful angle-closure treatment. One study was done over pseudoexfoliative glaucoma and concluded that micropulse trabeculoplasty demonstrated similar efficacy to SLT in PXE patients.[30] Overall, MLT likely has a similar efficacy profile across different patient populations as compared to SLT.

Predictive Factors for Success

In the study, "Comparison of successful outcome predictors for MicroPulse laser trabeculoplasty and selective laser trabeculoplasty at 6 months," the main goal was to identify and compare factors predictive of successful outcomes for MLT and SLT. There was no statistically significant association between degree of pigmentation in the TM, age, or glaucoma severity and the success rate for either SLT or MLT. Fewer number of shots were associated with success in MLT but not with SLT patients. Lastly, baseline IOP was not a statistically significant predictor of success for MLT patients but was in SLT patients at the six-month follow-up.[4]

How Long Does MicroPulse Laser Trabeculoplasty Last?

In a phase-II clinical trial, the treatment was successful in 75% at 12 months.[12] Similar articles by current MLT users have shown long-term efficacies comparable to SLT. SLT treatment efficacy is known to diminish with time, and the same is likely true with MLT. However, as shown in the LiGHT trial, 74.2% of patients were drop free three years after primary SLT treatment.[31] Proper patient education is advised to set up proper expectations. As with any laser trabeculoplasty, it does not guarantee a drop-free regimen or lasting effectivity. Overall, MLT duration of effectiveness is likely thought to have a similar profile to SLT.

Repeatability of MicroPulse Laser Trabeculoplasty

As MLT causes no structural damage to the TM, retreatment is a viable option as long as a clinically significant IOP reduction was achieved with the initial treatment. It is not advised to continue MLT as a treatment option if the IOP remains unchanged or progression continues with visual fields after the initial MLT treatment. Studies looking at the repeatability of SLT have shown a positive effect and have concluded that repeat treatment can continue as a first-line option if target IOP is met.[32,33] Therefore, since MLT parallels with SLT in a majority of characteristics, it is thought to be safe to repeat MLT as well.

Corneal Changes after MLT

In one study, central corneal thickness, endothelial cell count, hexagonal cell ratio, and coefficient of variation of the endothelial cell size showed no significant change between baseline and six months after MLT in both primary open-angle and pseudo-exfoliation glaucoma eyes.[30]

Incisional glaucoma surgery can often achieve lower IOP; however, there are greater risks and complications associated with surgery that are not seen with laser therapy. The concept behind pulsed laser delivery is to minimize thermal energy and, therefore its resultant physiological damage to ocular tissue. MLT offers advantages over other forms of laser trabeculoplasty and can be a great tool for any glaucoma practice. Thankfully lasers are becoming more of a first-line treatment option for glaucoma patients and can help alleviate previous problematic issues such as drop compliance and side effects.

CODING/BILLING

The CPT code 65855, *Trabeculoplasty by laser surgery*, is used for all trabeculoplasty procedures. Medicare assigns a ten-day postoperative period to laser trabeculoplasty, which makes laser trabeculoplasty a minor procedure according to Medicare. If both eyes are done in the same session, use modifier-50 after CPT code. Typically, it is recommended to perform one eye at a time unless patient factors necessitate bilateral same-day treatment. When treating the fellow eye during the global period of the first procedure, use modifier-79 after CPT code.

Common ICD-10 codes that support this procedure include the following:

H40.1111 to H40.1134 (primary open-angle glaucoma)
H40.011 to H40.029 (open angle with borderline findings)
H40.1310 to H40.1394 (pigmentary glaucoma)
H40.051 to H40.53 (ocular hypertension)
H40.1211 to H40.1294 (low-tension glaucoma)
H40.1411 to H40.1494 (capsular glaucoma with pseudoexfoliation of lens)
H40.2210 to H40.2294 (chronic angle-closure glaucoma)

REFERENCES

1. Gawęcki M. Micropulse laser treatment of retinal diseases. *J Clin Med*. 2019;8(2):242. Published 2019 Feb 13. doi:10.3390/jcm8020242
2. Iwach A. Micropulse laser trabeculoplasty. *Glacuoma Today* [Internet]. 2008 Jan [cited 2020 Dec 13]; Available from: https://glaucomatoday.com/articles/2008-jan-feb/GT0108_05-php
3. Mansour S. MicroPulse laser therapy of diabetic macular edema success in anti-VEGF non-responder [Internet]. Iridex. [cited 2020 Dec 13]. Available from: https://iridex.com/Portals/0/physician-education/pdf/Mansour,577 MP Anti-VEGF.pdf
4. Hirabayashi MT, Rosenlof T, An JA. Comparison of successful outcome predictors for MicroPulse laser trabeculoplasty and selective laser trabeculoplasty at 6 months. *Clin Ophthalmol* [Internet]. 2019 Jun 14 [cited 2020 Dec 17];Volume 13:1001–1009. Available from: https://www.dovepress.com/comparison-of-successful-outcome-predictors-for-micropulsereg-laser-tr-peer-reviewed-article-OPTH
5. Singh GM. Continuous-Wave and MicroPulse Modes, the IRIDEX IQ 577 Laser Provides Uncommon Versatility [Internet]. 2017 [cited 2020 Dec 18]. Available from: www.iridex.com
6. Ahmed I, Gossage D, Vold S. With years of SLT data, why consider MLT? [Internet]. 2013 Sep [cited 2020 Dec 18]. Available from: http://eyetube.net/?v=nohog

7. Sihota R. Lasers in primary open angle glaucoma. In: Indian Journal of Ophthalmology [Internet]. Wolters Kluwer--Medknow Publications; 2011 [cited 2020 Dec 13]. p. S114. Available from: /pmc/articles/PMC3038499/?report=abstract

8. Ahmed I, Gossage D, Vold S. MicroPulse laser trabeculoplasty [Internet]. [cited 2020 Dec 13]. Available from: http://eyetube.net/?v=nohog

9. Lee JWY, Yau GSK, Yick DWF, Yuen CYF. Micro pulse laser trabeculoplasty for the treatment of open-angle glaucoma. *Med (United States)* [Internet]. 2015 [cited 2020 Dec 13];94(49). Available from: https://pubmed.ncbi.nlm.nih.gov/26656331/

10. Detry-Morel M, Muschart F, Pourjavan S. Micropulse diode laser (810 nm) versus argon laser trabeculoplasty in the treatment of open-angle glaucoma: comparative short-term safety and efficacy profile. *Bull Soc Belge Ophtalmol.* 2008;(308):21–28. PMID: 18700451.

11. Lee JWY, Yau GSK, Yick DWF, Yuen CYF. Micro pulse laser trabeculoplasty for the treatment of open-angle glaucoma. *Med (United States)* [Internet]. 2015 [cited 2020 Dec 14];94(49). Available from: /pmc/articles/PMC5008476/?report=abstract

12. Fea A. Micropulse diode laser trabeculoplasty (MDLT): A phase II clinical study with 12 months follow-up. *Clin Ophthalmol* [Internet]. 2008 Jun [cited 2020 Dec 14];2(2):247. Available from: /pmc/articles/PMC2693967/?report=abstract

13. Narayanaswamy A, Leung CK, Istiantoro DV, Perera SA, Ho C, Nongpiur ME, et al. Efficacy of selective laser trabeculoplasty in primary angle-closure glaucoma: a randomized clinical trial. *JAMA Ophthalmol* [Internet]. 2015 Feb 1 [cited 2020 Dec 15];133(2):206–212. Available from: https://pubmed.ncbi.nlm.nih.gov/25429421/

14. Kennedy JB, SooHoo JR, Kahook MY, Seibold LK. Selective laser trabeculoplasty. *Asia-Pacific J Ophthalmol* [Internet]. 2016 [cited 2020 Dec 15];5(1):63–69. Available from: http://content.wkhealth.com/linkback/openurl?sid=WKPTLP:landingpage&an=01599573-201601000-00012

15. Koucheki B, Hashemi H. Selective laser trabeculoplasty in the treatment of open-angle glaucoma. *J Glaucoma* [Internet]. 2012 Jan [cited 2020 Dec 15];21(1):65–70. Available from: https://pubmed.ncbi.nlm.nih.gov/21278588/

16. Ayala M, Chen E. Comparison of selective laser trabeculoplasty (SLT) in primary open angle glau. *Clin Ophthalmol* [Internet]. 2011 [cited 2020 Dec 15];5(1):1469–1473. Available from: https://pubmed.ncbi.nlm.nih.gov/22069348/

17. Swan R, Foster CS. Incidence of inflammation following selective laser trabeculoplasty in uveitic eyes | IOVS | ARVO Journals [Internet]. Investigative Ophthalmology & Visual Science. 2015 [cited 2020 Dec 15]. Available from: https://iovs.arvojournals.org/article.aspx?articleid=2336225

18. Latina MA, Tumbocon JAJ. Selective laser trabeculoplasty: a new treatment option for open angle glaucoma [Internet]. Vol. 13, Current Opinion in Ophthalmology. *Curr Opin Ophthalmol;* 2002 [cited 2020 Dec 16]: 94–96. Available from: https://pubmed.ncbi.nlm.nih.gov/11880722/

19. Lee JWY, Chan JCH, Chang RT, Singh K, Liu CCL, Gangwani R, et al. Corneal changes after a single session of selective laser trabeculoplasty for open-angle glaucoma. *Eye* [Internet]. 2014 [cited 2020 Dec 16];28(1):47–52. Available from: /pmc/articles/PMC3890760/?report=abstract

20. Ong K, Ong L, Ong L. Corneal endothelial changes after selective laser trabeculoplasty. *Clin Experiment Ophthalmol* [Internet]. 2013 Aug 1 [cited 2020 Dec 15];41(6):537–540. Available from: http://doi.wiley.com/10.1111/ceo.12068

21. Alward W, Longmuir R. Principles of gonioscopy [Internet]. *American Academy of Ophthalmology.* 2017 [cited 2020 Dec 18]. Available from: https://www.aao.org/disease-review/principles-of-gonioscopy

22. Ritch Trabeculoplasty [Internet]. [cited 2020 Dec 18]. Available from: https://www.eyecareandcure.com/ECC-Products/SLT-Iridectomy-Capsulotomy/Ritch-Trabeculoplasty

23. Garg A, Gazzard G. Selective laser trabeculoplasty: past, present, and future. *Eye (Lond).* 2018 May;32(5):863–876. doi:10.1038/eye.2017.273. Epub 2018 Jan 5. Erratum in: *Eye (Lond).* 2020 Aug;34(8):1487. PMID: 29303146; PMCID: PMC5944654.

24. Johnson PB, Katz LJ, Rhee DJ. Selective laser trabeculoplasty: predictive value of early intraocular pressure measurements for success at 3 months. *Br J Ophthalmol.* 2006.

25. Valera-Cornejo D, Loayza-Gamboa W, Herrera-Quiroz J, Alvarado-Vlllacorta R, Cordova-Crisanto L, Valderrama-Albino V, et al. Micropulse trabeculoplasty in open angle glaucoma. *Adv Biomed Res* [Internet]. 2018 [cited 2020 Dec 21];7(1):156. Available from: /pmc/articles/PMC6319042/?report=abstract

26. Song J. Complications of selective laser trabeculoplasty: a review [Internet]. Vol. 10, Clinical Ophthalmology. Dove Medical Press Ltd; 2016 [cited 2020 Dec 21]: 137–143. Available from: /pmc/articles/PMC4716769/?report=abstract

27. Coombs P, Radcliffe NM. Outcomes of micropulse laser trabeculoplasty vs. selective laser trabeculoplasty. *Invest Ophthalmol Vis Sci* [Internet]. 2014 [cited 2020 Dec 13];55(13):6155. Available from: https://iovs.arvojournals.org/article.aspx?articleid=2271829

28. Hong Y, Song SJ, Liu B, Hassanpour K, Zhang C, Loewen N. Efficacy and safety of micropulse laser trabeculoplasty for primary open angle glaucoma. *Int J Ophthalmol* [Internet]. 2019 [cited 2020 Dec 21];12(5):784–788. Available from: /pmc/articles/PMC6520269/?report=abstract

29. Abramowitz B, Chadha N, Kouchouk A, Alhabshan R, Belyea DA, Lamba T. Selective laser trabeculoplasty vs micropulse laser trabeculoplasty in open-angle glaucoma. *Clin Ophthalmol* [Internet]. 2018 [cited 2020 Dec 22];12:1599–1604. Available from: /pmc/articles/PMC6124459/?report=abstract

30. Makri OE, Plotas P, Christopoulou E, Georgakopoulos CD. Effect of a single session of micropulse laser trabeculoplasty on corneal endothelial parameters. *Clin Exp Optom* [Internet]. 2020 Jul 16 [cited 2020 Dec 21];103(4):479–483. Available from: https://onlinelibrary.wiley.com/doi/abs/10.1111/cxo.12968

31. Gazzard G, Konstantakopoulou E, Garway-Heath D, Garg A, Bunce C, Wormald R, et al. Selective laser trabeculoplasty versus eye drops for first-line treatment of ocular hypertension and glaucoma (LiGHT): a multicentre randomised controlled trial. *Lancet* [Internet]. 2019 Apr 13 [cited 2020 Dec 21];393(10180):1505–1516. Available from: https://pubmed.ncbi.nlm.nih.gov/30862377/

32. Guo Y, Ioannidou A, Jute P. Selective laser trabeculoplasty: a review of repeatability. *Ann Eye Sci.* 2019;4:20. Available from: http://aes.amegroups.com/article/view/4834/html

33. Garg A, Vickerstaff V, Nathwani N, Garway-Heath D, Konstantakopoulou E, Ambler G, et al. Efficacy of repeat selective laser trabeculoplasty in medication-naive open-angle glaucoma and ocular hypertension during the LiGHT trial. *Ophthalmology* [Internet]. 2020 Apr 1 [cited 2020 Dec 22];127(4): 467–476. doi:10.1016/j.ophtha.2019.10.023

14 Peripheral Iridotomy and Iridoplasty

Jeff M. Miller

The concept of pupillary block is central to understanding the mechanism of a peripheral iridotomy (PI). As forward aqueous flow between the lens and posterior iris is impeded, pressure builds behind the iris. This distends the iris forward, narrows the anterior chamber angle, and reduces aqueous clearance through the trabecular meshwork.

An iridotomy is essentially a bypass mechanism allowing aqueous to escape to the anterior chamber from behind the iris. This equalizes the pressure between the anterior and posterior chambers and keeps the angle open. The first known attempt at this process was in the 19th century with a surgical iridectomy.[1] Laser peripheral iridotomy (LPI or PI) was introduced in the 1970s using an Argon laser, and by the 1980s, laser iridotomy had displaced surgical iridectomy as the more common procedure.[2,3]

Today, both the photodisruptive Q-switched Nd:YAG laser 1064 nm (usually shortened to just "YAG") and the photothermal Nd:YAG-KTP 532-nm laser (often referred to as a "Green laser" or, erroneously, an Argon laser) may be utilized with a PI. Typically, a PI is completed with a photodisruptive 1064-nm Nd:YAG while a green laser, if utilized, is used to pretreat the iris in order to thin the targeted tissue. Pretreating with a green laser is often beneficial for a thicker, brown iris as it reduces the amount of tissue to penetrate, reduces the amount of energy needed from the Nd:YAG, and often provides an easier PI procedure. However, the green laser's limited applications in other primary eye care procedures may not justify the additional expense.

INDICATIONS

Key Indications

- Primary angle-closure suspect (PACS)
- Primary angle closure (PAC)
- Primary angle-closure glaucoma (PACG)
- Acute, symptomatic PAC crisis
- Plateau iris configuration

The most common indication for an LPI is a prophylactic PI for primary angle closure suspects (PACS) who are judged to be at higher risk for angle closure than the average population. While effective in relieving pupil block, the practitioner must be judicious with patient selection when contemplating a prophylactic PI as most patients with narrow angle will not go on to develop angle closure.[4]

Findings that may indicate the need for a prophylactic PI in an angle-closure suspect include no visible structures on gonioscopy in at least 180°; angles of approximately 10° or less as judged by anterior segment optical coherence tomography (OCT); anterior chamber depth of less than 2.5 mm; and/or a family history of angle closure.

Primary angle closure (PAC) is an indication for a PI. PAC is defined as any of the previously mentioned findings along with increased intraocular pressure (IOP) and/or the presence of peripheral anterior synechiae. Primary angle closure glaucoma (PACG) demonstrates increased IOP and synechiae along with glaucomatous optic nerve head damage as indicated by visual field and OCT testing. A PI is generally indicated for PACG patients.

Laser PI is an effective treatment for patients with acute, symptomatic PAC along with medications. Any patient with acute angle closure in one eye should have a prophylactic PI in the contralateral eye due to the significantly increased risk for angle closure.[5]

Plateau iris is caused by anteriorly positioned ciliary body processes, which push the peripheral iris forward. Plateau iris configuration often has some pupil block present and therefore a PI is indicated. This also helps to clinically differentiate plateau iris configuration from plateau iris syndrome, which is a persistent angle closure despite a patent PI.[6,7] These patients may benefit from an iridoplasty, which will be discussed at the end of this chapter.

While primarily reserved for narrow-/closed-angle glaucomas, PI may be considered for pigmentary dispersion syndrome and pigmentary glaucoma, which are open-angle processes. These conditions often demonstrate an imbalance of IOP in the anterior and posterior chambers, with a higher pressure in the anterior chamber, which causes the iris to bow backward onto the lens zonules. The rubbing of the lens zonules on the back of the iris liberates the pigment, which then obstructs the trabecular meshwork. This phenomenon of backward iris bowing is known as reverse pupillary block. The pressure imbalance between the anterior and posterior chambers can be relieved by a PI and potentially decrease the irido-zonular friction and pigment liberation.

However, there is inconsistent evidence as to whether a PI slows pigmentary glaucoma disease progression.[8] Anterior segment imaging—ultrasound biomicroscopy or anterior segment OCT—should be performed before the PI to confirm evidence of posterior iris bowing. A PI will not reduce any pigment dispersion in the absence of posterior bowing and will only liberate additional pigment. Finally, caution should be used in pigmentary glaucoma patients with existing optic nerve head damage as a potential IOP spike could increase the patient's glaucomatous injury.

Other, less common, indications for a PI include an aphakic patient in need of an anterior chamber intraocular lens (IOL). Due to the high risk of pupil block with an anterior chamber IOL, a prophylactic PI is warranted. Similarly, an iridotomy before an implantable contact lens refractive surgery procedure provides for a safer surgical environment and reduces the risk of postoperative pupil block.

A subluxed posterior IOL or natural lens may also benefit from a PI. While a lensectomy may still need to be performed, relieving any pupil block will provide a safer surgical environment.

CONTRAINDICATIONS

Key Contraindications

- Secondary angle closures not involving pupil block
- Corneal opacities precluding view of the iris
- Extremely shallow anterior chamber
- Patient with unreliable fixation

The stronger contraindications to a PI include corneal opacities (edema, scar) prohibiting a clear view; a very shallow anterior chamber in which the corneal endothelium would be at risk from laser energy; or a patient unable to fixate and/or maintain posture in the slit lamp. Significant intraocular inflammation would also preclude the use of an ophthalmic laser. PIs should be avoided in secondary angle closure that does not feature pupil block such as neovascular glaucoma, irido-corneal endothelial syndrome, and inflammatory glaucoma. A PI is generally avoided in medication-induced angle closure (e.g., topiramate) due to the lack of efficacy.[9]

Relative contraindications include chronic corneal conditions (e.g., Fuchs endothelial dystrophy) and chronic retinal conditions (cystoid macular edema, epiretinal membrane). The risk–benefit ratio should be assessed for these patients. For mild and stable conditions, a PI may still be indicated after informed consent. For more severe disease, the underlying condition may need to be addressed first and/or other narrow-angle treatment options, such as cataract surgery, should be explored.

The presence of peripheral anterior synechiae, while not a contraindication, is related to the effectiveness of a PI. The amount of synechiae is inversely correlated with the expected amount of angle-opening post PI, and angle quadrants with peripheral anterior synechiae may not show appreciable opening after the PI.[10]

INFORMED CONSENT CONSIDERATIONS

Key Informed Consent Adverse Events Listed as Follows:

- IOP spike
- Inflammation
- Non-patency of the PI hole
- Transient blurring of vision
- Visual disturbances/glare/halos/lines in vision
- Floaters
- Bleeding/hyphema
- Cataract formation

Informed consent should include a description of the procedure in plain language. For example, "A laser will be used to create a small opening in the colored part of the eye (iris) to allow fluid to flow freely from behind the iris to the drainage system in the front of the eye. This will help reduce the risk of a certain type of glaucoma known as angle-closure glaucoma."

Potential alternative treatments, such as eye drops, monitoring, or invasive surgery, should be listed. Risks and complications inherent to any laser procedure include but are not limited to increased eye pressure, floaters, eye inflammation, irritation, and temporary blurring of vision. Complications more specific to PI include hyphema or microhyphema; the need for a repeat PI procedure; visual disturbances such as glare, halos, or lines in vision; as well as retinal detachment and permanent vision loss. While the incidence of retinal detachment after PI is very low, perhaps due to most eyes being hyperopic with a short axial length, it should still be considered for an informed consent.[11]

A note from the counseling physician should be included and phrased similar to, "I have counseled this patient as to the nature of the proposed procedure, the attendant risks involved, and the expected results." The patient's and doctor's names should be printed and signed with the date as well as a witness signature (typically a staff member).

PREOPERATIVE CARE

Key Preoperative Considerations

- Gonioscopy assessing for indications and contraindications
- Location—11:00, 1:00, 3:00, or 9:00 position, preferably in an iris crypt
- Preoperative drops: Alpha-agonist, pilocarpine, and proparacaine

If not already performed, angles should be viewed via gonioscopy to assess visible structures and any pathology such as peripheral anterior synechiae. Additionally, anterior segment OCT may be performed.

The iris should be examined for a suitable location for the PI. This should be near the limbus, at least two thirds (or more) the distance from the pupil to the limbus. Traditionally, the PI has been placed at the 11:00 or 1:00 position with the 12:00 position avoided in case air bubbles are encountered. Some studies indicated that PI placement near the temporal limbus actually resulted in less dysphotopsia; specifically, less complaints of line/streak images.[12] Subsequent studies have not shown a clear difference between superior and temporal placement of the PI.[13] Either approach—placing the PI superior or temporal—is appropriate and is a matter of doctor preference. If the PI is placed superiorly, a partially exposed PI, as opposed to a PI fully covered by the upper lid, has a higher chance of visual complaints by the patient.[14]

Once the general location for the PI has been determined, the doctor should attempt to identify a crypt or relatively thinner area of the iris for the exact placement of the PI. Of course, not all irides will have a thin crypt in an acceptable location. If not, then proceed with a suitable location based on the recommendations mentioned previously.

To increase iris tonicity and facilitate laser penetration of the iris, one drop of pilocarpine 1% or 2% is instilled into the selected eye approximately one-half hour before the procedure. Higher concentrations of pilocarpine have the potential to cause forward rotation of the lens and iris and should be avoided. In addition to pilocarpine, an alpha-agonist such as brimonidine (0.1%–0.2%) or apraclonidine 1% should be instilled into the selected eye to blunt any potential IOP spike. Immediately before the procedure, proparacaine should be instilled into both eyes; instillation in the fellow eye will help control blinking during the procedure.

SETTINGS AND PROCEDURE

Key PI Settings

- Green laser
  - Power—600 to 800 mW
  - Pulse duration—0.1 seconds
  - Spot size—50 to 100 microns
- Nd:YAG laser
  - Energy—3.0 to 4.0 mJ for blue irides, 4.0 to 6.0 mJ for brown irides, single or double shot
  - Offset—Zero microns
  - Spot size and pulse duration—Fixed/not adjustable

A laser (Abraham) lens is recommended (see Figures 14.1–14.3). While the procedure can be performed without a laser lens, use of a lens has several advantages: (1) it provides a 1.5× magnified view of the targeted tissue for the doctor; (2) it helps to focus and concentrate the laser energy; and (3) it provides an easy and inconspicuous method of staunching an iris bleed and potential hyphema. The most effective way to

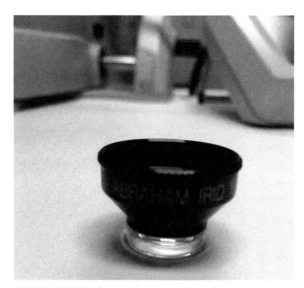

FIGURE 14-1 Abraham iridotomy contact lens.

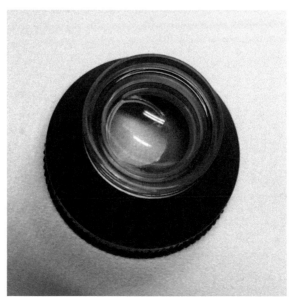

FIGURE 14-2 Abraham lens (patient perspective). Note the decentered 66D button.

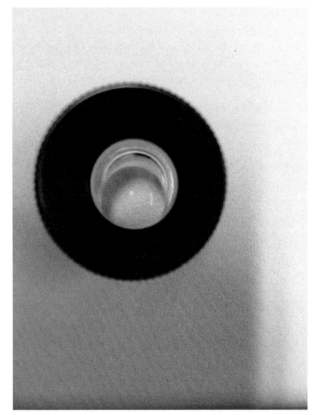

FIGURE 14-3 Abraham lens (doctor perspective). Note the decentered 66D button.

stop bleeding is to apply gentle pressure with the Abraham lens for 30 to 60 seconds. If a lens is not being utilized, digital pressure must be applied to the globe to stop the bleeding.

Additionally, the laser lens helps stabilize the eye and minimize eye movements and prevents the upper lid from blocking the doctor's view. The Abraham lens may also act as a heat sink—absorbing excess laser energy, which could potentially harm the cornea.

When using a laser lens, a small amount of cushioning agent should be instilled into the lens well. While 1% carboxymethylcellulose (Celluvisc) drops can be used, a gel formulation such as Genteal or Systane gel (both hypromellose 0.3%) has the advantage of better contact with the Abraham lens and less potential for air bubbles, thus providing a better view through the lens. After applying the laser lens to the patient's anesthetized eye, the magnifying button should be centered over the target area.

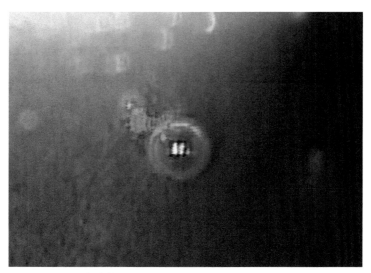

FIGURE 14-4 Air bubble seen with green laser application.

Green Laser Settings

Pretreatment with a green (532 nm) laser is especially beneficial in a thick, brown iris. If pretreating with a green laser, the energy is set to approximately 600 to 800 mW with a 50-micron spot size for a duration of 0.1 seconds per application. Typically, 10 to 15 shots are needed at the target area to adequately thin the iris. While having the advantage of thinning the iris and decreasing bleeding, the green laser does tend to cause more air bubbles which can be distracting to the doctor (Figure 14.4). These bubbles typically dissipate with additional applications of laser energy. After pretreating, the PI can then be completed with a standard 1064-nm Nd:YAG laser.

While not commonly done, the PI may be completed with the green laser. After thinning as described earlier, and using the same settings, burns are placed directly on top of each other until penetration occurs. Another method is the "drum technique". First, four to eight overlapping stretch burns are placed in a circle on the iris with a spot size of 200 μm, duration of 0.2 seconds, and a power of 200 mW. Then, aiming at the center of the stretch burns, penetration burns are applied directly over each other at a power of 600 to 800 mW, with a spot size of 50 μm, and a duration of 0.1 seconds. Burns are applied until the iris is penetrated.

Nd:YAG Settings

Energy settings have much more variability between patients than other laser procedures. Very generally, the energy of the Nd:YAG is set between 2.0 and 6.0 mJ on a single, double, or even triple burst. Spot size, at approximately 10 microns, and duration, at approximately 3–4 ns, are fixed with the 1064-nm Nd:YAG laser. Blue and other light-colored irides typically require less energy while thicker, darker irides require more energy and may need a double burst of energy to help penetrate the iris.

A very general starting point is 4.0 mJ with a single or double burst. Single versus double burst is strictly a doctor preference. Of note, when the Nd:YAG is set to a double burst or shot, the doctor only notices one laser application. However, two independent bursts of laser energy have been applied. So, at a 4.0-mJ double burst, a total of 8.0 mJ of energy is applied with every press of the button.

The energy setting can be lowered or raised based on the patient's iris color and/or the initial response of the tissue to the laser. Rarely is a triple burst needed as this compiles energy extremely fast and the same effect can be gained with a double-shot setting. The exception would be a patient with an active angle closure where the speed of the procedure is important. Then, a 5.0- or 6.0-mJ triple-shot setting may be appropriate.

THE PROCEDURE

Key Procedural Points

- Magnification—12.5 to 16× (medium magnification)
- Location—11:00, 1:00, 3:00, or 9:00 position, preferably in an iris crypt
- Pigment plume = full penetration
- PI final size approximately 0.25 to 0.5 mm in size

The approach to a PI differs somewhat from a capsulotomy or trabeculoplasty. In these procedures, great care is taken to avoid injury to the surrounding structures such as the IOL or trabecular meshwork. With an iridotomy, damage is the goal! The procedure is designed to create a patent hole through the iris tissue. Starting with an inappropriately low-energy setting will only complicate this process.

Using a moderate slit lamp magnification such as 12.5×, the laser should be focused at the iris plane with no offset. The target location will be near the limbus and, if possible, at a thinner area of an iris crypt. The location may be superior at the 11:00 or 1:00 position or temporal at the 3:00 or 9:00 position as described in the Preoperative Care section. A posterior offset is occasionally utilized with a shallow anterior chamber to help avoid the corneal endothelium; however, a very shallow chamber is a contraindication for a PI.

With the target area centered in the button of the Abraham lens, the initial shots should be placed in exactly the same position as much as possible. Poor initial centration usually complicates the procedure as the tissue responds to the laser. Penetration of the iris has occurred when an aggressive plume of pigment is seen coming forward

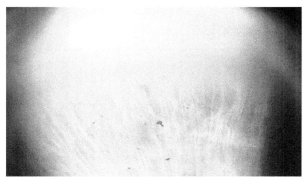

FIGURE 14-5 Pigment plume during a peripheral iridotomy.

(Figure 14.5). This is due to the aqueous in the posterior chamber now escaping to the anterior chamber. A "lazy" or mild plume indicates partial but incomplete penetration. Once a plume is noted, the procedure should be continued until the PI is an acceptable size (Figure 14.6).

The end goal is a patent PI approximately 0.25 to 0.5 mm. There is no universally accepted size for a PI. In general, the smaller the PI (<0.2 mm), the more likely that the PI will fibrose and close.[15] The larger the PI (>0.5 mm), the more likely that the PI will be partially exposed and cause increased dysphotopsia for the patient. Additionally, the Abraham lens button magnifies so the PI will appear larger while performing the procedure. The doctor should complete a careful inspection of the area without the lens after completing the PI.

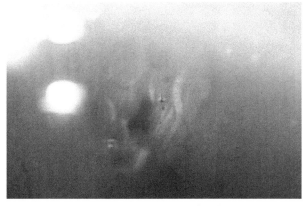

FIGURE 14-6 A newly opened peripheral iridotomy.

POSTOPERATIVE CARE/CO-MANAGEMENT (FOLLOW-UP SCHEDULE)

Key Postoperative Considerations

- Postoperative drops: Alpha-agonist in-office and anti-inflammatory prescribed
- IOP check 30 to 60 minutes post procedure
- IOP check and angle assessment one week post procedure

Immediately after completing the procedure and removing the Abraham lens, another one to two drops of brimonidine or apraclonidine should be instilled into the postoperative eye. After 30 to 60 minutes, IOP should be assessed and treated if a significant rise in IOP is noted.

The number of shots, energy per shot, and total amount of energy used should be recorded in the chart. A notation similar to "The patient tolerated the procedure well and left in no apparent distress" should be added to the chart.

Prednisolone acetate four times a day, or Durezol (difluprednate) twice a day, should be prescribed for the postoperative eye. A follow-up visit for one week is scheduled with instructions to the patient to return if any increased redness, increased pain, or decreased vision is noted.

At the one-week follow-up, the doctor should inspect the PI and assess the patency. IOP should be measured. Most importantly, gonioscopy (and anterior segment OCT, if available) should be performed to assess the effectiveness of the PI as it pertains to the angle anatomy.

POTENTIAL COMPLICATIONS AND THEIR TREATMENT

Key Potential Complications to Look for the Following:

- IOP spike
- Inflammation
- Non-patency of the PI hole
- Transient blurring of vision
- Visual disturbances/glare/halos/lines in vision
- Floaters
- Bleeding/hyphema
- Cataract formation

As with any laser procedure, one possible complication is ineffectiveness. A non-patent PI will have to be repeated or other interventions will have to be attempted.

One of the more common adverse events immediately following the iridotomy is a transient IOP spike due to the laser energy and/or the liberated pigment blocking aqueous outflow through the trabecular meshwork.[16] A relatively low rise (<10 mm Hg) can usually be treated with additional instillation of an alpha-agonist. Timolol or a timolol-combination drop could also be used. Prostaglandin analog medications such as latanoprost should be avoided as they have a very slow onset of action and could potentially increase inflammation.

For an IOP spike in excess of 10 mm Hg, supplementary IOP-lowering methods may be needed. In addition to the treatment previously mentioned, an in-office topical steroid and oral acetazolamide (two 250 mg tablets of acetazolamide) can be used. Instill topical drops every 15 to 20 minutes until the IOP is acceptable. Consider prescribing topical glaucoma drops and/or extended-release acetazolamide 500-mg tablets every 12 hours as well as following up with the patient sooner than the typical one-week post operative appointment.

Iris bleeding is noted in approximately 30% of peripheral iridotomies. This is stopped by pausing laser application and placing moderate pressure on the eye with the Abraham lens during the procedure for 30 to 60 seconds. Interestingly, anticoagulant or antiplatelet therapy does not increase the risk of bleeding during a PI and these medications do not need to be discontinued prior to the procedure (Figure 14.7).[16,17]

One other possible complication is the progression of cataracts due to lenticular injury from the Nd:YAG laser. This may be seen in 23% to 39% of patients over a course of one to six years.[15]

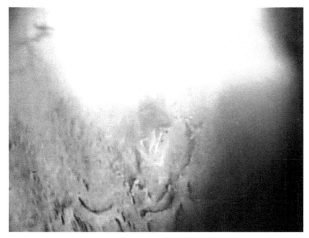

FIGURE 14-7 Small bleed during a peripheral iridotomy procedure.

VIDEOS OF PROCEDURE

Video 14.1—This PI was through a naturally thin iris (no pretreatment) with a power setting of a 3.5-mJ single shot with a 1064-nm Nd:YAG laser—duration and spot size are fixed. Note the pigment plume. The initial treated area is magnified by the Abraham lens and less than 0.25 mm. Additional treatment was added with care taken to avoid the adjacent blood vessel. Video courtesy of Nate Lighthizer.

Video 14.2—This PI was done with a Nd:YAG setting of a 4.5-mJ double shot as seen through the Abraham iridotomy lens. There was no ideal iris crypt to place the PI. This video is a good example of the iris collagen shifting with the laser energy. During a PI, it is common for a newly formed, small hole to "disappear" due to the changes in collagen. If this happens, the doctor should keep applying laser energy in that area and the hole will open back up. Video courtesy of Nate Lighthizer.

Video 14.3—A pretreatment with a 532-nm "Green" laser used to thin a brown iris through the Abraham lens. Thirteen shots were applied at 600 mW, 50-micron spot size, at a 0.1-second duration. This procedure is more likely to cause small air bubble formation. Immediately following the green laser pretreatment, a 1064-nm Nd:YAG laser was applied at a 3.6-mJ single shot (15 shots total) to complete the PI. Video courtesy of Nate Lighthizer.

Video 14.4—This video shows a bleed during a Nd:YAG peripheral iridotomy. If this is experienced, simply apply additional pressure with the Abraham iridotomy lens for 30–60 seconds until the bleeding has stopped and then continue the procedure. The blood may stay suspended and slowly dissipates after the procedure over a matter of days.

Video 14.5—(Iridoplasty video) Viewed through the Abraham iridotomy lens, this particular procedure used a 500-micron spot size with a 0.5-second burn duration and 250-mW power. Twenty-two burns were applied. Note the large laser spot size, peripheral placement, presence of a PI, and the iris contraction in response to the laser application. Video courtesy of Nate Lighthizer.

EFFICACY

Laser PI has been shown to improve anterior segment/angle morphology although this may regress over time due to lenticular changes.[18,19] Laser PI does seem effective in preventing acute, symptomatic angle closure in narrow-angle patients.[20] However, the more trabecular meshwork damage seen, as evidenced by significant peripheral anterior synechiae, the less effective a PI will be in IOP control and angle-closure prevention.[10,16]

Also unclear is the benefit for the PACS. One study suggested that while a PI can have significant prophylactic effect, an estimated 44 procedures would have to be completed to prevent one case of angle closure.[4] As with many conditions and treatments, this points to the doctor's responsibility of carefully measuring the patient's risk of disease progression (based on history, demographics, and exam data) and the risk/benefit of the PI procedure.

Finally, clear lens extraction (cataract surgery) has been shown to be superior to PI for IOP control (for pressures >30 mm Hg) and visual function.[21] Patients undergoing clear lens extraction are less likely to have anatomical changes to the angle over time as well. For any narrow-angle patient qualifying for cataract surgery, this approach should be strongly considered.

CODING/BILLING

For a PI, CPT code 66761 is used: "Iridotomy/iridectomy by laser surgery (e.g., for glaucoma) per session." This code has a ten-day postoperative global period. If both eyes are done in the same session (rarely done with PIs), use modifier-50 after the CPT code. Common ICD-10 codes that support this procedure include the following:

> H40.031 to H40.039 (anatomical narrow angle)
> H40.061 to H40.069 (primary angle closure without glaucoma damage)
> H40.1310 to H40.1394 (pigmentary glaucoma)
> H40.20X0 to H40.20X4 (unspecified primary angle-closure glaucoma)
> H40.211 to H40.219 (acute angle-closure glaucoma)
> H40.2210 to H40.2294 (chronic angle-closure glaucoma)
> H40.231 to H40.239 (intermittent angle-closure glaucoma)
> H40.241 to H40.249 (residual stage of angle-closure glaucoma)
> H40.831 to H40.839 (aqueous misdirection)

IRIDOPLASTY

Key Iridoplasty Points

- Main indication is plateau iris syndrome
- Green laser settings:
  - Power—200 to 300 mW
  - Spot size—400 to 500 microns
  - Pulse duration—0.5 seconds
- Twenty to 25 shots across the peripheral iris (about every 30 minutes on the clock dial)

Also known as gonioplasty, this procedure is most commonly performed on patients with plateau iris. This condition is more common in relatively younger patients (<50 years old) as compared to PAC. Plateau iris may have a pupil block component (configuration), so a PI is generally performed. However, iris crowding into the anterior chamber angle may persist despite a patent PI (plateau iris syndrome).

The goal of an iridoplasty is to contract the iris away from the trabecular meshwork causing a relative opening of the angle. This procedure, unlike a PI, exclusively uses a 532-nm green laser.

After informed consent, the preoperative protocol is identical to the PI protocol: brimonidine or apraclonidine to the selected eye as well as 2% pilocarpine. The Abraham laser lens is also used with moderate (12.5×) slit lamp magnification.

A large laser spot size is selected—400 or 500 microns with a duration of 0.5 seconds. A low-energy setting such as 250 mW can be used and increased in 50 mW increments if iris contraction is not noticed. If pigment release, air bubbles, or iris charring is noticed, the power should be decreased. Twenty to 25 burns are placed in the peripheral iris in a circular fashion—roughly 6 burns per quadrant.

Due to the relative rarity of plateau iris, there are limited data on the efficacy of iridoplasty. Nevertheless, available studies do suggest that it is an effective treatment for plateau iris syndrome.[22]

In theory, an iridoplasty could be of benefit for narrow-angle patients (PAC, PACG) by opening the angle and improving aqueous outflow. However, there is no strong evidence that an iridoplasty improves outcomes in these patients.[23]

CODING/BILLING

For an iridoplasty, CPT code 66762 is used: "Iridoplasty by photocoagulation— one or more sessions (e.g. for improvement of vision, for widening of anterior chamber angle)." This code has a 90-day post-op global period. Although this is typically done one eye per session, modifier-50 could be used for a bilateral procedure. ICD-10 H21.82, "Plateau iris syndrome (post-iridectomy) (post-procedural)," is commonly used.

REFERENCES

1. Razeghinejad MR, Spaeth GL. A history of the surgical management of glaucoma. *Optom Vis Sci.* 2011;88(1):39–47. doi:10.1097/OPX.0b013e3181fe2226
2. Khuri CH. Argon laser iridectomies. *Am J Ophthalmol.* 1973;76:490–493.
3. Rivera AH, Brown RH, Anderson DR. Laser iridotomy vs surgical iridectomy: have the indications changed? *Arch Ophthalmol.* 1985;103(9):1350–1354. doi:10.1001/archopht.1985.01050090102042
4. He M, Jiang Y, Huang S, et al. Laser peripheral iridotomy for the prevention of angle closure: a single-centre, randomised controlled trial. *Lancet.* 2019;393:1609–1618. doi:10.1016/S0140-6736(18)32607-2
5. See JS, Chew PK. Angle-closure glaucoma. In: Yanoff M, Duker JS, eds. *Ophthalmology.* 3rd ed. Philadelphia, PA; Mosby; 2009.
6. Ritch R. Plateau iris is caused by abnormally positioned ciliary processes. *J Glaucoma.* 1992;1:23–26.
7. Shukla S, Damji, KF, Harasymowycz P, et al. Clinical features distinguishing angle closure from pseudoplateau versus plateau iris. *Br J Ophthalmol.* 2008;92(3):340–344. doi:10.1136/bjo.2007.114876

8. Michelessi M, Lindsley K. Peripheral iridotomy for pigmentary glaucoma. *Cochrane Database* Syst Rev. 2016;2(2):CD005655. doi:10.1002/14651858.CD005655.pub2

9. Van Issum C, Mavrakanas N, Shutz JC, et al. Topiramate-induced acute bilateral angle closure and myopia: pathophysiology and treatment controversies. *Eur J Ophthalmol.* 2011;21(4):404–409. doi:10.5301/EJO.2010.5979

10. Lin Z, Liang Y, Wang N, et al. Peripheral anterior synechia reduce extent of angle widening after laser peripheral iridotomy in eyes with primary angle closure. *J Glaucoma.* 2013;22(5):374–379. doi:10.1097/IJG.0b013e318241ba1d

11. Behrendt S, Giess L, Duncker G. Incidence of retinal detachment after treatment with the Nd:YAG laser. *Fortschr Ophthalmol.* 1990;88(6):809–811.

12. Vera V, Naqi A, Belovay, GW, et al. Dysphotopsia after temporal versus superior laser peripheral iridotomy: a prospective randomized paired eye trial. *Am J Ophthalmol.* 2014;157(5):929–935. doi:10.1016/j.ajo.2014.02.010

13. Srinivasan K, Zebardast N, Krishnamurthy P, et al. Comparison of new visual disturbances after superior versus nasal/temporal laser peripheral iridotomy: a prospective randomized trial. *Ophthalmology.* 2018;125(3):345–351. doi:10.1016/j.ophtha.2017.09.015

14. Spaeth GL, Idowu O, Seligsohn A, et al. The effects of iridotomy size and position on symptoms following laser peripheral iridotomy. *J Glaucoma.* 2005;14(5):364–367. doi:10.1097/01.ijg.0000177213.31620.02

15. Fleck, BW. How large must an iridotomy be? *Br J Ophthalmol.* 1990;74(10):583–588. doi:10.1136/bjo.74.10.583

16. Radhakrishnan S, Chen PP, Junk AK, Nouri-Mahdavi K, Chen TC. Laser peripheral iridotomy in primary angle closure: a report by the American Academy of Ophthalmology. *Ophthalmology.* 2018;125(7):1110–1120. doi:10.1016/j.ophtha.2018.01.015

17. Golan S, Levkovitch-Verbin H, Shemesh G, Kurtz S. Anterior chamber bleeding after laser peripheral iridotomy. *JAMA Ophthalmol.* 2013;131(5):626–629. doi:10.1001/jamaophthalmol.2013.1642

18. Mansoori T, Balakrishna N. Anterior segment morphology after laser iridotomy in primary angle closure suspects. *Clin Exp Optom.* 2018;101:333–338. doi:10.1111/cxo.12631

19. Lee KS, Sung KR, Shon K, Sun JH, Lee JR. Longitudinal changes in anterior segment parameters after laser peripheral iridotomy assessed by anterior segment optical coherence tomography. *Invest Ophthalmol Vis Sci.* 2013;54:3166–3170. doi:10.1167/iovs.13-11630

20. Ang LP, Aung T, Chew PT. Acute primary angle closure in an Asian population: long-term outcome of the fellow eye after prophylactic laser peripheral iridotomy. *Ophthalmology.* 2000;107:2092–2096. doi:10.1016/s0161-6420(00)00360-2

21. Azuara-Blanco A, Burr J, Ramsay C, et al. Effectiveness of early lens extraction for the treatment of primary angle-closure glaucoma (EAGLE): a randomised controlled trial. *Lancet.* 2016;388:1389–1397. doi:10.1016/S0140-6736(16)30956-4

22. Ritch R, Tham CC, Lam DS. Long term success of argon laser peripheral iridoplasty in the management of plateau iris syndrome. *Ophthalmology.* 2004;111:104–108. doi:10.1016/j.ophtha.2003.05.001

23. Ng WS, Ang GS, Azuara-Blanco A. Laser peripheral iridoplasty for angle-closure. *Cochrane Database Syst Rev.* 2012;15;(2):CD006746. doi:10.1002/14651858.CD006746.pub3

15 Endoscopic Cyclophotocoagulation

Leonid Skorin, Jr.

In 1992, Martin Uram, MD, first published the effectiveness of the endoscopic cyclophotocoagulation (ECP) surgical laser in a group of 10 patients with intractable neovascular glaucoma.[1] ECP delivers laser energy in a titratable manner to the ciliary processes and produces coagulative necrotic damage to the secretory ciliary epithelium.[2] The clinical effect seen in all cycloablative procedures is mainly the reduction in the rate of aqueous humor formation (Fig. 15.1). ECP, the name of the surgical procedure, defines and describes the technique:

- Endoscopic: Intraocular visualization
- Cyclo: Circular pattern of application
- Photocoagulation: Laser energy ablation of ciliary tissue

Unlike other cycloablative laser procedures, such as transcleral cyclophotocoagulation (TCP), ECP is a more refined procedure. The ciliary processes are visualized directly and treated precisely to achieve the desired tissue effect (Fig. 15.2). This, in turn, prevents undesirable collateral tissue damage.[3] Collateral tissue damage and postoperative pain are more common with TCP. Patients may also experience more severe postoperative inflammation, cystoid macular edema, hypotony, and phthisis with permanent vision loss.[4] Because of these drawbacks, TCP has been reserved for eyes that have little or no vision potential, but required intraocular pressure (IOP) reduction because of severe pain from their intractable glaucoma. A new TCP laser system by IRIDEX known as the MicroPulse P3 Device uses repetitive micropulses of diode-laser energy delivered in an off-and-on cyclical manner to the ciliary body when applied to the external scleral surface 3 mm from the limbus. It is noninvasive and repeatable and, because of its increased precision, may potentially be used in primary glaucoma.

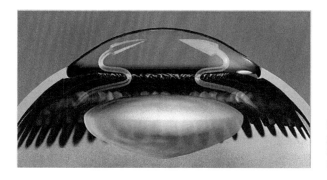

FIGURE 15-1 Ciliary processes produce aqueous humor. Image courtesy of BVI Medical.

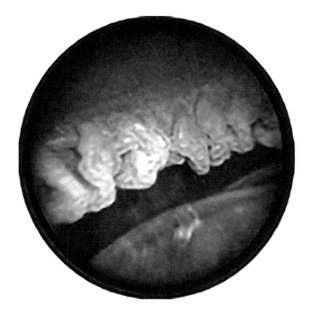

FIGURE 15-2 Endoscopic view of ciliary processes in a pseudophakic eye. Image courtesy of BVI Medical.

INDICATIONS

Key Indications

- Open angle glaucoma
- Pseudoexfoliative glaucoma
- Neovascular glaucoma
- Refractory glaucoma
- Pediatric glaucoma

ECP was initially used in the treatment of glaucoma refractory to maximal medical therapy and surgical treatment, which included trabeculectomy and tube shunt procedures.[5] Although ECP has shown efficacy in the treatment of refractory and neovascular glaucoma, it is most often used in open-angle and pseudoexfoliative glaucoma cases. Stand-alone ECP can readily be performed in these glaucoma patients. Most cases today are done as a combination surgery of ECP with cataract phacoemulsification.[6] The cataract surgery is completed first with the implantation of an intraocular lens (IOL) and then the ECP laser is performed. This combination surgery is a viable option for patients struggling with glaucoma medication compliance and want to reduce their dependence on multiple topical medications. Patients who have glaucoma medication intolerance are also excellent candidates for the combined cataract extraction and ECP surgery. Since phacoemulsification cataract surgery can be done with clear corneal incisions, there is no need to manipulate the conjunctiva. This preserves the conjunctiva for any future trabeculectomy or shunt valve implantation.[7]

ECP has also been used successfully in the treatment of pediatric glaucoma, although serious complications (retinal detachment, hypotony, progressive vision loss) are more common in this group.[8] ECP has also shown long-term efficacy in the management of pediatric glaucoma, following cataract surgery in children.[9]

CONTRAINDICATIONS

Key Contraindications

- Active uveitic glaucoma
- Patients with IOP greater than 40 mm Hg
- Vitreous in the anterior chamber

Since ECP is a targeted laser procedure under direct visualization, laser energy can be delivered in short titratable bursts with rest intervals, allowing for a tissue effect while minimizing collateral energy absorption.[4]

Even though ECP is a highly controlled procedure, laser energy that is delivered to the ciliary processes still has the potential to cause a significant amount of postoperative inflammation. The laser energy may also contribute to the breakdown of the blood-aqueous barrier, especially in cases of overly intensive treatment, mechanical trauma to intraocular tissue by endoscope manipulation, or other technical challenges.[6] Therefore, any patient who is already experiencing an active case of uveitic glaucoma or uveitis, in general, should not have the ECP procedure performed. The additional postoperative uveitis may make the patient's underlying inflammation much more difficult to control.

A more relative contraindication in doing ECP would be patients with IOP greater than 40 mm Hg. These patients would be considered to have severe glaucoma and would benefit most from trabeculectomy or tube shunt glaucoma surgery. If vitreous is present in the anterior chamber, it must be removed prior to the ECP procedure.[6] The vitreous will interfere with manipulation of the endoscope as the vitreous will get entangled around it.

Finally, eyes with end-stage glaucoma, and severely compromised outflow (e.g., eyes that have neovascular glaucoma with complete involvement of the angle) are also poor candidates for ECP.[10]

PREOPERATIVE CARE

Key Preoperative Considerations

- Lens status: Is the patient phakic, aphakic, or pseudophakic?
- Anterior or posterior segment approach
- Presence or absence of vitreous
- Combination surgery with phacoemulsification cataract extraction

The lens status, whether the patient is phakic, aphakic, or pseudophakic, dictates which surgical approach can be utilized. There are two main approaches to the ciliary processes. The anterior segment approach utilizes either a scleral tunnel or clear corneal incision. These are the typical surgical approaches used in combination ECP with phacoemulsification cataract extraction since these incisions have already been performed for the cataract extraction part of the combined surgery (Fig. 15.3).

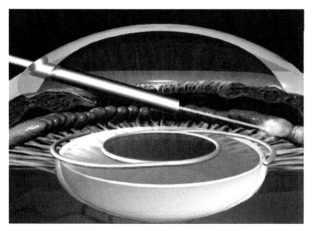

FIGURE 15-3 Endoscopic cyclophotocoagulation performed through clear corneal incision and over the intraocular lens implant. Image courtesy of BVI Medical.

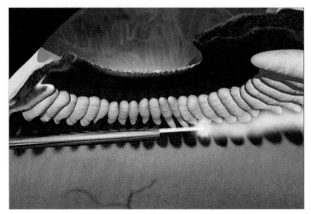

FIGURE 15-4 Endoscopic cyclophotocoagulation performed using the posterior segment approach (pars plana) in an aphakic eye. Image courtesy of BVI Medical.

As long as there is no vitreous in the anterior chamber, ECP can be performed as a stand-alone procedure in phakic, aphakic, or pseudophakic eyes.

The posterior segment approach accesses the ciliary processes from the pars plana (Fig. 15.4). This approach is amenable for both aphakic and pseudophakic eyes. It cannot be safely performed in phakic eyes since the natural lens interferes with access to the ciliary processes. The anterior vitreous must be removed with a vitrector before the endoscope can be introduced through the pars plana incision.[4] Further discussion of the posterior segment approach is beyond the scope of this chapter.

SETTINGS AND PROCEDURE

Key ECP Settings

- Laser power—0.25 to 0.35 W
- Laser duration—continuous
- Treatment area—270° (9 clock hours) to 360° (12 clock hours)
- Microendoscope—19-gauge curved cannula

The ciliary processes are very sensitive, so adequate anesthesia must be attained. General anesthesia is reserved for pediatric glaucoma patients. For all others and those having combination ECP with cataract extraction, the standard local anesthesia will suffice. This includes retrobulbar, peribulbar, or intracameral (non-preserved lidocaine injected into the anterior chamber).[3] Intracameral anesthesia helps the patient tolerate the surgical microscope light, in addition to reducing sensation in the ciliary body.[11] Purely topical anesthesia is insufficient.

Currently, the only commercially available glaucoma ECP device is the Endo Optiks E2 Ophthalmic Laser and Endoscopy System by BVI Medical. It consists of two components: the laser microendoscope and the laser endoscopy system (console) (Fig. 15.5). The most commonly used laser endoscope for the treatment of glaucoma contains a single, 19-gauge curved cannula (Fig. 15.6). There are two types of 19-gauge endoscopes: straight and curved. Both 20-gauge and 23-gauge cannula options are available but only as straight endoscopes. The clinician should be able to treat up to 180° of the ciliary body circumference using the straight endoscope, and up to 240° using the curved endoscope, through a single surgical incision (Fig. 15.7). To treat beyond 240° and up to 360° requires at least two surgical incisions. To achieve an adequate drop in IOP and derive a long-term benefit, at least 270° to 300° of treatment needs to be applied.[6]

The E2 Ophthalmic Laser and Endoscopy System incorporates an 810 nm diode-laser, which emits continuous energy, and a helium-neon red laser aiming beam (Fig. 15.8). The initial power setting is typically set at 0.25 W. If the treatment effect

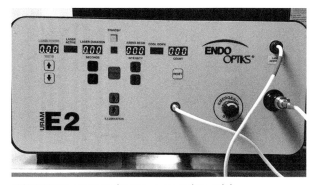

FIGURE 15-5 Laser endoscopy system (console).

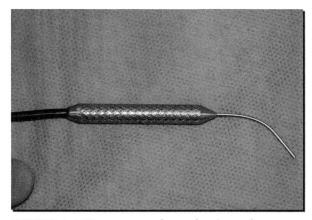

FIGURE 15-6 A 19-gauge curved cannula microendoscope.

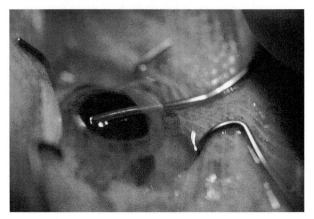

FIGURE 15-7 A 19-gauge curved cannula inserted through scleral tunnel in a combined phacoemulsification cataract extraction and endoscopic cyclophotocoagulation glaucoma surgery.

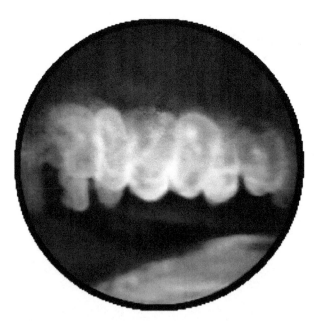

FIGURE 15-8 Note red helium-neon laser aiming beam focused on ciliary process to be treated. Image courtesy of BVI Medical.

is not adequate at this setting, the power level can be increased incrementally by 0.05 W until the desired tissue change is observed. The clinician controls the amount of total laser energy to be delivered by way of a footswitch. When the footswitch is depressed, the laser will fire and when it is released, laser delivery ceases.[6] The laser application is aimed at individual ciliary processes to produce a visible whitening and

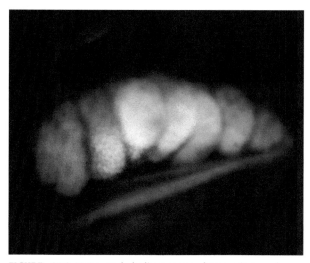

FIGURE 15-9 Note red helium-neon laser aiming beam focused on ciliary process. Ciliary processes to the right of the aiming beam are visibly white and shrunken from treatment. Process to the left of the aiming beam is still brown in color and untreated. Also note lens capsule below in this pseudophakic eye.

shrinkage of the entire anteroposterior extent of the process (Fig. 15.9).[12] Disrupted or scar tissue should not be treated. The average duration of direct laser application per ciliary process is around 0.5 to 2.0 seconds.[12] An alternative treatment approach is to "paint" the tissue by sweeping across the arc of the ciliary ring. Usually, several passes are required to treat most of the surface of each process.[6] Bubble formation and ciliary process "popping" is indicative of excessive energy application. This can result from holding the endoscope too close to the ciliary process or having the power setting turned up too high.[7] The ECP endoscope is usually held within 2 to 3 mm of the ciliary processes, allowing visualization of approximately four to six ciliary processes at a time (Fig. 15.10).[13] The 19-gauge endoscope incorporates a 17k pixel image fiber, with a 140° field of view and has a focus range from 1.5 mm to infinity. The image is delivered via the video camera and a 175 W xenon light source housed in the E2 system.[13,14] The clinician views the video monitor instead of looking through the operating microscope.

Prior to inserting the endoscope through the scleral tunnel or clear corneal incision, viscoelastic is injected into the anterior chamber. The viscoelastic is injected under the iris and over the ciliary processes.[4] This elevates the iris and expands the ciliary sulcus of the phakic, aphakic, or pseudophakic eye, which helps enhance visualization and maneuverability of the endoscope.[7] The viscoelastic helps position the natural lens in the phakic eye and the IOL in the pseudophakic eye more posteriorly, reducing the likelihood of natural lens or IOL damage.[15] Elevating the iris also minimizes the risk of thermal burn to the iris itself.[4]

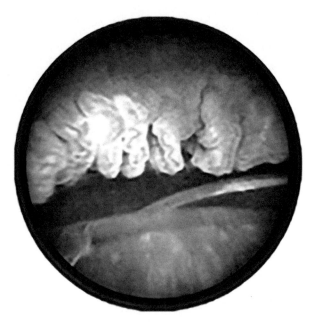

FIGURE 15-10 Six-seven processes visualized prior to treatment. Image courtesy of BVI Medical.

Once the image is focused on the video monitor, treatment can begin. As mentioned before, the physical goals of the treatment are to whiten the ciliary processes and shrink visible tissue.[12] More pigmentation of the ciliary processes will result in quicker and more extensive absorption of laser energy by the tissue. It is thought that laser energy absorbed by melanin in the ciliary pigmented epithelium causes thermal damage to the ciliary nonpigmented epithelium where aqueous humor production occurs.[5] The entire ciliary process including any vessels within the ciliary process, as well as the space between the processes (the "valleys" between the "hills"), must be treated for optimum effect (Fig. 15.11).[3,16] Treatment of the epithelium alone may control IOP temporarily, but the surviving vessels and stroma might allow the ciliary epithelium to regenerate, causing resumed aqueous humor production.[16] Treating only the anterior tips may miss 50% or more of the tissue, which could be producing the aqueous humor.[14]

A special yet common clinical case in point is patients with pseudoexfoliative glaucoma. Many of these patients will have unusual physical findings on video observation. The clinician will find variable amounts of white, flaky deposits present on the posterior aspect of the iris, which extend into the sulcus, covering the lens capsule and zonules.[6] The zonules themselves will appear thicker than normal and instead of appearing taut will often hang limply and droop. The ciliary processes appear blanched with little-to-no pigment on their surface. In addition, the ciliary processes appear stiff and do not readily shrink with laser energy application. This makes it difficult to titrate treatment. If there is a poor response, one can slowly increase the

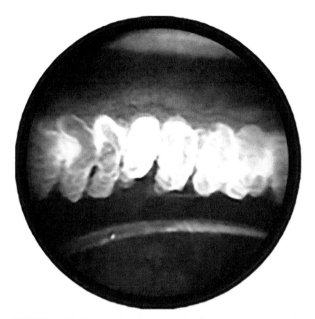

FIGURE 15-11 Appropriately treated ciliary processes on the right side of the image. The brown-colored ciliary processes on the left are yet to be treated. Image courtesy of BVI Medical.

power level until there is "tissue popping." This would indicate the threshold for overtreatment. The power level should be adjusted back down to the previous setting and then treatment can proceed in the usual manner.[6]

At the conclusion of the procedure, the endoscope is removed from the eye. A thorough viscoelastic removal is performed to avoid postoperative IOP spikes.[4]

POSTOPERATIVE CARE/CO-MANAGEMENT (FOLLOW-UP SCHEDULE)

Key Postoperative Considerations:

- Topical antibiotic QID for one to two weeks
- Topical nonsteroidal anti-inflammatory agent QID for one to two weeks
- Topical prednisolone acetate 1% every 2 hours while awake for one week, then slow taper over one month
- IOP check at one-day, one-week, and one-month post-ECP

The patient is seen at one day, one week, and one month after the procedure. They should avoid rubbing their eye, wear a plastic or metal eye shield at bedtime for 1 week, and use topical antibiotic and nonsteroidal anti-inflammatory drugs four times a day for one to two weeks. They will also need to start topical prednisolone acetate 1% every 2 hours while awake for one week. This can then be tapered slowly over the next month. This regimen seems to effectively control any postoperative inflammation.

Oral acetazolamide and subconjunctival or subtenon steroid injection may be used to provide supplemental IOP and inflammation control, if needed.[7] Acetaminophen may be recommended for pain.[12] Some patients may benefit from the short-term use of an ice pack.[12]

Maintain the patient on any preoperative glaucoma medications (except pilocarpine) for four to eight weeks postoperatively.[15,17] By this time, the patient's IOP should stabilize and the eye develops a new steady state.[6] Once the eye is fully stabilized, the patient can discontinue one of their glaucoma medications. If the IOP remains at an adequate level, the clinician can discontinue a second glaucoma eye drop medication if the patient is using more than one medication. Continue trialing the patient off any additional glaucoma eye drops until the IOP starts to rise or there are no more medications to stop using.

This also applies to oral glaucoma medications. In one study, about 75% of patients were using systemic carbonic anhydrase inhibitors preoperatively, but ultimately only about 10% required them as continued maintenance.[6]

POTENTIAL COMPLICATIONS AND THEIR TREATMENT

Key Potential Complications

- IOP spike
- Inflammation
- Hyphema
- Hypotony

As with any laser procedure, one possible complication is ineffectiveness. With ECP, this is usually due to inadequate treatment of the ciliary processes or inadequate amount of treated ciliary processes.

An IOP spike in the immediate postoperative time frame is probably the most frequently seen complication. This is usually due to retained viscoelastic.[6] The IOP can be lowered in most cases successfully by release of the anterior chamber fluid through one of the surgical incisions on the first postoperative day. Additional medical glaucoma management can be added if the IOP is quite high or the eye has substantial preexisting visual field loss.[6]

Inflammation will always be present postoperatively, especially if the patient had a combined ECP and phacoemulsification cataract extraction surgery. Topical prednisolone acetate 1% and a nonsteroidal anti-inflammatory agent will usually control the inflammation adequately. In cases that present with a fibrinous iritis, adding a topical cycloplegic agent may help. Most of these cases will require a subconjunctival or subtenon steroid injection.[7]

Hyphema can occur after ECP in up to 12% of cases.[18] The most likely source of this problem is bleeding from an abrasion of intraocular tissue by endoscope manipulation or overtreatment of one or more ciliary processes resulting in "popping" or tissue explosion.[6] Most of these hemorrhages clear spontaneously.

Postoperative IOP spikes, fibrinous iritis, and hyphema are the most common complications attributable to both stand-alone ECP and combined ECP with phacoemulsification cataract extraction surgery.[19] Other less common complications of ECP include cystoid macular edema (1.0%–3.0%), serous choroidal effusion (0.4%), retinal detachment (0.3%–0.7%), and hypotony with phthisis (0.1%).[5,20,21]

The higher rate of cystoid macular edema was recorded in cases where ECP was performed with phacoemulsification cataract extraction.[21] Cataract formation can also occur in phakic eyes that have undergone a stand-alone ECP.[5]

VIDEOS OF PROCEDURE

Video 15.1—Each ciliary process is treated individually to attain maximum whitening and shrinkage. Laser settings: laser power 0.25 W, laser duration continuous, duration (seconds) controlled by surgeon using footswitch. Video courtesy of Leonid Skorin, Jr., and Taylor Lauermann.

Video 15.2—Each ciliary process is treated individually to attain maximum whitening and shrinkage. Laser settings: laser power 0.25 W, laser duration continuous, duration (seconds) controlled by surgeon using footswitch. Video courtesy of Leonid Skorin, Jr., and Stephanie Norberg.

Video 15.3—Pseudoexfoliation glaucoma patient. Note white, thick, stiff, irregularly shaped, and spaced zonules. Ciliary processes are also abnormally shaped. Laser settings: laser power 0.30 W, laser duration continuous, duration (seconds) controlled by surgeon using footswitch. Video courtesy of Leonid Skorin, Jr., and Scott A. Bauer.

Video 15.4—Combined Procedure: ECP + Phaco. The limbal "over the PC-IOL" technique. Video courtesy of BVI Medical.

EFFICACY

The success of ECP has been evaluated since the first such published study in 1992 by Dr. Uram involving patients with intractable neovascular glaucoma.[1] Other authors feel that patients with greatly elevated IOP with poor outflow facility, as seen in neovascular glaucoma, are not appropriate candidates for ECP.[14]

A retrospective study that looked at patients who had at least one previous failed glaucoma surgery and presented with diverse forms of glaucoma (refractory open-angle, congenital, secondary) found that ECP alone decreased subjects' IOP by 10.7 mm Hg, with 90% of eyes achieving IOP ≤ 21 mm Hg and the mean number of glaucoma medications decreased from 3.0 to 2.0.[18]

ECP has been compared with both trabeculectomy and tube shunt implantation (Ahmed and Baerveldt).[22–25] All these studies found that ECP yielded comparable IOP-lowering results when compared with the aforementioned glaucoma surgical procedures. ECP can also be used for treating angle closure due to plateau iris. Laser applied to the ciliary body shrinks it more posteriorly, therefore opening the angle. This procedure is usually done with lens extraction surgery.[26]

As discussed previously, ECP is most commonly used in combination with phacoemulsification cataract extraction surgery.[6] Studies show the combination procedure, when performed in patients with mild-to-moderate glaucoma, can achieve an average IOP decrease between 2.6 and 3.3 mm Hg.[19–21,27,28] These studies have also found that the average number of postoperative glaucoma therapies decreased by one medication two years postoperatively.[20,21,28]

A financial cost-to-benefit analysis was done to see what patients could be saving by decreasing one medication each. An average savings of $1,504.00 a year per patient was calculated for those who underwent a combination surgery, while patients who only had phacoemulsification surgery had a slight increase in their expenditures.[29]

Another study looked at the efficacy of combination surgery in advanced glaucoma patients and found the reduction of IOP to be similar to that seen in patients with mild-to-moderate glaucoma.[30] The medication burden was also decreased.[30] Although this decline in IOP and medical burden would be considered a success in less-advanced glaucoma, it was considered to be insufficient to prevent further vision loss in those with advanced glaucoma.[5,30] The results were not convincing enough to replace phacoemulsification-tube shunt or phacoemulsification-trabeculectomy surgeries with combination phacoemulsification and ECP.[5]

CODING/BILLING

CPT codes: 66711—ciliary body destruction; cyclophotocoagulation; stand-alone ECP

CPT codes: 66987—complex cataract removal and ECP

CPT codes: 66988—routine cataract removal and ECP

Common ICD-10 codes that support ECP include the following:

H40.1111 to H40.1134 (primary open-angle glaucoma)

H40.011 to H40.029 (open angle with borderline findings)

H40.1310 to H40.1394 (pigmentary glaucoma)

H40.1211 to H40.1294 (low-tension glaucoma)

H40.1411 to H40.1494 (capsular glaucoma with pseudoexfoliation of lens)

REFERENCES

1. Uram M. Ophthalmic laser microendoscope ciliary process ablation in the management of neovascular glaucoma. *Ophthalmology.* 1992;99(12):1823–1828.
2. McKelvie PA, Walland MJ. Pathology of cyclodiode laser: a series of nine enucleated eyes. *Br J Ophthalmol.* 2002;86(4):381–386. doi:10.1136/bjo.86.4.381
3. Berke SJ. Endolaser cyclophotocoagulation in glaucoma management. *Tech Ophthalmol.* 2006;4(2): 74–81.
4. Dastiridou AI, Katsanos A, Denis P, et al. Cyclodestructive procedures in glaucoma: a review of current and emerging options. *Adv Ther.* 2018;35(12):2013–2027. doi:10.1007/s12325-018-0837-3
5. Cohen A, Wong SH, Patel S, et al. Endoscopic cyclophotocoagulation for the treatment of glaucoma. *Surv Ophthalmol.* 2017;62(3):357–365. doi:10.1016/j.survophthal.2016.09.004
6. Uram M. *Endoscopic Surgery in Ophthalmology.* Philadelphia: Lippincott Williams & Wilkins; 2003.
7. Rathi S, Radcliffe NM. Combined endocyclophotocoagulation and phacoemulsification in the management of moderate glaucoma. *Surv Ophthalmol.* 2017;62(5):712–715. doi:10.1016/j.survophthal. 2017.01.011
8. Neely DE, Plager DA. Endocyclophotocoagulation for management of difficult pediatric glaucoma. *JAAPOS.* 2001;5(4):221–229. doi:10.1067/mpa.2001.116868
9. Cantor AJ, Wang J, Li S, et al. Long-term efficacy of endoscopic cyclophotocoagulation in the management of glaucoma following cataract surgery in children. *JAAPOS.* 2018;22(3):188–191. doi:10.1016/j.jaapos.2018.01.014
10. Lin SC, Chen MJ, Lin MS, et al. Vascular effects on ciliary tissue from endoscopic versus trans-scleral cyclophotocoagulation. *Br J Ophthalmol.* 2006;90(4):496–500. doi:10.1136/bjo.2005.072777
11. Bahadur GG, Sinsky RM. *Manual of Cataract Surgery.* 2nd ed. Boston: Butterworth Heinemann; 2000.
12. Gaasterland DE. Diode laser cyclophotogoagulation. *Glaucoma Today.* 2009;7(2):35–37, 41.
13. Yu JY, Kahook MY, Lathrop KI, et al. The effect of probe placement and type of viscoelastic material on endoscopic cyclophotocoagulation laser energy transmission. *Ophthalmic Surg Lasers Imaging.* 2008;39(2):133–136.
14. Huang JY, Lin S. Endoscopic cyclophotocoagulation. *Glaucoma Today.* 2009;7(2):39–41.
15. Berke SJ. Endophotocoagulation. In: Shaarawy T, Sherwood M, Hitchings R, Crowston J, eds. *Glaucoma,* 2nd ed. Philadelphia: Elsevier, 2015:1160–1166.
16. Kahook MY, Noecker RJ. Endoscopic cyclophotocoagulation. *Glaucoma Today.* 2006;4(6):24–29.
17. Fallano KA, Conner IP, Noecker RJ, Schuman JS. Cyclodestruction procedures in glaucoma. In: Yanoff M, ed. *Ophthalmology,* 5th ed. Philadelphia: Elsevier; 2019:1131–1134.
18. Chen J, Cohn RA, Lin SC, et al. Endoscopic photocoagulation of the ciliary body for treatment of refractory glaucoma. *Am J Ophthalmol.* 1997;124(6):787–796.
19. Kahook MY, Lathrop KL, Noecker RJ. One-site versus two-site endoscopic cyclophotocoagulation. *J Glaucoma.* 2007;16(6):527–530.
20. Siegel MJ, Boling WS, Faridi OS, et al. Cyclophotocoagulation and phacoemulsification versus phacoemulsification alone in the treatment of mild to moderate glaucoma. *Clin Exp Ophthalmol.* 2015;43(6):531–539.
21. Clement C, Kampaugeris G, Ahmed F, et al. Combining phacoemulsification with endoscopic cyclophotocoagulation to manage cataract and glaucoma. *Clin Exp Ophthalmol.* 2013;41(6):546–551.
22. Gayton JL, Van Der Karr M, Sanders V. Combined cataract and glaucoma surgery: trabeculectomy versus endoscopic laser cycloablation. *J Cataract Refract Surg.* 1999;25(9):1214–1219. doi:10.1016/ s0886-3350(99)00141-8
23. Lima FE, Magacho L, Carvalho DM, et al. A prospective, comparative study between endoscopic cyclophotodcoagulation and the Ahmed drainage implant in refractory glaucoma. *J Glaucoma.* 2004;13(3):233–237. doi:10.1097/00061198-200406000-00011
24. Francis BA, Kawji AS, Vo NT, et al. Endoscopic cyclophotocoagulation (ECP) in the management of uncontrolled glaucoma with prior aqueous tube shunt. *J Glaucoma.* 2011;20(8):523–527. doi:10.1097/IJG.0b013e3181f46337

25. Murakami Y, Akil AS, Chahal J, et al. Endoscopic cyclophotocoagulation versus second glaucoma drainage device after prior aqueous tube shunt surgery. *Clin Exp Ophthalmol.* 2017;45(3):241–246. doi:10.1111/ceo.12828

26. Hollander DA, Pennesi ME, Alvarado JA. Management of plateau iris syndrome with cataract extraction and endoscopic cyclophotocoagulation. *Exp Eye Res.* 2017;158(5):190–194. doi:10.1016/j.exer.2016.07.018

27. Roberts SJ, Mulvahill M, SooHoo JR, et al. Efficacy of combined cataract extraction and endoscopic cyclophotocoagulation for the reduction of intraocular pressure and medication burden. *Int J Ophthalmol.* 2016;9(5):693–698.

28. Francis BA, Berke SJ, Dustin I, et al. Endoscopic cyclophotocoagulation combined with phacoemulsification versus phacoemulsification alone in medically controlled glaucoma. *J Cataract Refract Surg.* 2014;40(8):1313–1321.

29. Berke SJ. Data supports safety and efficacy of Phaco/ECP. *Rev Ophthalmol.* 2006. http://www.reviewofophthalmology.com/article/data-supports-safety-and-efficacy-of-phacoecp. Accessed 08-20-2020.

30. Morales J, Al Qahtani M, Khandekar R, et al. Intraocular pressure following phacoemulsification and endoscopic cyclophotocoagulation for advanced glaucoma: one-year outcomes. *J Glaucoma.* 2015; 24(6):e157–e162.

SUPPLEMENTAL READING

1. Asfeld LJ, Skorin L, Endoscopic cyclophotocoagulation for glaucoma. Modern Optometry. March 2021. Available at: https://collaborativeeye.com/articles/2021-mar/endoscopic-cyclophotocoagulation-for-glaucoma/?single=true

SECTION 4

Cataract and IOL

16 Femtosecond Laser-Assisted Cataract Surgery

John P. Berdahl • Justin A. Schweitzer • Adam R. Bleeker

Since its inception in the early 1980s, the neodymium-doped yttrium aluminum garnet (Nd:YAG) laser has played a pivotal role in clinical eye care. Its revolutionary nanosecond (10^{-9}) pulse rate allowed surgeon's to treat ocular pathology noninvasively with safe and predictable results. However, the Nd:YAG laser lacked precision, preventing its use in corneal and refractive procedures.

In 1990, Dr. Juhasz and his colleagues at the University of Michigan College of Engineering Center for Ultra-fast Optical Sciences developed a means of shortening the pulse duration of the Nd:YAG laser from the nanosecond (10^{-9}) to femtosecond (10^{-15}) range.[1] This decreased energy output and increased peak intensity, leading to micron precision and less surrounding tissue injury.[2] In 2008, Nagy et al. described the use of the femtosecond laser during cataract surgery.[3] Initial outcomes were promising as all anterior capsulotomies were appropriately sized/centered, and laser-assisted lens fragmentation resulted in less overall phacoemulsification time.[3] By 2010, the procedure known as femtosecond laser-assisted cataract surgery (FLACS) had received approval from the United States Food and Drug Administration (FDA).[4]

While conventional cataract surgery is safe and effective, there remains room for improvement. The femtosecond laser replaces several of the manual steps of cataract surgery, with the goal of improving safety and reproducibility. However, its implementation into primary ophthalmologic care has been slow due to the ongoing debate regarding its advantages over traditional phacoemulsification techniques. Nonetheless, it remains a viable option for ophthalmology practices seeking to offer premium refractive cataract surgery.

INDICATIONS

Key Indications

- Anterior capsulotomy
- Lens fragmentation and liquefaction
- Corneal incisions
- Astigmatic keratotomy

259

Anterior Capsulotomy

Creating a continuous circular capsulorhexis is one of the more difficult aspects of traditional cataract surgery. If the capsulorhexis is too large, the intraocular lens (IOL) implant can tilt or decenter, producing posterior capsule opacification and greater higher-order aberrations. If the capsulorhexis is too small, the IOL can shift posteriorly, resulting in hyperopic shift and capsular phimosis.[5] A properly centered and sized capsulorhexis is essential for successful refractive outcomes.

Although skilled surgeon's generate consistent results, anterior capsulotomies cut by the femtosecond laser have demonstrated less deviation in size, superior centration, and greater circularity (Figure 16.1).[5] There is, however, disagreement regarding the safety of laser-assisted anterior capsulotomy. Two small prospective studies evaluating the safety of laser-assisted anterior capsulotomy demonstrated a similar number of adverse events, compared with manual capsulotomy.[5,6] Yet meta-analysis data suggest that capsular tears and tags may be more common than initially reported.[4] Despite this discordance, laser-assisted capsulotomy is a step toward a safer and more standardized approach.

Lens Liquefaction and Fragmentation

At present, phacoemulsification is the standard of care for cataract extraction. Over the past half-century, the safety of phacoemulsification has greatly improved, yet corneal endothelial cell loss and posterior capsular rupture still occur. The femtosecond laser seeks to alleviate these risks, given its micron precision and reliability.

Lens fragmentation occurs through a complex set of molecular reactions (Figure 16.1). Femtosecond laser energy gives rise to free electrons and ionized molecules, which, in turn, create a rapidly expanding wave of plasma. Similar to an acoustic shock wave, this plasma liquifies and dissects through optically transparent tissue.[7] For patients with softer cataracts, central liquification of the opacified lens is recommended. As nuclear sclerosis progresses, a hybrid pattern consisting of central liquification and peripheral fragmentation is favored.[7] Various sequences have been developed for the purpose of reducing phacoemulsification time and corneal endothelial cell loss.[8] Therefore, as surgeon's push for zero effective phacoemulsification time, the femtosecond laser presents one possible solution.[6,8]

Corneal Incisions

Irregular corneal wounds are more susceptible to aqueous leak, infection, and surgically induced astigmatism (SIA).[7] Historically, clear corneal incisions pass along a single plane, creating an opportunity for bacteria to enter the eye and often requiring stromal hydration at the end of the case.[7] Laser-assisted corneal incisions are highly customizable, theoretically reducing the complication risk. The femtosecond laser offers multiplanar, trapezoid wounds, which demonstrate better integrity and predictability (Figure 16.1).[9] Yet like traditional cataract surgery, laser-assisted corneal incisions result in SIA and higher-order aberrations.[10] The rate of SIA correlates directly with docking issues and tends to decrease with experience.

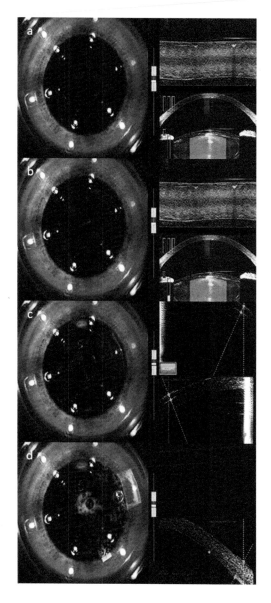

FIGURE 16-1 FLACS laser sequence. (a) 360 capsulorhexis, (b) lens fragmentation, (c) arcuate incisions, and (d) clear corneal incisions.

Astigmatic Keratotomy

Between 33% and 50% of eyes possess one diopter of corneal astigmatism at the time of cataract surgery.[11] An armamentarium of surgical options exists for astigmatism correction, including toric IOLs, astigmatic keratotomy (AK), limbal relaxing incisions, and light-adjustable IOLs. Femtosecond laser-assisted AK possesses many advantages over manual incisional techniques (Figure 16.1). Traditional AK incisions are open, placing eyes at risk for scarring and infection along the visual axis.

Femtosecond laser-assisted AK incisions are intrastromal, reducing the risk of post-operative infection and pain. Though adverse outcomes have been reported, laser-assisted AK is a safe and effective treatment for astigmatism, which can be completed at the time of cataract surgery.[11,12]

CONTRAINDICATIONS

Key Contraindications

- Small, non-dilating pupil (relative)

The only relative contraindication to FLACS is a small, non-dilating pupil.[7] Pupil dilation is measured preoperatively and should be greater than 6.0 mm. While laser-assisted anterior capsulotomy is possible with a pupil diameter less than 6.0 mm, there is increased risk of injury to the iris (Figure 16.2). Furthermore, if an already small pupil experiences intraoperative miosis following laser pretreatment, subsequent phacoemulsification and lens extraction can be challenging. The size of anterior capsulotomy can be adjusted to accommodate for a small, non-dilating pupil. However, smaller anterior capsulotomies (i.e., less than 4.0 mm in diameter) are at increased risk of capsular phimosis.

INFORMED CONSENT CONSIDERATIONS

Key Informed Consent Adverse Events

- Complications of ocular surgery may include blindness, double vision, loss of corneal clarity, infection, iritis, droopy eyelid, glaucoma, hyphema, pupillary dysfunction, lens dislocation, loss of eye, retinal swelling, and retinal detachment.
- Complications due to anesthesia or drug reactions of other factors may involve other parts of the body, including the possibility of brain damage or even death.
- Complications for presbyopia correction include halos, ghost images, night glare, double vision, blurry vision, trouble with depth perception, trouble with nighttime driving, and glasses may still be needed.

The introduction of several new technologies in the cataract surgery space has led to an increased importance of the informed consent process. In order to reduce medicolegal risk associated with cataract surgery, it is important to manage patient

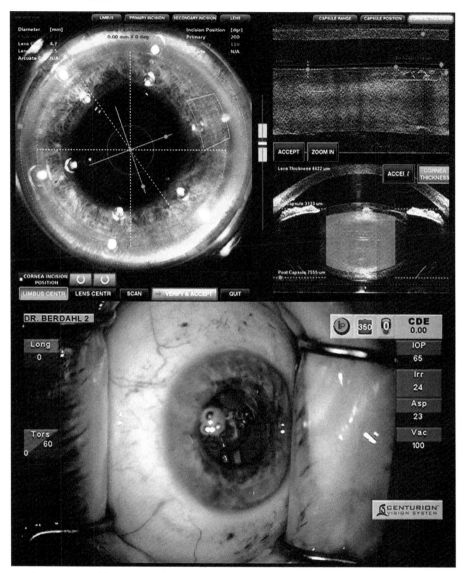

FIGURE 16-2 Poor dilation is a relative contraindication for FLACS. In the example cited earlier, a 4.7-mm diameter capsulorhexis was cut due to poor dilation.

expectations and have documents that support it. The informed consent is intended to promote patient safety and reduce liability exposure when cataract surgery is performed. The decision to proceed with cataract surgery is acceptable once the informed consent process has been shown to be well documented in the patients' medical record, and the risk/benefits of the procedure are documented on the informed consent.

PREOPERATIVE EVALUATION

> **Key Preoperative Considerations**
>
> - Dilated slit lamp and fundus exam assessing for indications and contraindications
> - Preoperative drops: cyclopentolate 1%, phenylephrine 10%, ketorolac 0.5%, and tropicamide 1%

A standard cataract evaluation is required prior to FLACS. This includes a thorough review of the patient's past medical and surgical history. Notably, patients with dry eye may experience worsening of symptoms after FLACS.[13] Thus, treating the ocular surface before the procedure is important. This can be achieved in a variety of ways, including artificial tears, topical pharmaceutical agents, punctal plugs, meibomian gland treatments, and nutraceuticals. An algorithm for the treatment of dry eye prior to cataract surgery has been described elsewhere.[14] Current medications should also be reviewed as blood thinners may compound the intraoperative bleeding risk. However, discontinuation of these medications is not required.

Visual acuities, manifest refraction, and glare testing are useful in determining the visual significance of the cataract. Undilated slit lamp examination of the anterior segment provides an overall health assessment. Dilated fundus examination establishes baseline vitreoretinal disease and helps to assess pupillary dilation. Surgical planning is completed following ocular biometry, optical coherence tomography, and corneal topography, which aid in selection of the IOL and calibration of the femtosecond laser. On the day of surgery, mydriasis is achieved via the instillation of either of a combination of cyclopentolate 1%, phenylephrine 10%, ketorolac 0.5%, and/or tropicamide 1%.

SETTINGS AND PROCEDURE

There are currently four FDA-approved FLACS systems commercially available in the United States. Each laser differs in terms of the patient and physician interfaces. Additionally, most surgeon's have personal preferences regarding energy settings, anterior capsulotomy size, and lens fragmentation pattern. Due to the inherent variability between laser systems and surgeon's, an in-depth analysis of the procedure itself extends beyond the scope of this book. If more comprehensive study is desired, the authors suggest referring to the Supplemental Readings section.

POSTOPERATIVE CARE/CO-MANAGEMENT (FOLLOW-UP SCHEDULE)

Key Postoperative Considerations

- Postoperative drops: topical antibiotic, topical corticosteroid, and topical nonsteroidal anti-inflammatory (NSAID)
- Routine follow-up appointments at 1-day, 1-week, 1-month postoperative, and 3 months postoperative

Postoperative care is identical to traditional cataract surgery with phacoemulsification. Patients are prescribed a combination drop regimen consisting of topical antibiotic, topical corticosteroid, and topical nonsteroidal anti-inflammatory. Follow-up visits are scheduled at 1-day, 1-week, 1-month postoperative, and 3 months postoperative.

POTENTIAL COMPLICATIONS AND THEIR TREATMENT

Key Potential Complications:

- Subconjunctival hemorrhage
- Intraoperative miosis
- Capsular blockage syndrome
- Incomplete capsulotomy and fragmentation
- Surgically induced astigmatism

Subconjunctival Hemorrhage

Subconjunctival hemorrhage is a familiar complication seen following the application of suction to the eye during the docking procedure.[15] Notably, the type of patient interface dictates the frequency and pattern of subconjunctival hemorrhage. Rigid corneal applanation interfaces are responsible for the majority of cases, producing a ring-like pattern around the limbus (Figure 16.3). In contrast, subconjunctival hemorrhage is more diffused with liquid immersion interfaces.[16] Though not medically significant, patients should be informed of the potential for postoperative redness. This is especially pertinent in patients on anticoagulants or antiplatelets. While subconjunctival hemorrhage typically resolves spontaneously within a few days, it can be a source of concern and should be addressed.

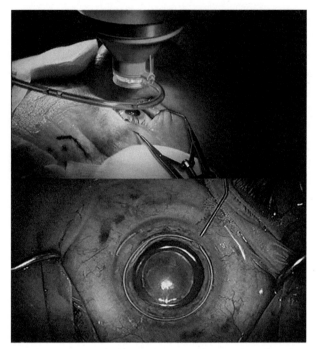

FIGURE 16-3 Laser docking using a rigid corneal applanation interface. Note the ring-like subconjunctival hemorrhage.

Intraoperative Miosis

Intraoperative miosis occurs in 9.5% to 32.0% of FLACS.[15,17,18] The application of intraocular laser is thought to trigger a release of cytokines from the iris, trabecular meshwork, and corneal endothelium, leading to an influx in inflammatory mediators, which constrict the pupil. A study published by Schultz et al. noted an increased concentration of prostaglandin E_2 (PGE_2) in the anterior chamber following femtosecond laser pretreatment. However, no relationship existed between PGE_2 levels and the incidence of intraoperative miosis.[19]

Pupillary constriction during surgery presents a daunting challenge as visualization of the anterior capsulotomy and crystalline lens can be obstructed. On average, the pupillary area decreases by approximately 29.7% after pretreatment. This directly correlates with the amount of laser exposure during lens fragmentation and primary incision creation.[17] Therefore, intraoperative miosis is an important component of preoperative planning.

Nagy et al. mitigated this via the administration of sympathomimetic and parasympatholytic dilating agents.[16] He also noted beneficial results with less suction during patient docking.[15] To counterbalance the action of PGE_2, topical NSAIDs have been added to the standard dilating regimen with tremendous success.[20,21] In resistant eyes, a Malyugin Ring (MicroSurgical Technology, Redmond, Wash.) can be utilized, but this requires specialized surgical technique.[7]

Capsular Blockage Syndrome

Capsular blockage syndrome is an avoidable complication seen predominantly during the learning curve of FLACS. It occurs as a result of increased intracapsular volume secondary to residual intralenticular cavitation bubbles created during lens fragmentation. During rapid hydrodissection, the anterior capsulotomy can become partially occluded, resulting in high pressure within the capsular bag, ultimately leading to posterior capsule rupture or posterior dislocation of the crystalline lens.

The first two cases of capsular blockage syndrome associated with FLACS were reported by Roberts et al.[22] Note that both cases were older patients with mature cataracts, which is a known risk factor of capsular blockage syndrome. Implementation of various surgical techniques has been shown to significantly reduce the incidence of capsular blockage syndrome (Figure 16.4).[22]

Incomplete Anterior Capsulotomy

Incomplete anterior capsulotomy and anterior capsular tags are intraoperative complications of FLACS (Figure 16.5).[18] These issues are often missed and predispose additional complications throughout the remainder of the case. Surgeon's should assume an incomplete capsulorhexis in all FLACS cases, carefully lifting and removing the cut capsular edge.[5] Many cases of incomplete capsulorhexis can be attributed to early femtosecond laser technology, improper docking, or patient movement. However, with experience, the incidence of incomplete anterior capsulotomy decreases.

Surgically Induced Astigmatism

The amount of SIA associated with FLACS is debated.[10] However, it is an important consideration as patients electing for laser-assisted cataract surgery often seek

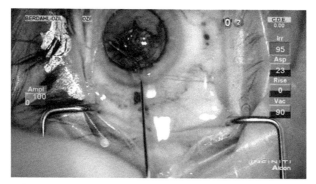

FIGURE 16-4 Hydrodissection following FLACS. Two surgical techniques—decompression of the anterior chamber and lens capsule—help to blunt the rapid change in capsular pressure during hydrodissection.

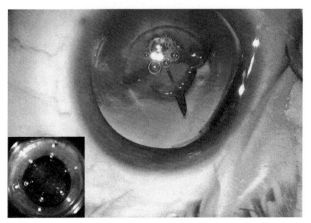

FIGURE 16-5 Incomplete capsulotomy occurs as the result of numerous factors. It is recommended that a surgeon manually tear the remainder of the capsulorhexis.

postoperative spectacle independence. Proper patient docking is critical to avoid SIA. If the patient is not centered, the corneal wounds can be displaced centrally, resulting in visually significant astigmatism.[7] As a surgeon becomes more confident operating the laser, the incidence of docking complications has been shown to decrease.[23]

VIDEOS OF PROCEDURE

Video 16.1—This FLACS case highlights laser-assisted creation of the anterior capsulorhexis. In this example, the anterior capsule was thick due to pseudoexfoliation, which produced capsular flatting as depicted by real-time OCT. A perfectly symmetric anterior capsulotomy was established, and the patient proceeded to the operating room for cataract removal. Trypan blue was used to stain the dense anterior capsulotomy before it was removed using capsulorhexis forceps.

Video 16.2—This FLACS case demonstrates the benefit of the femtosecond laser in complicated cataract extraction. In particular, this patient exhibited a small pupil and dense cataract. A number of different patterns can be used to break up the lens. This video depicts the creation of a liquified central cylinder and two peripheral chops. Additionally, a trip-planar 2.4 mm clear corneal incision and paracentesis are cut.

Video 16.3—This FLACS case notes one potential complication, incomplete capsulorhexis. If this is experienced, do not reattempt laser-assisted anterior capsulotomy. Proceed to the operating room. In this example, capsulorhexis forceps were used to mobilize the anterior capsule flap, and the capsulorhexis was manually torn to completion.

Video courtesy of John P. Berdahl.

SAFETY AND EFFICACY

By automating the critical steps of manual cataract surgery, the femtosecond laser aims to improve patient outcomes. Several randomized clinical trials have examined the safety and efficacy of FLACS, yet heterogeneity among endpoints has hindered meaningful conclusions.[4,24] A meta-analysis conducted in 2015 analyzed the results of 989 eyes, finding no significant difference in surgical complication rate (anterior capsule tears, macular edema, and elevated intraocular pressure) between traditional cataract surgery and FLACS.[24] This dataset was expanded by a subsequent meta-analysis which included 14,567 eyes from 15 small randomized controlled trials and 22 observational cohort studies.[4] Safety outcomes were similar; however, posterior capsular ruptures were higher with FLACS. This difference could be explained by the higher complication rate seen during the learning curve, yet even experienced surgeon's report a slightly greater number of complications with FLACS.[23,25] While the safety profile of laser-assisted cataract surgery is likely equivalent to that of conventional cataract surgery, further testing is required.

Initial studies reported reduced effective phacoemulsification time and cumulative dissipated energy (CDE) in laser-assisted cataract surgery.[26,27] It was theorized that FLACS could spare the corneal endothelium, resulting in less postoperative corneal edema and faster visual recovery. Pooled data published in 2016 demonstrated less surgically induced corneal endothelial cell loss following FLACS.[4] Though statistically significant, the difference in endothelial cell loss was small and lacked clinical significance.[28] Recent prospective studies have drawn mixed conclusions.[29,30] Nonetheless, there exists a nonlinear correlation between CDE and endothelial cell loss with an inflection point occurring at 10 ultrasound units (U/S) of CDE. CDE is equivalent to the total phacoemulsification time in minutes multiplied by the average phacoemulsification power divided by 100. Under 10 U/S CDE, FLACS demonstrated more endothelial cell loss than traditional cataract surgery, suggesting a limited overall benefit.

Refractive outcomes following FLACS are controversial due to differences in potential bias. Now that a decade has passed since the introduction of FLACS, long-term, cumulative data are beginning to emerge. Three meta-analyses, a Cochrane Review, and three randomized clinical trials have evaluated refractive outcomes between FLACS and traditional cataract surgery. A Cochrane Review article published in 2016 concluded that current evidence was insufficient and failed to define the refractive equivalency of FLACS.[31] Interestingly, all three meta-analyses found no significant difference in refractive endpoints between the two procedures.[4,24,32] One of the randomized clinical trials noted slightly better uncorrected visual acuities in the FLACS arm; however, the difference was not statistically significant.[33] The Femtosecond Laser-Assisted Cataract Trial determined that FLACS was not inferior to traditional cataract surgery at 3 months postoperative, citing the results of 785 randomized participants.[34] These results agreed with the femtosecond laser-assisted versus phacoemulsification cataract surgery (FEMCAT) trial, which demonstrated little-to-no overall refractive advantage despite additional cost.[35]

CODING/BILLING AND MODIFIERS

Coding and billing for FLACS includes two parts. CPT code 66984 (Cataract surgery, extracapsular, with insertion of IOL) is billed for the medical portion of the cataract surgery with an appropriate ICD-10 cataract diagnosis code. CPT code 66999 (Other procedures of the anterior segment of the eye) is billed for the refractive component with an appropriate ICD-10 code for refractive error (i.e., presbyopia or astigmatism).

The patient is responsible for payment of the refractive component of the procedure with the medical portion traditionally applied to their insurance.

H25.011-H25.019 (cortical age-related cataract)
H25.031-H25.039 (anterior subcapsular polar age-related cataract)
H25.041-H25.049 (posterior subcapsular polar age-related cataract)
H25.091-H25.099 (other age-related incipient cataract)
H25.10-H25.13 (age-related nuclear cataract)
H25.20-H25.23 (age-related cataract, Morgagnian type)
H25.811-H25.819 (combined forms of age-related cataract)
H26.001-H26.009 (unspecified infantile and juvenile cataract)
H26.011-H26.019 (infantile and juvenile cortical, lamellar, or zonular cataract)
H26.031-H26.039 (infantile and juvenile nuclear cataract)
H26.041-H26.049 (anterior subcapsular polar infantile and juvenile cataract)
H26.051-H26.059 (posterior subcapsular polar infantile and juvenile cataract)
H26.061-H26.069 (combined forms of infantile and juvenile cataract)
H26.101-H26.109 (unspecified traumatic cataract)
H26.111-H26.119 (localized traumatic opacities)
H26.121-H26.129 (partially resolved traumatic cataract)
H26.131-H26.139 (total traumatic cataract)
H26.20 (unspecified complicated cataract)
H26.211-H26.219 (cataract with neovascularization)
H26.221-H26.229 (cataract secondary to ocular disorders [degenerative] [inflammatory])
H26.231-H26.239 (glaucomatous flecks [subcapsular])
H26.30-H26.33 (drug-induced cataract)

RETURN ON INVESTMENT

The cost-effectiveness of FLACS is controversial, given the initial monetary investment. However, it may be a worthwhile option for practices seeking to offer a broad variety of refractive cataract surgery options. Few studies have compared the financial implications between FLACS and traditional cataract surgery. Given its high start-up cost, it is reasonable to assume a slow return on investment. The FEMCAT trial analyzed the cost-effectiveness of FLACS versus standard phacoemulsification finding an incremental cost-effectiveness ratio in favor of traditional cataract surgery.[35] These results agreed with the findings of Abell and Vote.[36] Though the financial implications of FLACS remain undefined, it represents an exciting avenue within the field.

REFERENCES

1. Soong HK, Malta JB. Femtosecond lasers in ophthalmology. *Am J Ophthalmol.* Feb 2009;147(2): 189–197.e2. doi:10.1016/j.ajo.2008.08.026

2. Ratkay-Traub I, Ferincz IE, Juhasz T, Kurtz RM, Krueger RR. First clinical results with the femtosecond neodynium-glass laser in refractive surgery. *J Refract Surg.* 2003 Mar–Apr 2003;19(2):94–103.

3. Nagy Z, Takacs A, Filkorn T, Sarayba M. Initial clinical evaluation of an intraocular femtosecond laser in cataract surgery. *J Refract Surg.* Dec 2009;25(12):1053–1060. doi:10.3928/1081597X-20091117-04

4. Popovic M, Campos-Möller X, Schlenker MB, Ahmed II. Efficacy and safety of femtosecond laser-assisted cataract surgery compared with manual cataract surgery: a meta-analysis of 14 567 eyes. *Ophthalmology.* 10 2016;123(10):2113–2126. doi:10.1016/j.ophtha.2016.07.005

5. Friedman NJ, Palanker DV, Schuele G, et al. Femtosecond laser capsulotomy. *J Cataract Refract Surg.* Jul 2011;37(7):1189–1198. doi:10.1016/j.jcrs.2011.04.022

6. Reddy KP, Kandulla J, Auffarth GU. Effectiveness and safety of femtosecond laser-assisted lens fragmentation and anterior capsulotomy versus the manual technique in cataract surgery. *J Cataract Refract Surg.* Sep 2013;39(9):1297–1306. doi:10.1016/j.jcrs.2013.05.035

7. Nagy ZZ. New technology update: femtosecond laser in cataract surgery. *Clin Ophthalmol.* 2014;8:1157–1167. doi:10.2147/OPTH.S36040

8. Conrad-Hengerer I, Hengerer FH, Schultz T, Dick HB. Effect of femtosecond laser fragmentation of the nucleus with different softening grid sizes on effective phaco time in cataract surgery. *J Cataract Refract Surg.* Nov 2012;38(11):1888–1894. doi:10.1016/j.jcrs.2012.07.023

9. Masket S, Sarayba M, Ignacio T, Fram N. Femtosecond laser-assisted cataract incisions: architectural stability and reproducibility. *J Cataract Refract Surg.* Jun 2010;36(6):1048–1049. doi:10.1016/j.jcrs.2010.03.027

10. Serrao S, Giannini D, Schiano-Lomoriello D, Lombardo G, Lombardo M. New technique for femtosecond laser creation of clear corneal incisions for cataract surgery. *J Cataract Refract Surg.* 2017;43(1):80–86. doi:10.1016/j.jcrs.2016.08.038

11. Day AC, Lau NM, Stevens JD. Nonpenetrating femtosecond laser intrastromal astigmatic keratotomy in eyes having cataract surgery. *J Cataract Refract Surg.* Jan 2016;42(1):102–109. doi:10.1016/j.jcrs.2015.07.045

12. Day AC, Stevens JD. Predictors of femtosecond laser intrastromal astigmatic keratotomy efficacy for astigmatism management in cataract surgery. *J Cataract Refract Surg.* Feb 2016;42(2):251–257. doi:10.1016/j.jcrs.2015.09.028

13. Yu Y, Hua H, Wu M, Yu W, Lai K, Yao K. Evaluation of dry eye after femtosecond laser-assisted cataract surgery. *J Cataract Refract Surg.* Dec 2015;41(12):2614–2623. doi:10.1016/j.jcrs.2015.06.036

14. Starr CE, Gupta PK, Farid M, et al. An algorithm for the preoperative diagnosis and treatment of ocular surface disorders. *J Cataract Refract Surg.* 2019;45(5):669–684. doi:10.1016/j.jcrs.2019.03.023

15. Nagy ZZ, Takacs AI, Filkorn T, et al. Complications of femtosecond laser-assisted cataract surgery. *J Cataract Refract Surg.* Jan 2014;40(1):20–28. doi:10.1016/j.jcrs.2013.08.046

16. Talamo JH, Gooding P, Angeley D, et al. Optical patient interface in femtosecond laser-assisted cataract surgery: contact corneal applanation versus liquid immersion. *J Cataract Refract Surg.* Apr 2013;39(4):501–510. doi:10.1016/j.jcrs.2013.01.021

17. Jun JH, Hwang KY, Chang SD, Joo CK. Pupil-size alterations induced by photodisruption during femtosecond laser-assisted cataract surgery. *J Cataract Refract Surg.* Feb 2015;41(2):278–285. doi:10.1016/j.jcrs.2014.10.027

18. Bali SJ, Hodge C, Lawless M, Roberts TV, Sutton G. Early experience with the femtosecond laser for cataract surgery. *Ophthalmology*. May 2012;119(5):891–899. doi:10.1016/j.ophtha.2011.12.025
19. Schultz T, Joachim SC, Kuehn M, Dick HB. Changes in prostaglandin levels in patients undergoing femtosecond laser-assisted cataract surgery. *J Refract Surg*. Nov 2013;29(11):742–747. doi:10.3928/1081597X-20131021-03
20. Yeoh R. Intraoperative miosis in femtosecond laser-assisted cataract surgery. *J Cataract Refract Surg*. May 2014;40(5):852–853. doi:10.1016/j.jcrs.2014.02.026
21. Diakonis VF, Kontadakis GA, Anagnostopoulos AG, et al. Effects of Short-term preoperative topical ketorolac on pupil diameter in eyes undergoing femtosecond laser-assisted capsulotomy. *J Refract Surg*. Apr 2017;33(4):230–234. doi:10.3928/1081597X-20170111-02
22. Roberts TV, Sutton G, Lawless MA, Jindal-Bali S, Hodge C. Capsular block syndrome associated with femtosecond laser-assisted cataract surgery. *J Cataract Refract Surg*. Nov 2011;37(11):2068–2070. doi:10.1016/j.jcrs.2011.09.003
23. Roberts TV, Lawless M, Bali SJ, Hodge C, Sutton G. Surgical outcomes and safety of femtosecond laser cataract surgery: a prospective study of 1500 consecutive cases. *Ophthalmology*. Feb 2013;120(2):227–233. doi:10.1016/j.ophtha.2012.10.026
24. Chen X, Xiao W, Ye S, Chen W, Liu Y. Efficacy and safety of femtosecond laser-assisted cataract surgery versus conventional phacoemulsification for cataract: a meta-analysis of randomized controlled trials. *Sci Rep*. Aug 2015;5:13123. doi:10.1038/srep13123
25. Abell RG, Darian-Smith E, Kan JB, Allen PL, Ewe SY, Vote BJ. Femtosecond laser-assisted cataract surgery versus standard phacoemulsification cataract surgery: outcomes and safety in more than 4000 cases at a single center. *J Cataract Refract Surg*. Jan 2015;41(1):47–52. doi:10.1016/j.jcrs.2014.06.025
26. Conrad-Hengerer I, Hengerer FH, Schultz T, Dick HB. Effect of femtosecond laser fragmentation on effective phacoemulsification time in cataract surgery. *J Refract Surg*. Dec 2012;28(12):879–883. doi:10.3928/1081597X-20121116-02
27. Abell RG, Kerr NM, Vote BJ. Toward zero effective phacoemulsification time using femtosecond laser pretreatment. *Ophthalmology*. May 2013;120(5):942–948. doi:10.1016/j.ophtha.2012.11.045
28. Zhu DC, Shah P, Feuer WJ, Shi W, Koo EH. Outcomes of conventional phacoemulsification versus femtosecond laser-assisted cataract surgery in eyes with Fuchs endothelial corneal dystrophy. *J Cataract Refract Surg*. May 2018;44(5):534–540. doi:10.1016/j.jcrs.2018.03.023
29. Krarup T, Ejstrup R, Mortensen A, la Cour M, Holm LM. Comparison of refractive predictability and endothelial cell loss in femtosecond laser-assisted cataract surgery and conventional phaco surgery: prospective randomised trial with 6 months of follow-up. *BMJ Open Ophthalmol*. 2019;4(1):e000233. doi:10.1136/bmjophth-2018-000233
30. Dzhaber D, Mustafa O, Alsaleh F, Mihailovic A, Daoud YJ. Comparison of changes in corneal endothelial cell density and central corneal thickness between conventional and femtosecond laser-assisted cataract surgery: a randomised, controlled clinical trial. *Br J Ophthalmol*. 2020;104(2):225–229. doi:10.1136/bjophthalmol-2018-313723
31. Day AC, Gore DM, Bunce C, Evans JR. Laser-assisted cataract surgery versus standard ultrasound phacoemulsification cataract surgery. *Cochrane Database Syst Rev*. Jul 2016;7:CD010735. doi:10.1002/14651858.CD010735.pub2
32. Ye Z, Li Z, He S. A meta-analysis comparing postoperative complications and outcomes of femtosecond laser-assisted cataract surgery versus conventional phacoemulsification for cataract. *J Ophthalmol*. 2017;2017:3849152. doi:10.1155/2017/3849152
33. Shaheen MS, AbouSamra A, Helaly HA, Said A, Elmassry A. Comparison between refractive outcomes of femtosecond laser-assisted cataract surgery and standard phacoemulsification. *BMC Ophthalmology*. 2020;20(1):1. doi:10.1186/s12886-019-1277-9
34. Day CA, Burr MJ, Bennett K, Balaggan SK, Wilkins RM. Femtosecond laser-assisted cataract surgery versus phacoemulsification cataract surgery (FACT): a randomized noninferiority trial. *Ophthalmology*. 2020;127(8):1012–1019.

35. Schweitzer C, Brezin A, Cochener B, et al. Femtosecond laser-assisted versus phacoemulsification cataract surgery (FEMCAT): a multicentre participant-masked randomised superiority and cost-effectiveness trial. *Lancet.* 2020;395(10219):212–224. doi:10.1016/S0140-6736(19)32481-X
36. Abell RG, Vote BJ. Cost-effectiveness of femtosecond laser-assisted cataract surgery versus phacoemulsification cataract surgery. *Ophthalmology.* Jan 2014;121(1):10–16. doi:10.1016/j.ophtha.2013.07.056

SUPPLEMENTAL READING

Krueger R, Talamo J, Lindstrom R. *Textbook of Refractive Laser Assisted Cataract Surgery (ReLACS).* 1st ed. Springer; 2013:289.

17

Nd:YAG Capsulotomy

Jason Ellen • Sophia Leung

The use of a quick-pulsed neodymium-doped yttrium aluminum garnet (Nd:YAG) laser (1064 nm) for capsulotomy dates back to the early 1980s. A plasma microexplosion is created by the Nd:YAG laser and the resulting shockwave allows for photodisruption of ocular tissue.[1] A directional offset is often used to aim the shockwave volume away from adjacent structures to avoid unwanted damage. Nd:YAG laser capsulotomy (Nd:YAG capsulotomy) is the standard treatment for posterior capsular opacification (PCO), replacing manual discission and its associated risks of endophthalmitis and vitreous loss.[2]

Development of PCO is mainly caused by remaining residual lens epithelial cells (LECs), which migrate and spread along the inner face and surface of the capsular bag after cataract removal. LECs transdifferentiate into myofibroblasts, which proliferate and cause fibrosis, resulting in capsular opacification. The innate immune system has also been implicated in the fibrosis process.[3]

Multiple forms of PCO exist. Fibrotic PCO occurs when LECs undergo fibrous metaplasia appearing as folds and wrinkles. The presence of posterior subcapsular cataracts can lead to plaque-like PCO, which appears hard, white, and dense. Elschnig pearls or Soemmering rings occur when LECs undergo crystalline-expressing lenticular fiber regeneration or when residual cortical cells proliferate.[4,5] This appears as clear "droplets" and is best seen in retroillumination. Posterior capsular distension syndrome occurs when residual lens remnants are trapped and absorb fluid. The resulting appearance is focally thick and dense at the posterior capsule. Mechanical PCO results from intraoperative folds and tears that lead to posterior capsular irregularities and can have variable presentations.[4] While specific classification of PCO types does not necessarily change the treatment, certain types may require higher-energy settings and specific treatment considerations, which will be discussed later (Fig. 17.1).

At five years from cataract surgery, PCO occurs in up to 29% of patients.[2] Factors associated with increased PCO development include the following:

Cataract Severity at the Time of Surgery

Higher chances for residual LECs that lead to PCO formation are associated with advanced posterior subcapsular cataracts, nuclear sclerotic cataracts, and mature cataracts.[5] For example, a dense posterior subcapsular cataract (PSC) may be partially

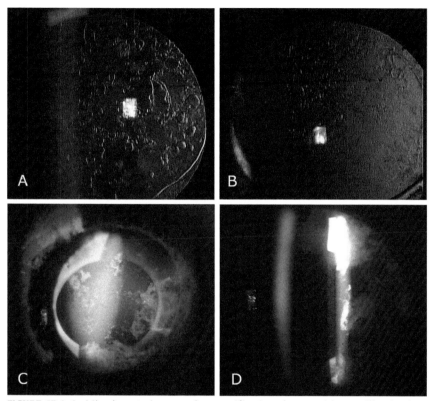

FIGURE 17-1 A. Mixed posterior capsular opacification shown with retroillumination; fibrotic plaques and Elschnig pearls or Soemmering rings are present. **B.** Elschnig pearls observed by retroillumination. **C.** Posterior capsular distension syndrome with significant fluid accumulation surrounding trapped lenticular debris. **D.** Optic section showing thickness of posterior capsule and backward bowing of posterior capsular distension syndrome.

embedded into the posterior capsule risking posterior capsular rupture during extraction. Less posterior capsule polishing during surgery may be performed to mitigate the risk of posterior capsular rupture. This often leads to increased PCO. In certain cases, conversion from phacoemulsification to extracapsular cataract extraction (ECCE) may be necessary, which also increases the risk of PCO development.[6]

Surgical Technique

ECCE is associated with higher occurrences of PCO.[6] In contrast, the use of phacoemulsification, irrigation and aspiration, continuous curvilinear capsulorhexis, smaller incision sizes, and less disruption to the blood–aqueous barrier have been reported to result in lower rates of PCO formation.[4,7]

Intraocular Lens Implant Design

Intraocular lenses (IOL) that have blunt edges will have a higher rate of PCO formation, whereas IOL designs that have sharper edges are thought to disrupt LEC migration thereby reducing PCO formation.[3] Hydrophilic acrylic lens materials (such as in Akreos) are more prone to posterior capsular pearl formation. Single-piece intraocular lens (IOL) designs have been observed to allow more PCO development than three-piece IOL designs.

Younger Age

This is likely due to more rapid cellular restructuring and healing in younger patients.[4]

Inactive or Active Uveitis

Twenty percent of patients with a history of uveitis develop PCO within the first year after cataract surgery.[3]

Anterior capsular opacification or anterior phimosis occurs with similar pathophysiology to PCO, but at the anterior capsulorhexis edge instead. Anterior capsular contraction syndrome occurs more often in patients with pseudoexfoliation syndrome, retinitis pigmentosa, primary angle closure, and diabetic retinopathy.[8] Such contraction from anterior phimosis can result in visual disturbance, IOL decentration, and/or flexion. This can occur with or without the use of capsular tension rings (Fig. 17.2).[9]

INDICATIONS

Key Indications

- Decreased vision, subjective visual complaints, and increased glare complaints caused by capsular opacification
- Capsular contraction syndromes
- Refractive shifts in plate haptic or pseudo-accommodating IOLs
- Prior to refractive enhancements in pseudophakic patients

For insurance qualifications, decreased vision must be confirmed by decreased visual acuity of two lines or more, in normal lighting or by Brightness Acuity Testing (BAT). However, it is important to note that a subjective visual decrease may not involve the loss of visual acuity and, nonetheless, be visually significant to the patient. The decision to treat may be independent of whether the procedure will be reimbursed by insurance or not. Monocular diplopia and impaired contrast sensitivity are often reported symptoms as well.[10] Visual acuity with multifocal IOL technology is more likely to be affected, reported, and visually symptomatic in earlier stages of capsular opacification.

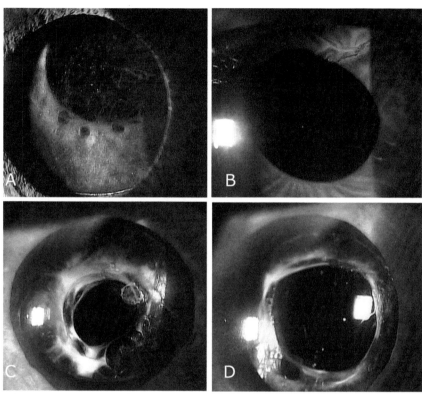

FIGURE 17-2 A. Anterior phimosis covering inferior half of IOL and affecting visual axis. **B.** Anterior capsular contraction syndrome with tension lines shown. **C.** Anterior phimosis with shrunken capsulorhexis diameter noticeable by the patient. **D.** The same patient with widened anterior capsulorhexis after Nd:YAG anterior capsulotomy. Visual symptoms were improved.

Anterior capsular contraction syndrome results when anterior phimosis results in lens flexing. Treatment to reduce tension is necessary. Anterior phimosis also warrants treatment if opacification is observable within the pupil margin, which affects visual acuity or causes subjective visual complaints. In posterior capsular contraction syndrome, early signs of Z formation of an IOL (as seen with Crystalens) warrant Nd:YAG capsulotomy. Z formation presents as an asymmetric vaulting where one plate haptic is bent forward while the other is bent backward, resulting in astigmatic and myopic shifts. It is now standard to perform early Nd:YAG capsulotomy in all Crystalens patients as soon as fibrosis or lenticular astigmatism is observed.[11] If Nd:YAG capsulotomy is insufficient, surgical correction may be required (Fig. 17.3).

A "pre-refractive" Nd:YAG capsulotomy may be warranted prior to corneal refractive surgery enhancement for pseudophakic patients so that future lens flexion and refractive error changes from capsular contraction syndromes are prevented. This is more commonly considered in "refractive cataract surgery" patients.

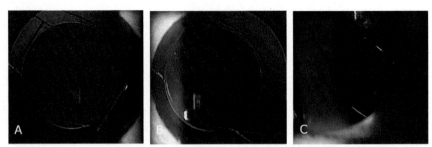

FIGURE 17-3 A. Early Z formation in a patient with Crystalens IOL in OS. The inferior temporal haptic is vaulted anteriorly while the superior nasal haptic is vaulted posteriorly due to capsular contraction syndrome. Notice the slightly larger appearance of the inferior temporal haptic due to its anterior position and the slight tilt of the IOL optic. **B.** The same Z formation shown with retroillumination at a different angle. **C.** The tension lines from capsular contraction syndrome behind the inferior temporal haptic is shown here.

CONTRAINDICATIONS

Key Relative Contraindications

- If visual complaints are due to other treatable ocular pathology
- Corneal scars and opacities that prevent capsular opacifications to be clearly visible
- If the patient is unable to fixate stably or sit stably for the procedure
- Active intraocular inflammation (uveitis, cystoid macular edema) or high risk of intraocular inflammation (history of cystoid macular edema, diabetes, epiretinal membrane)
- Patients with high risk of retinal detachment

Key Absolute Contraindications

- Glass intraocular lens implants[12]
- Significant calcification of IOL surface (older silicone and hydrogel materials)[13]

Despite the presence of capsular opacification, other treatable ocular pathology that is more responsible for patient complaints ought to be addressed first and expectations set appropriately.

Use caution if performing Nd:YAG capsulotomy in an eye where visibility is hindered by corneal pathology (previous radial keratotomy, epithelial basement membrane dystrophy (EBMD), Fuchs dystrophy, corneal edema, and scars). Using a

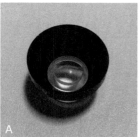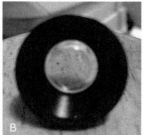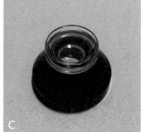

FIGURE 17-4 A. Abraham Nd:YAG capsulotomy contact laser lens is shown here. B. Central lens button provides 1.8× magnification. C. Lens well shown requires coupling solution for stability on the patient's eye and higher optical quality during treatment.

contact capsulotomy laser lens helps to improve visualization through corneal opacities. It also provides better focusing and concentration of the Nd:YAG laser beams.[12] However, in patients who have advanced EBMD, a laser lens may not be appropriate due to a higher risk of unintentional corneal debridement from suction upon laser lens removal. Corneal opacities may also necessitate an increase in overall energy level, which may increase the risk of inflammation, intraocular pressure (IOP) spike, cystoid macular edema (CME), and potentially retinal detachments.[14]

For patients who have trouble with stable fixation, a contact laser lens is extremely helpful. A laser lens provides 1.8× magnification, which is especially helpful in the presence of anterior segment opacities. As previously mentioned, it also helps concentrate the laser energy through corneal opacities.[12] A laser lens also provides stabilization of the patient's eye during treatment by negating the blink reflex. In addition, a contact laser lens is useful with heavy breathers as it helps maintain the IOL on a single plane as the patient breathes (Fig. 17.4).

For patients who are unable to sit still for the procedure, utilization of head straps or having an assistant help stabilize a patient's head position at the laser can be effective. This increases accuracy and ease during the procedure. In certain situations, an oral sedative may be helpful to decrease uncontrollable movement and tremors, and a pinhole capsulotomy may be sufficient enough to improve functional vision. If stability is not possible, Nd:YAG capsulotomy should not be performed. Surgical disscission under general anesthesia performed by a retina or cataract surgeon may be required in such cases. This may be warranted in patients with nystagmus, for example.

Active intraocular inflammation should be treated and managed prior to performing Nd:YAG capsulotomy. This includes postoperative inflammation from cataract surgery. Generally, one should wait at least three months after cataract surgery before doing a Nd:YAG capsulotomy. Although limited evidence is found for this recommendation, general consensus for the three-month postoperative period is to conservatively allow for IOL exchange if necessary. Some recommendations also include waiting at least one month after intraocular inflammation has resolved.[10]

The presence of CME is also a relative contraindication and CME should be treated, stable, or resolved prior to the procedure. In patients who are at higher risk of developing

CME (i.e., diabetic, presence of epiretinal membrane, previous vitrectomy),[15] pretreatment with a topical nonsteroidal anti-inflammatory agent (NSAID) or topical corticosteroid the week prior to the procedure may be warranted, per doctor's discretion.[2]

Patients with a high risk of retinal detachment must be monitored carefully during the postoperative period. These include patients who have a history of retinal detachments, lattice degeneration, axial length greater than 24 mm, vitreoretinal pathology, and intraoperative complications.[2]

Especially in patients with risk of CME and retinal detachments, while Nd:YAG capsulotomy is not absolutely contraindicated, low total energy should be prioritized. Studies are somewhat inconclusive on the direct relationship between energy levels and complications.[12] Bhargava et al. reported more complications associated with total energy levels between 60 to 80 mJ.[14]

Glass intraocular implants are exceptionally rare in the context of today's available IOL technology. The interaction of the Nd:YAG with glass can result in fracturing and should be avoided. Surgical discission may be more appropriate in this particular situation.[12]

Although rare with current IOL technology and materials, older silicone and hydrogel materials (such as the Hydroview IOL) have been reported to result in significant crystalline deposition and calcification of the lens surface. In many of such cases reported, Nd:YAG capsulotomy did not resolve visual impairment and required IOL exchange.[13,16]

INFORMED CONSENT CONSIDERATIONS

Key Adverse Effects to Include

- Transient iritis
- Transient floaters and visual disturbances/blurring
- IOP increase
- CME
- Retinal detachment

Informed consent via paper or electronic means should address risks, benefits, and complications of the procedure in plain language. This should include a simple explanation of the Nd:YAG capsulotomy procedure, its indications and purpose, and potential alternative treatments. Typical postoperative expectations and adverse effects should be listed. A statement outlining that the counseling clinician discussed the procedure, risks involved, and expected results should be included, with signatures from the patient, the counseling clinician, and a witness (typically a staff member).

The patient should be informed about what to expect during the procedure. This includes audible "pops" and "clicks" as the laser fires and the potential for a "sensation" behind the eye or at the back of the patient's head during the procedure.

PREOPERATIVE CARE

Key Preoperative Considerations

- Pre-dilation pupil size should be noted to give the treating clinician an idea of how large to make the capsulotomy opening.
- A full exam including dilated fundus exam to fully examine the level of capsular opacification as well as rule in/out other pre-existing ocular pathology.
- Preoperative drops: Alpha-agonist and proparacaine.

Visual acuity and/or glare testing, also known as BAT, should be acquired. Anterior segment evaluation with dilated pupils should be performed to assess the level of capsular opacification, position of IOL, and the presence of corneal opacities that may affect visibility. Intraocular inflammation should also be ruled out. Posterior segment examination should also be performed to assess for risk of retinal detachment, CME, and other adverse postoperative events. Other ocular pathology that may be attributable to the patient's visual complaints should also be assessed. Once Nd:YAG capsulotomy is determined appropriate, informed consent should be obtained. Topical proparacaine should be instilled in both eyes to control blink reflexes. A topical alpha-agonist, such as brimonidine (0.1%–0.2%) or apraclonidine (0.5%–1%), should be instilled into the eye being treated.

SETTINGS AND PROCEDURE

Key Nd:YAG Capsulotomy Settings

- Energy
  - 1.0 to 1.8 mJ (typical starting energy range).
  - Dense opacification may necessitate higher-energy levels, while mild opacification may allow lower-energy levels.
- Offset
  - 100- to 250-µm posterior offset for posterior capsulotomies.
  - 0- to 100-µm anterior offset for anterior capsulotomies.
- Spot size and pulse duration
  - Internally fixed and cannot be adjusted by the treating clinician.

1. Check laser settings
   a. Offset: The actual center of the shockwave created is typically offset from the targeted plane to avoid undesired damage to adjacent structures such as the IOL. For posterior capsulotomy, typically 100- to 250-µm posterior offset is used. For anterior capsulotomy, 0- to 100-µm anterior offset is typically used.

    b. Energy: 1.0 to 1.8 mJ as a starting point.

        Denser opacification requires higher energy, and starting energy level varies depending on the specific laser model and age of the Nd:YAG crystal. Mean starting energy ranges of 1.5 to 2.5 mJ have been reported in treating denser opacification.[14]

    c. Pulse: Single. Double and/or triple pulse settings are typically reserved for other procedures such as Nd:YAG laser peripheral iridotomy and are generally not recommended for use during Nd:YAG capsulotomy.

2. Focus oculars.

3. If using a contact laser lens, instill a coupling solution such as 1% carboxymethyl-cellulose (Celluvisc) or 2.5% hydroxypropyl methylcellulose (Goniosol) into the lens well. Then, place on the patient's anesthetized eye.

    If *not* using a laser lens, artificial tears may be helpful in patients with ocular surface disease to create a smoother corneal surface to see and treat through. In a 2015 survey, 53% of ophthalmologists reported using a contact laser lens for acrylic and collamer lenses, whereas 47% did not. This was also similar for Crystalens and silicone lenses.[17]

4. Advise the patient to focus on the fixation light or target and hold steady. If a fixation light is not available, use the clinicians' contralateral ear lobe or earring as a target. If a laser lens is not used, remember to allow patients time to blink in between laser shots. Having someone to assist by stabilizing the patient's head may be helpful. Some laser systems have a strap that can be used to stabilize the patients head. If the patient is a heavy breather, laser shots may need to be timed with the patient's breathing to ensure aiming accuracy. A laser lens would be beneficial in a patient who is a heavy breather.

5. For posterior capsulotomy:

    a. Cruciate pattern: Follow a cruciate pattern from 12 o'clock to 6 o'clock and then dissect the horizontal working central to peripherally on each side shooting across capsular tension lines. Typically, the first laser shots should be taken outside of the visual axis to determine how the capsule and laser are going to react (which can vary widely) so that both the doctor and patient are more comfortable and familiar when the visual axis area is being treated. Treat the flaps that remain in the visual axis to allow a larger opening (stop sign or octagon pattern). The capsular tissue should "peel away" as the tension is loosened after each shot. The recommended capsulotomy size should be larger than the patient's undilated pupil.

    b. Circular pattern or "Can Opener" method: Start at 7 o'clock and treat peripherally in a clockwise fashion to allow the inner capsular tissue to "fall" inferiorly/posterior. In this technique, one never treats along the visual axis. This may be beneficial for patients with increased risk of CME or previous retinal conditions.

        For anterior capsulotomy: Either three or four anterior capsule relaxing, equidistantly placed laser shots, are made to release the capsular tension. If anterior phimosis is denser or involving the visual axis, circumferential treatment may be necessary to enlarge the capsulorhexis margin.

6. Additional laser shots can be used to clean up any attached or residual strands. Any remaining posterior capsular striae responsible for IOL tilt should be treated.

7. Maintain at least 1 to 1.5 mm of untreated capsule from the edge of the IOL optic. IOL optics vary in size and is dependent on pupil size. Leaving the capsulotomy too small may allow proliferation of LECs at the capsulotomy edge back into the visual axis.

The number of laser shots and resultant total laser energy is highly variable depending on the severity of capsular opacification and individual patient circumstances. A grossly general estimate of the average number of shots for a Nd:YAG capsulotomy is typically between 15 and 50 laser shots. Multiple studies have shown lower complication rates associated with total energy levels around 30 to 40 mJ whereas higher complication rates have been associated with total energy levels around 60 to 80 mJ.[14]

POSTOPERATIVE CARE/CO-MANAGEMENT (FOLLOW-UP SCHEDULE)

Key Postoperative Considerations

- Postoperative drops: Alpha-agonist in-office and anti-inflammatory prescribed
- IOP check 30 to 60 minutes post-procedure
- IOP check and anterior segment/capsular opening assessment one to two weeks post-procedure

After the procedure, another drop of topical alpha-agonist may be instilled in the treated eye. IOP should be checked within 1 hour of the procedure. Increased IOP should be treated. Topical NSAID or topical corticosteroid is prescribed for one to two weeks following the procedure, which has been reported to control postoperative inflammation.[2] Some clinicians elect to not prescribe anti-inflammatory therapy in the postoperative period based on their clinical experience of low amounts of inflammation usually seen following Nd:YAG capsulotomy. The patient should have vision and IOP checked at the one- to two-week follow-up. It should be explained to the patient that floaters may be more noticeable within the first few days after the procedure and will decrease eventually.

Document Treatment

The eye treated, number of shots, and energy settings (per shot and total) should be documented in the operative report including any issues that arose during the procedure. One should also document the post-laser IOP reading.

POTENTIAL COMPLICATIONS AND THEIR MANAGEMENT

Key Potential Complications

- Damage or "pitting" of IOL
- Increased IOP
- Iritis and/or vitritis
- IOL movement and refractive error changes (especially with larger plate haptic IOLs or with pseudo-accommodating IOLs).
- CME
- Retinal detachment
- Corneal injury, hyphema, pupil blockage, vitreous prolapse

Pitting of the IOL can occur when the shockwaves occur too close to the IOL. Patient movement, misaligned ocular focus, and IOL material can contribute to this.[2] Silicone material is more susceptible to pitting than others while other IOL materials are more forgiving. Pitting in multifocal IOLs may be more visually disruptive as well. Adjusting the offset and starting the treatment outside of the visual axis help to minimize visually significant IOL pitting.

Transient-increased IOP results after a Nd:YAG capsulotomy likely due to deposition of debris in the trabecular meshwork and inflammation of the ciliary body.[2] This has been reported in 12.5% of cases.[14,18] This is typically worse with anterior phimosis treatment. Some studies have suggested higher IOP increases with higher total energy levels.[2,10] Prophylactic use of IOP-lowering medications substantially decreases the occurrence of postoperative IOP spikes.[10] To avoid uncontrolled IOP spikes that can result in permanent damage, IOP-lowering medications may be warranted in high-risk patients such as advanced glaucoma or known steroid-responders.

Transient iritis and vitritis can occur, resolving within a few days especially with the use of topical steroids or NSAIDs during the postoperative period. Postoperative uveitis has been reported to occur in 10% of cases.[14,18] Persistent inflammation is rare[2] and must be aggressively treated if present at the one-week postoperative follow-up.

Studies suggest that there is a posterior movement of the IOL after Nd:YAG capsulotomy, especially with larger posterior capsulotomies.[2,10] However, studies disagree on the significance of such slight changes in effective lens positioning on refractive error.[10] IOL dislocation or tilt may occur if the posterior capsulotomy edge extends beyond the optic, or causes a large split beyond the edge of the optic or to the capsule bag equator. This is more likely in capsules that are tighter and less opaque, such as in posterior capsular distention syndrome or with thickened or dense Elschnig pearls without other opacification.

CME has been reported to occur in 0.2% to 7.9% of cases.[2,18] Vitreous cavity movement and damage to the blood–aqueous barrier result in inflammatory mediators being released which leads to CME development.[10] Occurrences are low especially if Nd:YAG capsulotomies are performed more than six months after cataract surgery[2] but should be treated aggressively with topical NSAID and topical corticosteroids synergistically if noted on postoperative assessments. As previously discussed, preexisting retinal conditions are considered higher risk, and despite strong evidence of prophylactic treatment benefit in low-risk situations, pretreatment with topical NSAID and/or corticosteroids should be strongly considered when risk factors have been identified.[19]

Retinal detachment is a rare but significant potential complication of Nd:YAG capsulotomy. However, occurrences have been reported in as high as 4% to 8% of cases.[2,10,18] The mechanism for the increased risk is unknown but the risk can continue for years after Nd:YAG capsulotomy is performed.[10] To reiterate the importance of identifying risk factors, patients at higher risk include those with previous history of retinal detachment, lattice degeneration, axial lengths greater than 24 mm, and complex cataract surgeries with intraoperative complications.[2] These patients should be monitored carefully. A thorough peripheral exam should have been performed prior to performing Nd:YAG capsulotomy to identify these patients, and ensure that treatable preoperative retinal defects have been addressed.

Corneal injury, hyphema, and pupil blockage are extremely rare. Vitreous prolapse, albeit rare, is more common when anterior or posterior capsulorhexis is larger than the IOL optic allowing vitreous to "escape" through. Vitreous prolapse is also more common when the anterior capsule is not in contact with the anterior surface of the IOL (common in pseudo-accommodating IOLs). Such complications should be treated if observed at postoperative follow-ups.

VIDEOS OF PROCEDURE

Video 17.1—This Nd:YAG posterior capsulotomy was performed without a contact laser laser lens and with a power setting of 1.8 to 2.0 mJ per pulse and a total of 21 shots for a maximum total energy of 42 mJ. The posterior offset was set at 250 μm. This patient had mild-to-moderate PCO with mainly glare symptoms.

Video 17.2—This Nd:YAG posterior capsulotomy was performed with a contact laser lens and with a power setting of 0.8 to 1.0 mJ per pulse and a total of 71 shots for a maximum total energy of 71 mJ. The posterior offset was set at 125 μm. This patient had dense fibrotic plaques. Certain denser areas of opacification required higher-energy settings per pulse.

Video 17.3—This Nd:YAG posterior capsulotomy was performed with contact laser lens and with a power setting of 1.8 mJ per pulse and a total 31 shots for a total energy of 55.8 mJ. The posterior offset was set at 150 μm. A laser lens was used to counteract a strong blink reflex.

Video 17.4—This Nd:YAG posterior capsulotomy was performed with contact laser lens and with a power setting of 1.5 mJ per pulse and a total 27 shots for a total energy of 40.5 mJ. The posterior offset was set at 125 μm. This was in a patient with moderate PCO; mainly fibrotic plaques. A lens was used for stability due to strong blink reflexes.

Video 17.5—This Nd:YAG posterior capsulotomy was performed with a contact laser lens and with a power setting of 1.0 mJ per pulse and a total 151 shots for a total energy of 151 mJ. The posterior offset was set at 125 μm. This was in a patient with a silicone IOL and with densely fibrotic PCO positioned very close to the IOL back surface. A "pie-cutting" technique was used to break away sections of PCO. Low energy per pulse was used in this case to avoid pitting this highly susceptible lens material.

Video 17.6—This Nd:YAG posterior capsulotomy was performed without a contact laser lens and with a power setting of 2.0 to 2.3 mJ per pulse and a total 80 shots for a total energy of 187 mJ. The posterior offset was set at 250 μm. This was in a patient with 4+ PCO with Elschnig pearls. Due to a well-formed bleb, lid holding required frequent breaks to minimize discomfort. Preoperative unaided visual acuity was 20/200, and immediate postoperative unaided visual acuity was 20/30. The fluid outflow after the initial shot resembles that which would occur with posterior capsular distension treatment.

Video 17.7—This early pinhole Nd:YAG posterior capsulotomy was performed without a contact laser lens and a power setting of 1.8 to 2.3 mJ per pulse and a total of 13 shots for a total energy of 35.3 mJ. The posterior offset was set at 125 μm. Due to high visual disruption from dense PCO (history of an advanced cataract and significant postoperative inflammation), a pinhole Nd:YAG was performed to significantly improve vision at the one-month postoperative visit. It is often beneficial to perform this procedure through an undilated pupil to ensure the capsule opening is centered. This patient had a history of retinal detachment and extensive retinal surgery. Therefore, low-energy settings were prioritized.

Video 17.8a—This Nd:YAG posterior capsulotomy was performed without a contact laser lens and with a power setting of 1.0 mJ per pulse and a total of 68 shots for a total energy of 68 mJ. The posterior offset was set at 150 μm. This patient had a Crystalens IOL and an early Nd:YAG capsulotomy was performed to reduce risk of capsular contraction syndrome risking Z-formation.

Video 17.8b—This Nd:YAG posterior capsulotomy was performed without a contact laser lens and with a power setting of 1.2 mJ per pulse and a total of 47 shots for a total energy of 56.4 mJ. The posterior offset was set at 150 μm. In contrast to video YC-8a, this was in a patient with a Crystalens IOL where early capsular contraction syndrome was causing the inferior temporal haptics to vault anteriorly and the superior nasal haptics to vault posteriorly. The tension was relieved just posterior to the haptics to restore proper IOL alignment and position. It is prudent to avoid making the focal capsule opening at the vaulted haptics too large and risking posterior IOL shifting or anterior vitreous herniation. The remaining central Nd:YAG capsulotomy was performed on a separate day to prevent early contraction syndrome at the untreated haptic area.

Video 17.9—This Nd:YAG anterior capsulotomy was performed without a contact laser lens and with a power setting of 1.5 mJ per pulse. The offset was set at 0 μm. The "can-opener" technique was used here, and the large capsular debris was split into smaller pieces at the end of the video. Posterior capsulotomy was also performed following the anterior phimosis treatment with a total energy of 153.5 mJ for both procedures combined.

EFFICACY

Nd:YAG capsulotomy is extremely effective for PCO and anterior phimosis. Visual improvement occurs in up to 96% of patients who receive the procedure.[10,12] Guarded prognosis or limited efficacy results from preexisting ocular conditions. For significant lens tilt or IOL decentration from capsular contraction syndromes, Nd:YAG capsulotomy may not be sufficient in severe cases and, as such, warrants surgical repositioning.

CODING AND BILLING

For a Nd:YAG capsulotomy with a laser, CPT code *66821* should be used: *Discission of secondary membranous cataract (opacified posterior lens capsule and/or anterior hyaloid); laser surgery (e.g., Nd:YAG laser) (one or more stages)*. If an exam is performed and Nd:YAG capsulotomy is performed within three days of the exam, the *57* modifier code (*Decision for surgery*) should be applied to the appropriate level of the examination. If the second eye is done at the one-week follow-up, the *79* modifier code (*Unrelated procedure or service by the same physician during the post-op period*) should be used. If comanaged with a physician outside of the facility where the procedure was performed, the *54* modifier code (*Surgery only*) should be used.[20]

Common ICD-10 codes that support this procedure include[20] the following:

H24.411—Soemmering's ring, right eye
H26.412—Soemmering's ring, left eye
H26.413—Soemmering's ring, bilateral
H26.491—Other secondary cataract, right eye
H26.492—Other secondary cataract, left eye
H26.493—Other secondary cataract, bilateral
T85.21XA—Breakdown (mechanical) of intraocular lens, initial encounter
T85.22XA—Displacement of intraocular lens, initial encounter
T85.29XA—Other mechanical complication of intraocular lens, initial encounter

CAUTIONARY TALES AND SPECIAL CASES

In posterior capsular distension syndrome, it is beneficial to treat from 6 o'clock first to allow fluid exit to occur inferiorly. This will minimize view obstruction due to the gravitational pull. Due to the density of this type of PCO, the energy per pulse and total energy will be higher.

With sulcus-fixated IOLs, caution must be taken as the posterior capsule may not be juxtaposed to the IOL. There is increased risk for vitreous prolapse. This is the same consideration for an anterior chamber IOL.

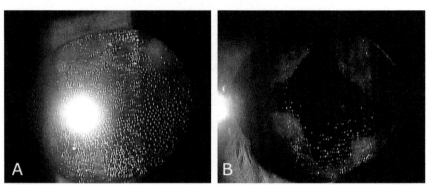

FIGURE 17-5 A. Trapped residual silicone oil from previous complex vitrectomy and retinal surgery performed prior to cataract surgery. High energy per pulse was required for photodisruption due the presence of silicone oil. **B.** Due to high total energy, Nd:YAG capsulotomy treatment was divided into two parts to control postoperative inflammation. Posterior capsular opacification appearance after the first half of treatment is shown here.

When treating Z formation, which is likely with pseudo-accommodating IOLs (Crystalens) and plate haptic IOLs (Starr), treatment of the hinge or separate posterior capsulotomies at the haptics may be required to release contraction of the lens (Fig. 17.5).[21]

ACKNOWLEDGMENTS

All laser procedures were performed on the NIDEK YC-200 S Plus Laser System. All video recordings were captured by the TelScreen *Eye*Res Digital Imaging System. A special thanks to both of these companies for their support and excellent technology.

REFERENCES

1. Vogel A, Busch S, Jungnickel K, Birngruber R. Mechanisms of intraocular photodisruption with picosecond and nanosecond laser pulses. *Lasers Surg Med.* 1994;15(1):32–43. doi:10.1002/lsm.1900150106

2. Karahan E, Er D, Kaynak S. An overview of Nd:YAG laser capsulotomy. *Med Hypothesis Discov Innov Ophthalmol J.* 2014;3(2):45–50. http://www.ncbi.nlm.nih.gov/pubmed/25738159%0Ahttp://www.pubmedcentral.nih.gov/articlerender.fcgi?artid=PMC4346677.

3. Chen HC, Lee CY, Sun CC, Huang JY, Lin HY, Yang SF. Risk factors for the occurrence of visual-threatening posterior capsule opacification. *J Transl Med.* 2019;17(1):1–8. doi:10.1186/s12967-019-1956-6

4. Wu S, Tong N, Pan L, et al. Retrospective analyses of potential risk factors for posterior capsule opacification after cataract surgery. *J Ophthalmol.* 2018;2018. doi:10.1155/2018/9089285

5. Mootha VV, Tesser R, Qualls C. Incidence of and risk factors for residual posterior capsule opacification after cataract surgery. *J Cataract Refract Surg.* 2004;30(11):2354–2358. doi:10.1016/j.jcrs.2004.03.038

6. Chakrabarti A, Nazm N. Posterior capsular rent: prevention and management. *Indian J Ophthalmol.* 2017;65(12):1359. doi:10.4103/ijo.IJO_1057_17

7. Sinha R, Shekhar H, Sharma N, Titiyal J, Vajpayee R. Posterior capsular opacification: a review. *Indian J Ophthalmol.* 2013;61(7):371. doi:10.4103/0301-4738.115787

8. Hayashi K, Yoshida M, Hirata A, Hayashi H. Anterior capsule relaxing incisions with neodymium: YAG laser for patients at high-risk for anterior capsule contraction. *J Cataract Refract Surg.* 2011; 37(1):97–103. doi:10.1016/j.jcrs.2010.07.027

9. Zaugg B, Werner L, Neuhann T, et al. Clinicopathologic correlation of capsulorhexis phimosis with anterior flexing of single-piece hydrophilic acrylic intraocular lens haptics. *J Cataract Refract Surg.* 2010;36(9):1605–1609. doi:10.1016/j.jcrs.2010.06.029

10. Parajuli A, Joshi P, Subedi P, Pradhan C. Effect of Nd:YAG laser posterior capsulotomy on intraocular pressure, refraction, anterior chamber depth, and macular thickness. *Clin Ophthalmol.* 2019;13: 945–952. doi:10.2147/OPTH.S203677

11. Page T, Whitman J. A stepwise approach for the management of capsular contraction syndrome in hinge-based accommodative intraocular lenses. *Clin Ophthalmol.* June 2016:1039. doi:10.2147/OPTH.S101325

12. Steinert R. Nd:YAG laser capsulotomy. American Academy of Ophthalmology. https://www.aao.org/munnerlyn-laser-surgery-center/ndyag-laser-posterior-capsulotomy-3. Published 2013. Accessed July 8, 2020.

13. Izak AM, Werner L, Pandey SK, Macky TA, Trivedi RH, Apple DJ. Calcification on the surface of the Bausch Lomb Lomb Hydroview Intraocular Lens. *Int Ophthalmol Clin.* 2001;41(3):63–77. doi:10.1097/00004397-200107000-00007

14. Bhargava R, Kumar P, Phogat H, Chaudhary K. Neodymium-yttrium aluminium garnet laser capsulotomy energy levels for posterior capsule opacification. *J Ophthalmic Vis Res.* 2015;10(1):37. doi:10.4103/2008-322X.156101

15. Schaub F, Adler W, Enders P, et al. Preexisting epiretinal membrane is associated with pseudophakic cystoid macular edema. *Graefes Arch Clin Exp Ophthalmol.* 2018;256(5):909–917. doi:10.1007/s00417-018-3954-4

16. Altaie R, Loane E, O'Sullivan K, Beatty S. Surgical and visual outcomes following exchange of opacified Hydroview(R) intraocular lenses. *Br J Ophthalmol.* 2007;91(3):299–302. doi:10.1136/bjo.2006.095414

17. Gossman M. YAG Capuslotomy, part 1. EyeWorld. https://www.eyeworld.org/article-yag-capsulotomy--part-1. Published 2015.

18. O'Boyle D, Perez Vives C, Samavedam S, et al. Post-Nd:Yag laser complications in cataract patients treated for posterior capsular opacification: a systematic literature review. *Value Heal.* 2018;21(Cv):S243. doi:10.1016/j.jval.2018.09.1450

19. Russo A, Costagliola C, Delcassi L, et al. Topical nonsteroidal anti-inflammatory drugs for macular edema. *Mediators Inflamm.* 2013;2013:1–11. doi:10.1155/2013/476525

20. American Academy of Ophthalmic Executives. Chapter 7: Eye and Ocular Adnexa. In: American Academy of Ophthalmology, ed. *Coding Coach: Complete Ophthalmic Reference.* 2020:93.

21. Katsev DA, Piracha A, Talamo J, Whitman J. Z syndrome after laser cataract surgery. *Cataract Refract Surg Today.* 2015;(May):29–31.

SECTION 5

Retina and Vitreous

18 Laser Floater Treatment (Vitreolysis)

I. Paul Singh

Like most providers, I downplayed floaters in the past because I felt there was nothing I could do. Now, after performing more than 5,000 laser-based floater treatments over the past seven years, I have come to appreciate the impact floaters can have on a patient's daily functioning. They often return for their posttreatment visits with improvement in their daily life similar to post-cataract surgery patients; "I can drive again," "I can read again," "I can perform in the orchestra again." It is clearly evident that, in symptomatic patients, the visual symptoms associated with floaters are a growing concern and warrant more than merely observation. Until I started treating floaters, I thought of floaters as just a nuisance and counseled patients to live with them. Because they are part of the normal aging process, I felt there was no need to address them. Indeed, I dismissed my floater patients as there was no safe, in-office treatment option. I'm sure many of you have also said these words to your patients, "Get used to them," "They will eventually go away," "They are normal and don't harm you." But have you stopped and thought: "Why are we so quick to dismiss these patients?"

In medicine, our decision to treat or not to treat has been based on the risk–benefit ratio involved with the treatment. Basically, the higher the risk, the more severe the symptoms must be before the surgeon is willing to perform the surgery. As technology has advanced and techniques have evolved, the risk profile of many treatments has improved. Not only does this offer obvious benefits for the patient, but it also allows treatment earlier in the disease process—and for patients who would have historically been ignored. For instance, the old paradigm of cataract surgery has changed. Today, our definition of "clinically significant" cataract has changed. A 20/40 cataract, once considered not suitable for treatment 20 years ago due to the risk and limitations of surgery, is now considered treatable. Advances in glaucoma procedures, and more specifically the advent of micro-invasive surgery (MIGS), have changed the glaucoma treatment paradigm, with surgery now offered earlier in the disease process due to its enhanced safety profile. This, in turn, has redefined the patient type and the justification for surgery. Now, quality of life is a key definition of "uncontrolled glaucoma." One would rarely consider a trabeculectomy for a patient with mild glaucoma on 1 or 2 medications, but with the advent of MIGS, the "ideal" patient for glaucoma surgery has changed. The same can be said for dry eye. Until recently, many of us ignored this condition, minimizing its impact on daily functioning due to a lack of options to treat, or even to diagnose. Once new treatment options and diagnostic devices became available, we as a profession recognized the impact ocular surface disease has on patient quality of life, and as a result, more and more options are becoming available.

Historically, the only treatment offered for vitreous floaters was a pars plana vitrectomy (PPV). This procedure works well to eliminate the symptoms associated with floaters, but there are significant risks involved with the procedure, such as cataract formation and retinal detachment.[1] Although recent advances in technology have improved the safety profile of vitrectomy, there is still the challenge of postoperative healing time, during which patients may be off of work for a few days to weeks and on eye drops for a few weeks to months. For many surgeon's and patients, the overall risk and cost from a PPV is greater than the issues caused by floaters. Therefore, a majority of doctors decide to observe many of the common types of floaters, such as a Weiss ring or other solitary vitreous opacities. Unfortunately, these floaters can still negatively affect patient's quality of life.

A study by Wagle et al. addressed the impairment on functional quality associated with floaters in 311 outpatients.[2] The utility values of floaters were equal to age-related macular degeneration, and similar to glaucoma, mild angina, stroke, and asymptomatic human immunodeficiency virus (HIV). This demonstrates that floaters do have a significant impact on quality of life, similar to other ocular and systemic diseases. Further, a study by Webb et al. found that floaters are very common in the general population, irrespective of age, race, gender, and eye color. In a review of 603 smartphone users, 76% (n = 458) indicated that they notice floaters, with 199 of these individuals citing noticeable vision impairment as a result of their floaters. Furthermore, myopes and hyperopes were 3.5 and 4.4 times more likely, respectively, to report moderate-to-severe floaters.[3] A 2016 study by Garcia et al. showed that there was a 52.5% reduction in contrast sensitivity function following posterior vitreous detachment (PVD). In a survey of approximately 600 smartphone users, 33% of respondents reported that their floaters caused noticeable visual impairment.[4]

Now, with advances in laser technology, laser lenses, and new treatment protocols, the adverse event profile associated with laser-based floater treatment is favorable. It also offers the benefit of a simplified postoperative course. As a result, the definition of clinically significant vitreous opacity (CSVO) has changed: symptomology does not have to be as severe as that for a vitrectomy. Smaller floaters, such as Weiss rings and other types of floaters (amorphous clouds and strings), that were often considered to be not clinically significant to warrant surgery, are now able to be treated. We don't have to minimize the impact of these floaters and tell patients to "just deal with it."

It is important to note that laser floater treatment (LFT) is not intended to replace or compete with vitrectomy. The ideal patient for LFT is very different from that of a vitrectomy patient. These patients often have been told they are not good candidates for a vitrectomy. This can be the case in a phakic patient, or in patients with a smaller type floater.

LFT for symptomatic floaters, also known as vitreolysis, is actually not new. It was first introduced in 1993, when Tsai et al. described a series of patients undergoing Nd:YAG vitreolysis. It was later popularized by Dr. Karickhoff. Despite their work, which demonstrated good efficacy and safety, other older data sets, which suggested only modest efficacy and possible safety concerns, led many doctors to be skeptical about the procedure. It is important to note these older studies were using laser technology not optimized for LFT. Further, the treatment protocol was not optimized. For instance, Delaney et al. in 2002 published a study reporting 38.3% success using a non-randomized questionnaire. The study was performed using older Nd:YAG technology with average energy settings of 1.2 mJ. This energy is too low to vaporize and sufficiently reduce the size of the floater. A fear of complications and an overall lack of understanding of Nd:YAG laser delivery of energy have also contributed to the skepticism surrounding LFT. Colleagues often fear LFT will cause retinal detachment, inflammation, and other serious complications. Recent data based on new technology, and new protocols, addresses these fears. The reason for the variable outcomes in some earlier studies was due to the limitations of traditional Nd:YAG lasers. There were three main limiting factors when performing LFT with traditional Nd:YAG lasers: (1) Lack of visualization of the entire vitreous and necessary spatial awareness between lens and retina; (2) suboptimal power usage during the procedure thus limiting vaporization of the floater (3) inability to fire sufficient number of shots due to older cooling cavities and thus the instability and inconsistency of energy delivery through the entire procedure.

INDICATIONS

Patient selection is extremely important. Like any procedure, not all patients are good candidates or qualified for the procedure. First and foremost, I recommend performing the laser on symptomatic patients, those where the floaters are disabling to daily functioning (regardless of visual acuity on the Snellen chart) and do not resolve over time. For instance, patients often describe a Weiss ring not always affecting clarity of vision, but as distracting and thereby affecting reading and driving. In general, solitary opacities tend to have the best outcomes.

I pay attention to these key variables:

1. Patient symptoms—how long have they been present, are they disabling to daily functioning, where are the floaters coming from, and do they have a specific shape per patient perception?
2. Where in the vitreous is the floater?—if too close to the retina or lens, the patient may not be a good candidate. If close to the lens, especially in a pseudophakic patient, we may need to observe or limit the number of shots (usually less than 500 per session to prevent an IOP spike).
3. Size and density of the floater—if the floater is thin and more like a fibril, it may be difficult to laser. If the floaters are larger and denser, it may require higher number of shots and multiple sessions.

CONTRAINDICATIONS

It is important for surgeon's to know when to say no. Following are some key contra-indication considerations:

- If there is any active vitreoretinal pathology, address it first.
- Relative contraindication is glaucoma—IOP spikes can happen from the procedure.
- If the patient has a floater that is too close to the lens or too close to the retina, recommend observation. We want to keep at least 2 mm from the retina if possible. A clinical pearl: if the floater and the retina are in focus at the same time, it is too close.
- If the patient has a recent PVD with symptoms of a floater or flashes, I recommend observation and repeat a dilated examination within three to six months. It is important to give patients time to neuroadapt before setting up for a laser.
- I would suggest holding off on younger patients with thin strings or who have symptoms you cannot correlate with your clinical exam.
- Those with large amounts of asteroid hyalosis or a vitreous full of opacities may be difficult to treat unless there is a consolidated clumping of calcium that can be broken up.
- Patients with unreasonable expectations should be accounted for as well.

INFORMED CONSENT CONSIDERATIONS

Key Informed Consent Adverse Events Listed as Follows:

- IOP rise (immediate or delayed)
- Pain/discomfort during and/or after the procedure (mostly from the contact lens)
- Transient blurring of vision
- Ineffectiveness of the procedure
- Need for multiple sessions
- Corneal haze/edema
- Retinal hemorrhage
- Retinal detachment
- Lens opacity from hitting the lens

Informed consent should allow for a patient to attest the floaters are disabling to daily functioning, may require multiple sessions, and may not be able to be completely resolved.

Yes/No My floaters do affect my vision and daily functioning.

Yes/No I realize more than one treatment may be necessary to improve symptoms.

Yes/No I realize all symptoms may not be completely resolved even after multiple treatments.

Often, patients with cloud-like, more diffuse amorphous opacities tend to need multiple treatment sessions whereas those with a solitary opacity may have resolution of their symptoms after 1 to 2 treatment sessions.

Also, a description of the procedure should be included. For example, "The eye is dilated and anesthetized, a special contact lens is put in place, and the laser is focused through the pupil on individual floaters. The laser will be used to break up (fractionate) and/or vaporize the floaters in the vitreous (hollow space in the back of the eye) to reduce the impact of the floater on your vision. The laser doesn't have the power to vaporize a large amount at one time therefore may require hundreds of shots."

Potential alternative treatments, such as observation, dilating eye drops, or vitrectomy, should be listed. Risks and complications inherent to any laser procedure, including vitreolysis, include but are not limited to increased eye pressure, irritation or pain during or after the procedure, cataract formation, retinal hemorrhage, temporary blurring of vision, and ineffectiveness of the procedure.

PREOPERATIVE CARE

Key Preoperative Considerations:

- It is important to detail a thorough history of patient symptoms, onset, duration, and location. This history can be helpful when trying to correlate the symptoms to the clinical exam since many patients have multiple floaters on exam but are only bothered by a select few.
- A full dilated examination, including an IOP check, is a must. It is important to rule out active retinal pathology and document location, size, and density of the floaters. It is also important to explain to the patients, although extremely rare, the risks of the procedure including increased IOP, retinal hemorrhage, hitting the lens, and retinal detachment.
- Education and setting expectations are paramount: Explain the laser works by fractionating the floater into smaller pieces and then vaporizing those smaller pieces. The amount of vaporization per shot is extremely small and to prevent complications, such as IOP spikes, we limit the number of shots. Therefore, certain types of floaters, such as diffuse clouds and strings, may require multiple sessions over time to significantly reduce symptoms. Symptoms can vary postoperatively based on how the remaining floaters come back together.
- Document floaters if possible, with a slit lamp picture, ultrasound, or fundus photograph. This allows a chance to educate the patient and help document for payors

if billing insurance. Can you see an opacity that could correlate to the patient's symptoms? If not, then the procedure may not be warranted.

- Document how close the floater is to the lens or retina. If the floater is seen without a 78- or 90-D lens, the floater is likely closer to the phakic lens (Figure 18.1). If too close to the lens, observation is usually recommended, especially early in the treating clinician's experience with the procedure. Once more experienced, one can consider treating behind the floater to "loosen" the vitreous attachments in order to move the floater posteriorly. Conversely, if the floater can be seen in focus at the same time as the retina, observation is recommended, although one can consider treating anterior to the floater to move the floater away from the retina. You can have the patient look up and down during the exam to observe the behavior of the floater; there are times when the forces of eye movement bring the floater more anteriorly or posteriorly and may change your decision to treat.

- Document if the floater is solitary or diffuse/amorphous. Consolidated and more solitary floaters tend to require less number of shots/sessions whereas more diffuse floaters require a greater number of shots and sessions (Fig. 18.2). In some cases, a vitrectomy might be a better option for the diffuse floaters.

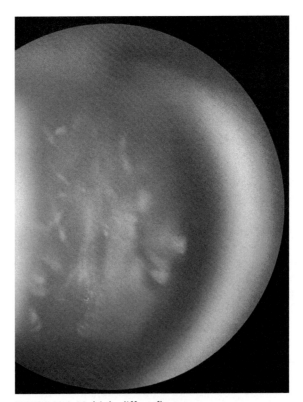

FIGURE 18-1 Multiple diffuse floaters.

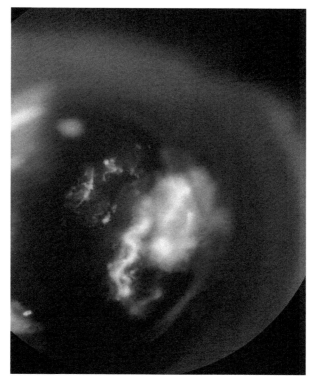

FIGURE 18-2 Consolidated amorphous clump behind the phakic lens located more posterior.

- Place dilating drops in the procedure eye (tropicamide 1% and phenylephrine 10% recommended).

SETTINGS AND PROCEDURE

- At first, give yourself 20 to 30 minutes to perform the procedure. It takes time to feel comfortable "finding" the floater and feeling comfortable firing at a more rapid pace. For certain solitary types of floaters, the time can be as short as 5 minutes once you develop a high comfort level.
- Ask the patient to describe where the floater resides in their visual field right before you start. Often times, they will draw their symptoms on a piece of paper. This allows you to focus your attention in the area where the symptomatic floater resides and treat the ones causing the patient's symptoms (especially if they have multiple opacities in the vitreous).

- The use of a lens is recommended to visualize the entire vitreous to the retina. Lenses help to stabilize the eye and help to manipulate the eye if needed to bring the floater in position, while also helping to focus and concentrate the laser energy. Try and use the new vitreous lenses available, such as the Volk—Singh MidVitreous lens (Fig. 18.3) or the Ocular Instruments—Karickhoff vitreous lenses (Fig. 18.4). Practice using them in the exam room during your consult to get used to the view you will expect to see when at the laser. The Karickhoff lenses come in an 18-, 21-, and 30-mm lens. The 21-mm lens seems to be used for a broad range of floater locations whereas we use the 30-mm lens to reach more peripherally located floaters due to the built-in prism.
- A small amount of coupling agent should be instilled into the lens well. While 1% carboxymethylcellulose (Celluvisc) drops can be used, a gel formulation such as Genteal or Systane gel (both hypromellose 0.3%) has the advantage of better contact with the lens and less potential for air bubbles thus providing a better view through the lens and less irritating to the cornea.
- Even if performing the treatment in one eye, consider applying a topical anesthetic (proparacaine or tetracaine) in both eyes to help decrease the blink reflex and potential for squeezing the non-procedure eye.

Visualization with the laser:

Visualization is key to performing LFT. Appreciating spatial context is crucial for safety and efficacy. Without the proper technology, it is very difficult to identify many of the symptomatic floaters and confirm a safe distance from the

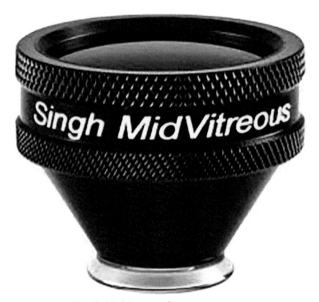

FIGURE 18-3 Singh MidVitreous lens.

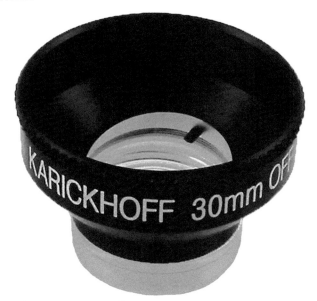

FIGURE 18-4 Karickhoff Vitreous lens.

posterior capsule and the retina. The illumination systems on traditional Nd:YAG lasers were not optimized to visualize and treat floaters in the middle or posterior vitreous. This is because Nd:YAG lasers have primarily been indicated for capsulotomies and laser peripheral iridotomy, procedures requiring visualization of the anterior chamber (AC) only. These Nd:YAG lasers utilize non-coaxial illumination towers, in which the illumination is coming from one pathway of the optical system and the laser and oculars are coming from a different optical pathway, converging at the posterior capsule (Fig. 18.5). Therefore, one could not see beyond a few millimeters from the posterior capsule. Thus, we were not able to identify many of the symptomatic floaters that reside in the middle-to-posterior vitreous (such as a Weiss ring). In addition, surgeon's need to be able to determine where they are within the vitreous in relation to other ocular structures, such as the retina and lens. This limitation of visualization is a reason why some of the earlier studies demonstrated variable efficacy and safety; often they were only treating floaters right behind the lens.

USING NEW LASER TECHNOLOGY

Visualization: Coaxial Illumination

Due to the limitations of previous Nd:YAG lasers, new Nd:YAG laser illumination systems in the form of a flipping mirror system, known as True Coaxial Illumination or TCI (Ellex/Lumibird), a dual mirror system, known as the Smart V System

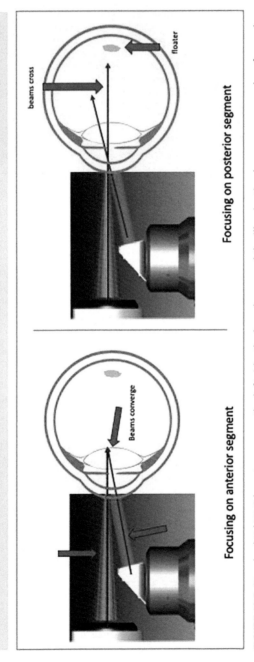

Standard YAG Laser - Illumination Position

Focusing on anterior segment

Focusing on posterior segment

FIGURE 18-5 Standard Nd:YAG laser tower—on the left side, the laser beam and the illumination beam converge when focused on the posterior capsule. On the right side, the laser beam and illumination beam cross when attempting to focus on a floater in the posterior vitreous, thus not allowing a view of the floater and the relationship between the floater and the retina.

(Lumenis), and a similar system used by Lightmed have been developed. Also, using new mid-vitreous contact lenses, these illumination systems provide surgeon's with full visualization of the entire vitreous from the lens to the retina. The TCI system achieves coaxial illumination by using a retractable, reflecting mirror designed to move out of the laser pathway during the treatment. The laser, the oculars, and the illumination tower use the same optical pathway, allowing for simultaneous visualization of both the retina and the floater (Fig. 18.6). This is important to prevent inadvertently hitting the retina. The dual mirror systems achieve a view from lens to retina by incorporating two converging light beams directed at 2 mirrors that converge the light to the retina.

Both the flipping mirror and dual mirror systems enable titration of the red reflex by moving the slit lamp obliquely or off-axis, since the laser can fire at any position of the slit lamp. The TCI design does allow for slightly more titration with less "skip" areas than the dual mirror systems. For the illumination examples described in the rest of this chapter, we will be referring to the TCI design. For example, a floater in the middle of the vitreous that is seen using coaxial positioning with a full red reflex can occasionally have a lot of glare or too much light entering the eye (Fig. 18.7). In order to maximize the contrast in the vitreous to best visualize this type of floater, yet still have enough coaxial illumination to view where the retina is, we can titrate the degree of illumination by moving the slit lamp illumination tower slightly oblique, around 5° to 10°. This allows us to limit the amount of glare, while also maintaining enough illumination to know where we are in the middle or posterior vitreous. This technique is not possible with standard Nd:YAG lasers.

By moving the laser slit lamp illumination tower to an oblique or off-axis position, we are able to allow ourselves better contrast of the anterior floater by titrating off some of the glare and minimize axial red reflex, but still providing enough illumination to determine if the floater is located a safe distance from the retina (Fig. 18.8).

An important clinical pearl: if the floater is in focus and the retina is also in focus, do not fire. Conversely, if the floater is in focus and retina is out of focus, you have enough spatial distance from the retina to fire (Fig. 18.9).

Moreover, it is vitally important for the surgeon to understand how far behind the lens one can treat, which is of great concern when treating phakic patients. The on-axis slit lamp position can be used to first visualize the floater against the red-glow background (to help visualize floaters in the middle and posterior vitreous), then go further off-axis to determine how far behind the lens it is. If the floater is hard to see in off-axis position, then it is safe to treat because the off-axis position only allows for visualization of floaters a few millimeters behind the lens. Using off-axis slit lamp position allows the surgeon to identify the posterior capsule with more clarity than when the slit lamp is the center (on-axis) position (Figs. 18.10 and 18.11).

Other key procedural pearls:

- Using a 16× magnification at the laser can help optimize the view of the floater.
- Having a technician hold the patient's head while doing the procedure protects from inadvertent movement from the patient forward or backward.

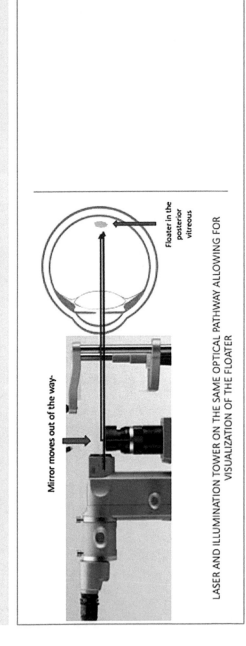

Reflex Tower –True Co-Axial Illumination

Mirror moves out of the way-

Floater in the posterior vitreous

LASER AND ILLUMINATION TOWER ON THE SAME OPTICAL PATHWAY ALLOWING FOR VISUALIZATION OF THE FLOATER

FIGURE 18-6 Reflex laser tower—the mirror moves out of the way of the laser beam allowing for coaxial illumination. The laser, aiming beam, and illumination tower are on the same optical pathway, thus allowing for visualization of the floater in the posterior vitreous.

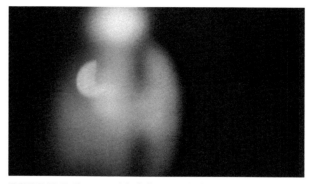

FIGURE 18-7 Picture with full coaxial illumination. Slit lamp illumination tower is in the center position. Notice the nice red reflex demonstrating retina is not in focus, but the floater is a little obscured by the glare of the red reflex.

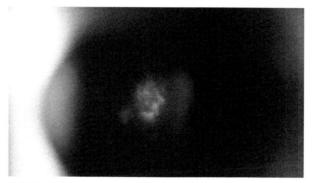

FIGURE 18-8 Picture shows the same patient as Figure 7 but with the slit lamp illumination tower moved 10° oblique (off-axis). This titrates off some of the anterior illumination and glare while keeping enough posterior illumination to see if the retina is in focus or not. This helps to maximize contrast with the floater and still provide spatial context, which helps to ensure the retina is far enough away.

- Often times for a Weiss ring, you might have to direct the patient to look nasally and a little downward to find the opacity.
- Try to keep a 2- to 3-mm distance between the lens and the floater. To determine the distance the floater is from the lens, one can use the analogy of AC depth. When determining AC depth, we use the slit lamp in the oblique position and then determine the space between the endothelium and the iris. I use the same idea for the floater. With the slit lamp in the oblique position (off-axis), I focus on the posterior capsule and then move posteriorly to the floater. The distance between the lens and floater is analogous to the AC depth (which is usually 3 mm). If the patient is pseudophakic, I tend to be less concerned about the distance from the

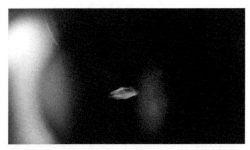

FIGURE 18-9 Photo demonstrates the view achieved for a Weiss ring using the reflex tower providing true coaxial illumination. Slight titration of the illumination tower helps to maximize the view of the opacity and provide spatial context of where the retina is located. In this picture the floater is in focus, but retina is not clearly seen, indicating safe distance to fire.

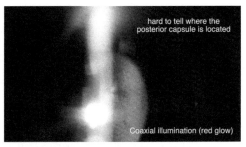

FIGURE 18-10 Picture shows a rope like floater behind the lens. Due to the full red glow of the coaxial beam (slit lamp in the center position), it is hard to tell where the posterior capsule is located. It is not recommended to fire until the surgeon identifies the posterior capsule.

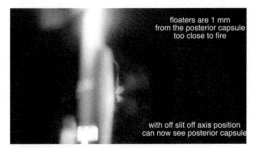

FIGURE 18-11 Picture demonstrates the view when the laser slit lamp illumination tower is in a slightly oblique (off-axis) position thus decreasing the glare and also allowing for visualization of the posterior capsule and the floater. In this case, the floater is too close to the posterior capsule and one would not want to fire.

lens since a small pitting of the lens, if it does occur, is not clinically significant. Also, you can gain experience and learn from the pseudophakic patient LFT cases how close to fire behind the lens.
- For floaters close to the retina, if the floater and retina are in focus at the same time, do not fire.

Energy

> **Key Vitreolysis Settings**
>
> - Energy
>   - 4 to 5 mJ (good starting point)
>   - Lower energy closer to the lens (3–4 mJ)
>   - Higher energy more posteriorly (5–7 mJ)
> - Pulses per burst
>   - Start with 1 pulse per burst, but for larger amorphous clouds in the middle of the vitreous, consider multiple pulses per burst to improve efficiency.
> - Offset
>   - Start with zero offset.
>   - The more anterior the floater, consider 100 microns posterior offset or greater to protect from hitting the lens.
>   - The more posterior the floater, use an anterior offset to protect from hitting the retina. An anterior offset also helps to focus the energy due to parallax.

Understanding Energy Delivery:

Previous studies, which reported marginal results with Nd:YAG laser vitreolysis, often set the energy level to 1 to 2 mJ,[5] which is much less than the 4 to 8 mJ typically required to vaporize floaters. When the laser is fired into the vitreous, plasma is formed. A small acoustic wave of energy is circumferentially emitted surrounding the plasma, with some of the energy moving anteriorly toward the laser source. An "energy shield" develops, preventing further propagation of energy posteriorly. The total energy "shock wave," from the furthest anterior to posterior extent, is known as the convergence zone. A key relationship to understand is the nonlinear rise in convergence zone as the energy level is increased. This is an important safety concept to understand when setting the laser to generate enough energy to vaporize floaters. For Nd:YAG lasers, the growth of plasma as a function of power is a LOG law phenomenon, and consequently the increase in size of plasma (convergence zone) between 1 mJ and 10 mJ is less than 50%. For instance, at 1 mJ, the convergence zone (shock wave) is around 110 microns, whereas at 10 mJ, the convergence zone increases to only 210 microns. Therefore, a 10× increase in energy on the laser translates to less than a 50% rise in dispersion of energy in the vitreous. So, when firing at 5 or 6 mJ (the average for most treatments), the convergence zone is less than 200 microns (Fig. 18.12).

We conducted a study in which we held a B scan probe temporally while performing LFT (using the Ultra Q Reflex laser) to observe the behavior of the vitreous surrounding the plasma creation.[6] We found, even with energy at 7 mJ per shot fired, no movement of vitreous was evident even 1 mm from the plasma formation. No traction or pulling of the posterior hyaloid face was seen. This is why we feel comfortable using energy settings well above what was used in the past or for Nd:YAG capsulotomies. Without generating a plasma spark, one will merely push the floater away, rather than causing optical breakdown and vaporization of the collagen fibers.

Recent refinements in Nd:YAG laser technology have resulted in a narrow ultra-Gaussian beam that has a fast pulse rise time of 3-ns and a small spot size. This is in contrast to other conventional Nd:YAG lasers, which produce a wider beam profile. The new truncated beam profile allows for 50% air breakdown at 1.88 mJ. Put simply, less energy is required in order to achieve the optical breakdown necessary to effectively vaporize the floater(s) (Fig. 18.13).

Remember, plasma is the 4th state of matter, solid to gaseous state. Therefore, despite perception, there is true vaporization of the floater, but it occurs in a small area, which necessitates a larger number of shots to fully remove the opacity. We are often initially breaking up the opacity into smaller pieces then vaporizing the smaller pieces. We often use 200 to 300+ shots when treating a Weiss ring floater, and even more for an amorphous cloud. Due to the 3-ns pulse, heat is dissipated before the next shot is fired and therefore there is no accumulation of energy. This nonlinear rise with increasing laser energy allows us to achieve higher power density and tightly controlled plasma, with fewer shots and less cumulative energy being delivered to the patient.

Some lasers (Ellex) also feature a specially designed active cooling cavity. When firing several hundred shots in one sitting, standard laser cavities can overheat. The active cooling cavity of newer Nd:YAG lasers has been shown to decrease the risk of the cavity overheating. Further, the stable energy output of these lasers is vastly improved (Fig. 18.14).

Other key settings and procedural pearls:

- Don't be afraid to use energy settings higher than a Nd:YAG capsulotomy. The average power we use per shot is 5 mJ. The closer the floater is to the lens, the less power you need, and the further posterior the floater, the higher the energy. Incidentally, we have not seen a significant clinical benefit using energy settings above 8 mJ per shot.
- If you do not see a plasma spark form, despite high energy settings, check to make sure your lens on the cornea is perpendicular to the laser. If the patient is looking to one side and the lens is tilted, one of the aiming beams of the laser can be cut off and no reaction will occur.

Convergence Zone

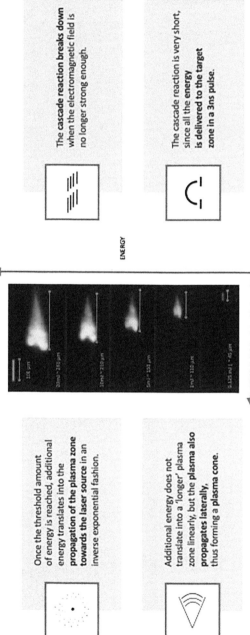

Once the threshold amount of energy is reached, additional energy translates into the **propagation of the plasma zone towards the laser source** in an inverse exponential fashion.

Additional energy does not translate into a "longer" plasma zone linearly, but the **plasma also propagates laterally,** thus forming a plasma cone.

The **cascade reaction breaks down** when the electromagnetic field is no longer strong enough.

The cascade reaction is very short, since all the **energy is delivered to the target zone in a 3ns pulse.**

ENERGY

PLASMA CONE EXTENSION

FIGURE 18-12 Picture demonstrates that the size of the convergence zone increases in a nonlinear fashion as the power on the laser is increased. At 1 mJ, the size of the convergence zone is 110 microns, and increasing power to 10 mJ increases the size to 210 microns (less than a 50% increase).

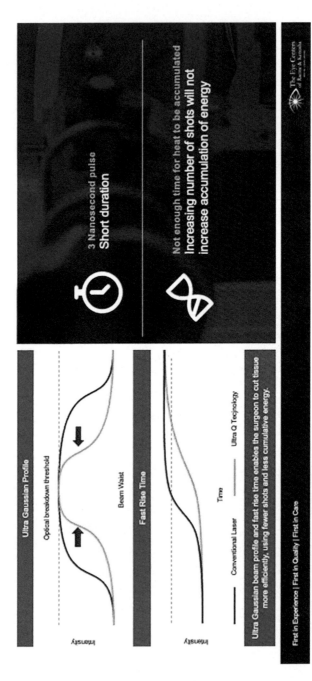

FIGURE 18-13 Arrows in the picture point to the narrow Gaussian curve of the energy delivery using the new reflex cavity. There is a sharper rise and fall of the energy therefore limited wasting of energy.

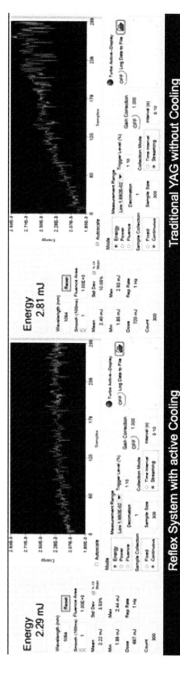

FIGURE 18-14 Graph on the left side demonstrates a stable delivery of energy over hundreds of shots when using an active cooling cavity, whereas on the right using a passive cooling cavity the delivery of energy is not stable over hundreds of shots fired.

- Learn to play with the offset on the laser. Some surgeon's keep the offset at zero and adjust anteriorly or posteriorly with the joystick as the plasma forms. The closer the floater is to the lens, the more posterior offset typically used. Due to parallax, the more posterior the floater, the more anterior the offset typically used along with adjusting the joystick as needed.
- Since it is much easier to produce a plasma spark when the opacity is directly in front and in the middle of the vitreous, if the floater starts to move away, have the patient look up or down, left or right, then back to the middle to "move" the floater into a better position.
- Let the patient know ahead of time the vision will be dark for 5 to 10 minutes posttreatment and they will likely see "bubbles" in the lower half of their vision for a day or so (this is from the gas induced by the plasma formation). Floaters may reappear after a day or two once the dilation wears off.
- The number of shots required per session can depend on the size, location, and density of the floater. As a general rule, solitary, more consolidated floaters tend to respond best to the laser and require the least number of shots and sessions. The more amorphous/cloud like the floater the less efficient the vaporization, and therefore it more often requires a higher number of shots. For example, a Weiss ring type floater may take 200 to 300 shots to sufficiently break and vaporize whereas a more amorphous cloud or rope-like floater may take 500 to 600 shots and require multiple sessions. The more anterior the floater, the more efficient the vaporization and thus less power and number of shots is typically needed.

POSTOPERATIVE CARE/CO-MANAGEMENT (FOLLOW-UP SCHEDULE)

Key Postoperative Considerations

- Immediately after completing the procedure, wash the eye out with sterile water or balanced salt solution (BSS) to remove gel. The patient's vision will be "dark" for 10 to 15 minutes post-procedure. Also, they may notice "bubble" floaters in the bottom of their vision due to the gasses rising up from the plasma creation.
- Instill 1 to 2 drops of brimonidine or apraclonidine to protect from an immediate IOP spike.
- An IOP check is performed 30 to 60 minutes post-procedure. IOP should be treated if a significant rise (>10 mm Hg) in IOP is noted.
- The number of shots, energy per shot, and total amount of energy used should be recorded in the chart. A notation similar to "The patient tolerated the procedure well and left in no apparent distress" should be added to the chart.

- Postoperative take home drops: No drops are necessary, but one can consider a topical antihypertensive such as an alpha agonist to prevent an IOP spike.
- Recommend an IOP check and dilated exam assessment one-week post-procedure; however, once you feel comfortable, you can consider waiting for a month before checking IOP and performing a dilated fundus exam (DFE).
- At the one-month follow-up, repeat IOP check and DFE. This is the time to assess the efficacy of the treatment. Often patients will describe the floaters "coming back." This is due to the fact that the residual pieces that were broken up but not vaporized were likely pushed to the periphery. After a few weeks, they consolidate and can often times migrate toward the visual axis. Although patients notice floaters again, they are often less dense and less noticeable than before the treatment. At this time, if they are overall seeing an improvement and there are no safety issues, one can set up another treatment session.

POTENTIAL COMPLICATIONS AND THEIR TREATMENT

Key Potential Complications

- IOP spike, immediate or delayed
  - Topical antihypertensive drops, such as brimonidine or apraclonidine, typically work well for a mild-to-moderate IOP spike ($\approx$10–20 mm Hg rise).
  - Acetazolamide 500 mg PO BID works very well for an immediate severe IOP spike (>20 mm Hg rise).
  - IOP rise can last months. If controlled on topical medications, do not suddenly remove all topical medications once the IOP is down, rather slowly reduce drops one class at a time.
  - In those cases where IOP is controlled with topical medications, selective laser trabeculoplasty (SLT) works well to reduce drop burden.
- Immediate blurred vision (from gas bubbles and dilation)—observe.
- Retinal hemorrhage (when the floater is too close to the retina). It is OK to observe if outside the fovea.
- Lens opacity (when the floater is too close to the lens). If the patient is asymptomatic, then it is OK to observe. If the patient is symptomatic, then we need to consider lens removal. If the posterior capsule is compromised from the laser hit, then use a similar lens removal technique as a posterior polar cataract.
- Retinal detachment (rare and mostly theoretical)—send to retina accordingly.

Please see Efficacy/Studies section for further details on complication data.

VIDEOS OF PROCEDURE

Video 18.1—This is a Nd:YAG LFT being done using the Singh MidVitreous lens with the laser power set to 5 mJ and no offset. The laser slit lamp illumination tower is in the center position (on-axis) to achieve full coaxial illumination in order to view the floater and the retina. For this Weiss ring type floater, you will notice the laser is fired only when the floater is in focus and the retina is out of focus. This is a key pearl. If the floater and retina are in focus at the same time, it is important not to fire since the floater is too close to the retina. One can also see the floater is breaking up into smaller pieces, but the end point is visual confirmation the pieces are gone. Unlike a Nd:YAG capsulotomy, we will keep firing at the smaller pieces until they are no longer visible, which can require hundreds of shots. The pieces also are staying relatively close to the plasma creation, which is in part due to the efficiency of energy delivery.

Video 18.2—This is a Nd:YAG LFT for a symptomatic amorphous cloud-like opacity located in the anterior vitreous. Since the floater is closer to the phakic lens, you see how we can move the slit lamp illumination tower from the center position (on-axis illumination) to an oblique position (off-axis illumination) in order to remove the coaxial illumination and allow greater contrast of the floater and appreciation of the distance from the floater to the lens. This is a similar technique to when we assess the AC depth where we move the exam room slit lamp oblique to view the corneal endothelium, then moving the slit lamp posteriorly to the iris we get a feel for the AC depth, which usually is close to 3 mm. Using this distance as a comparison, we can appreciate the distance between the lens and the anterior floater, trying or keep a 2 mm or greater distance if possible.

Video 18.3—This is a Nd:YAG LFT for a symptomatic amorphous cloud-like opacity located in the middle of the vitreous. To maximize contrast of the floater while still appreciating the distance from the retina, this video demonstrates the titration of illumination technique. Since full coaxial illumination can result in significant glare, you can move the slit lamp illumination tower 15° to 20° oblique (partial off-axis position of the slit lamp) to reduce the amount of illumination anteriorly to improve the view of the floater, but still keep enough coaxial illumination posteriorly to provide sufficient view of the retinal vessels to appreciate distance from floater to the retina.

EFFICACY—VITREOLYSIS STUDY DATA

The recently published paper by Shah and colleagues (JAMA, July 2017) was the first randomized placebo-controlled trial evaluating the safety and efficacy of LFT using advanced Nd:YAG technology specifically designed for laser-based floater treatment.[7] This study involved 52 eyes, of which 36 patients were treated with the Reflex Technology platform (Ellex Medical, Australia). The study concluded that 54% of patients in the Nd:YAG laser group experienced symptomatic improvements compared to 9% of patients in the control group. The Nd:YAG laser group also showed greater improvement in the 10-point visual disturbance score than the control group.

Improved symptoms were reported by 53% of patients in the Nd:YAG laser group and 0% in the sham arm. Although there were improvements in the Nd:YAG laser group in terms of general and peripheral vision, role difficulties, and dependency, neither group showed changes in best corrected visual acuity. That is important to note and emphasizes that we cannot use the Snellen chart alone to define if patients are clinically symptomatic.

This study also demonstrated no retinal adverse events in the treatment group, although a retinal defect was seen in the control group. This is an important point because the cause of retinal defects is often the result of vitreous traction. According to the American Academy of Ophthalmology, the definition of Nd:YAG vitreolysis is the "severing of vitreous strands and opacities with a laser." There is no evidence that the LFT causes traction on the retina. Also, skeptics argue that literature points to an increased risk of retinal defects in patients undergoing Nd:YAG capsulotomy, therefore the assumption is there must be an increased risk with LFT. It is important to understand that LFT and Nd:YAG capsulotomy are two entirely different procedures working on different anatomical structures. When breaking the posterior capsule during capsulotomy, there is a transfer of forces/energy to the zonules, which is in turn transferred to the attached vitreous base. With LFT, the collagen fibers that are being lasered do not have the same connection directly to the vitreous base, and as such the risk of retinal breaks is markedly less. There also have been no reports of increasing cataract formation after LFT if the lens was not directly hit at the time of the procedure.

Some skeptics point to a psychological or adaptive component to floaters. Doctors may say the laser did not have an effect, but rather there was a placebo effect or neuroadaptation. The Shah study addresses that issue as subjects in the study did not know whether they were in the treatment group or control group. There was a significant difference in patient satisfaction between the control group and the treatment group. This study showed significant subjective improvement in the treatment group; however, there were some who still noticed symptoms. This study was not designed for a follow-up treatment session. It is important for doctors to realize that multiple sessions are common; the plasma or vaporization is occurring in such a small area; thus, it is not able to always vaporize the entire floater in one session.

Another paper recently published demonstrated Nd:YAG laser vitreolysis decreased the amount of vitreous floater opacities seen on color fundus imaging and improved related symptoms according to the NEI VFQ-25 responses.[8] Thirty-two patients (32 eyes; 13 men and 19 women) with symptomatic vitreous floaters were enrolled in this study (mean age: 59.4 years). All study patients were followed up for six months. Following the laser vitreolysis, there was a statistically significant improvement in both the near visual function ($z = -2.97$; $p = 0.003$; $r = 0.633$) and visual disturbance rate ($z = -3.97$; $p < 0.001$; $r = 0.84$). Distance visual function did not show statistically significant difference after the laser procedure ($p = 1.00$). Color fundus photography did reveal vitreous opacity improvement over time in 93.7% of study eyes (partial improvement in 37.5% and total improvement in 56.2% of study eyes).

During the follow-up period, recurrence of vitreous floaters, best corrected visual acuity (BCVA) deterioration and adverse events were not observed.

In 2016, we presented a paper at the American Society of Cataract and Refractive Surgery (ASCRS) meeting, which investigated patient satisfaction, complication rates, and treatment specifics associated with LFT in a prospective review of patients undergoing the procedure.[9] This observational study included 130 patients (mean age, 61 years [range, 28–92 years]) who underwent LFT with the Ultra Q Reflex system (Ellex, Australia). Patient satisfaction was assessed with a 1 to 10 self-rated scale, with higher values indicating greater patient satisfaction, as well as a "Yes" or "No" indicating whether they were satisfied with improvement in daily functioning. Information on complications was recorded for all patients. We found 91% of patients stated that they were satisfied with their improvement in daily visual functioning. The noted average degree of improvement was 8.5 out of 10 (after multiple sessions in some patients). Patients with a Weiss ring required 1.3 sessions to sufficiently vaporize the floater as compared to 3.2 sessions in patients with amorphous clouds. The number of laser shots to sufficiently vaporize amorphous cloud floaters was 568 shots as compared to 186 shots for Weiss rings. Power settings also varied depending on floater type with the average setting at 5.8 mJ (range 2.9–9 mJ). Best results and higher patient satisfaction scores were notably seen with solitary Weiss rings versus amorphous clouds. The adverse event profile included 2 phakic lenses that were hit, 3 IOP spikes, and one retinal hemorrhage. The 2 lenses were hit (both in the first 50 cases of surgeon experience) before we appreciated the importance of using the laser slit lamp in the oblique position to view the posterior capsule and appreciate the distance of the floater from the lens (Fig. 18.15). The retinal hemorrhage occurred due to the fact the retina was in focus at the same time as the floater. It was not the laser that was dangerous or misfired, rather the retina was in focus at the same time as the floater and therefore the laser should not have been fired at that moment. The 3 IOP spikes occurred in post-Nd:YAG capsulotomy patients where the amorphous clouds were right behind the lens. It correlated not with energy settings, rather with number of shots. Therefore, we now decrease the number of shots to 300 or less if the floaters are close to the lens in a post-Nd:YAG capsulotomy patient to help decrease the chance of a post-laser IOP spike.

At ASCRS 2017, we also presented our analysis of all consecutive patients who underwent Nd:YAG laser vitreolysis for the treatment of symptomatic floaters and had at least one to four years of follow-up. This retrospective study included 1272 procedures performed in 680 patients.[10] In all cases, the Ellex Ultra Q Reflex Nd:YAG laser was employed to vaporize floaters. An average power of 6 mJ per laser shot was used with an average of 564 shots per treatment session. Patients with both amorphous clouds and solitary Weiss ring type of floaters were included. Ten adverse events were recorded, comprising seven cases of intraocular pressure (IOP) spikes, two cases of hitting the phakic lens (Figure 18.15) and one retinal hemorrhage (this included the adverse events from the 130 cases in the 2016 prospective paper), representing a total adverse event rate of 0.8%. Patients with IOP spikes were placed on topical antihypertensive medications, and the average post-medication IOP was

Hitting the Lens...happened early in learning

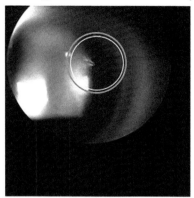

Nucleus was hit in the periphery. Patient asymptomatic and is being observed.

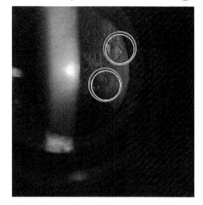

Posterior capsule was hit near center of the visual axis. Patient was symptomatic and underwent lens removal with IOL

FIGURE 18-15 Two cases of a phakic lens being hit with the laser. On the left, the patient is asymptomatic and being observed. On the right, the patient was symptomatic and ended up with cataract removal with intraocular lens (IOL) implant.

19 mm Hg. One of the phakic patients subsequently required cataract surgery and achieved a corrected visual acuity of 20/20. The other patient, whose lens was hit in the periphery, is still being observed. The case of retinal hemorrhage resolved in three months with no long-term negative effects. There were no inflammatory issues faced, no AC or vitreous cell or flare seen. No exacerbation of diabetic retinopathy nor progression of epiretinal membrane or cystoid macular edema was seen. Postoperative regimen for all cases included IOP checks immediately after the procedure, at one week, and at one month. No anti-inflammatory drops or topical antihypertensive medications were given. Preoperative, one-month, and three-month macular optical coherence tomography (OCT's) were obtained on all patients.

Objective Data

Qualitative analysis of the effects of LFT have been achieved with spectral domain OCT and scanning laser ophthalmoscopy by comparing shadows on the retina created by floaters before and after treatment. A recent study published in Ophthalmic Surgery, Lasers, and Imaging (OSLI) Retina in October 2018 on novel OCT applications, including shadow changes on a 5-line raster scan following vitreolysis, described cases where patients had complained of a scotoma that would not go away.[11] Multiple initial testing from other doctors did not reveal an etiology. After further examination of the vitreous and evidence on spectral domain optical coherence tomography (SD-OCT) of the shadow being cast by a large floater over the macula, Nd:YAG vitreolysis was performed. Posttreatment, patients described resolution of the floater and the SD-OCT scans revealed resolution of the shadow that was cast on the retina (Figs. 18.16 and 18.17).

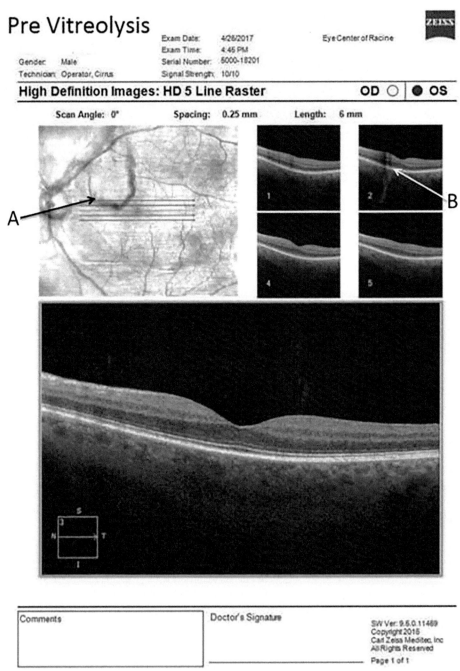

FIGURE 18-16 Arrow A—large vitreous opacity over the macula region. Arrow B—shadow is seen being cast over the macula on the 5-line raster scans.

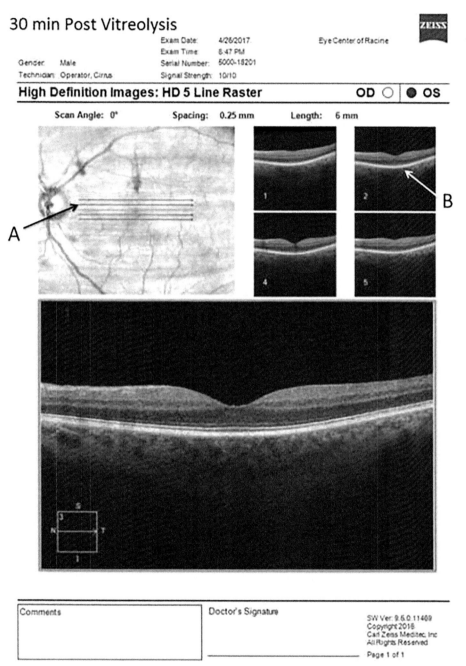

FIGURE 18-17 Arrow A—most of the vitreous opacity has been removed with the laser. Arrow B demonstrates the shadow now gone on the 5-line raster scan.

Ray-tracing aberrometry, using the iTrace by Tracey Technologies, offers true quantitative analysis of floaters and the objective benefits of vitreolysis. Ray-tracing uses a laser beam parallel to the line of sight through the pupil to the retina. It measures the exact retinal location by retroreflected light captured by reference sensors. Aberrations caused by ocular structures result in a measurable shift in the perceived retinal location (point spread function). Aberrations are measured repeatedly and sequentially in multiple locations (256 points for the iTrace), until a reconstruction of the ocular wavefront error is created.

The maps produced show color-coded total and higher-order aberrations (HOA) including coma, spherical aberration, and trefoil. It can measure internal quality of vision, displayed to the user by the dysfunctional lens index (DLI), which measures quality of the optical system from behind the cornea to the retina. This can be used to compare wavefront and refractive information with a differential prior to and after surgery. Due to the ability of the machine to determine the size and intensity of the 256 rays hitting the retina, it can also determine contrast sensitivity (modulation transfer function (MTF) curve). With respect to vitreolysis, with all things being equal (the cornea, the lens, and the retina), this same index can be used to measure the impact of floaters before and after vitreolysis, effectively providing a dysfunctional "vitreous" index. If 10 is considered a perfectly clear media and 0 is considered opaque, many patients with floaters measure an index of between 3 and 6, which can be significantly improved with vitreolysis. We presented a paper on this topic at ASCRS 2017 demonstrating these findings in the following section.[12] We found a significant improvement in HOA, MTF area under the curve and DLI score post-LFT (Figs. 18.18–18.22).

Pre-op DLI is 3.79

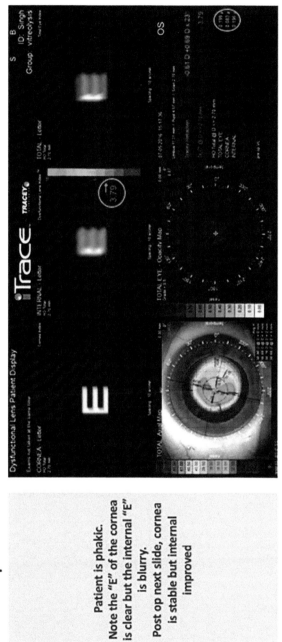

Patient is phakic.
Note the "E" of the cornea is clear but the internal "E" is blurry.
Post op next slide, cornea is stable but internal improved

FIGURE 18-18 Pre op LFT case showing DLI of 3.79 and HOA of the internal optical system is 0.195. Autorefraction and topography are also shown.

Next Day Post-op

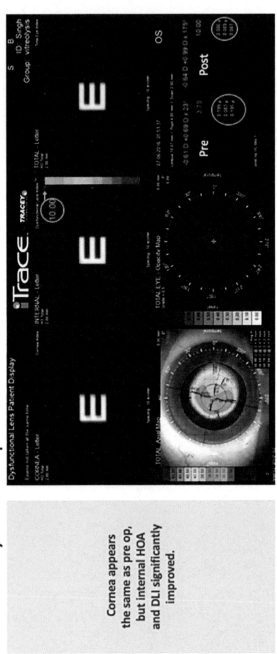

Cornea appears the same as pre op, but internal HOA and DLI significantly improved.

FIGURE 18-19 iTrace scan of the patient is now post-LFT. The DLI increased to 10 and the internal HOA improved from 0.195 to 0.087 with no change in corneal aberrations, topography, or autorefraction.

Pre and Post MTF Comparison

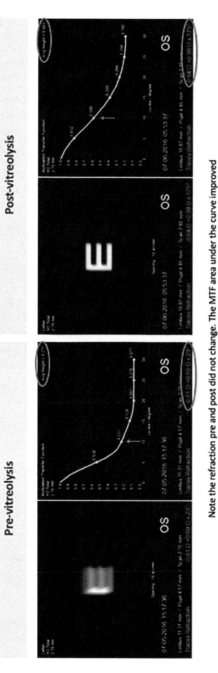

FIGURE 18-20 Evaluating MTF curves in the same LFT patient. MTF area under the curve increased from 0.271 to 0.483. The representative "E" has cleared posttreatment and the autorefraction has not changed, indicating the only change to the optical system was the removal of the floater from the visual axis.

DLI AND/OR HOA	33/36 EYES NOTED IMPROVEMENT
Average DLI improvement	3.1 • Pre-Op DLI: 5.2 • Post-Op DLI: 8.3
Average HOA improvement	0.16 • Trefoil demonstrated the biggest difference
MTF curve height	0.217 average change

FIGURE 18-21 Chart providing the improvement data seen for DLI, HOA, and MTF in the study presented at ASCRS 2017.

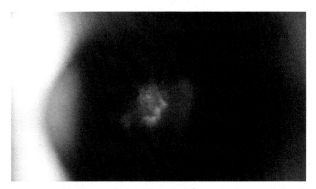

FIGURE 18-22 Picture is an example of a typical central cloud like floater included in the study.

CODING/BILLING AND MODIFIERS

- Diagnostic ICD 10 codes to be used are as follows:
  - H43.391 to H43.399 (Other vitreous opacities)
  - H43.811 to H43.819 (Vitreous degeneration)
- There are two CPT codes that are often used:
  - 67031 (Severing of vitreous strands, vitreous face adhesions, sheets, membranes or opacities, laser surgery, one or more stages)
  - 67299 (Unlisted procedure, posterior segment)
- It has been suggested to use CPT 67031 when the goal of treatment is to sever the vitreous opacity from its attachment, allowing it to sink to the bottom of the vitreous and out of the line of sight. When the goal is to "vaporize" and not sever, CPT 67031 does not apply. Instead, one should use CPT 67299 to describe photoablation, destruction, or vaporization of a vitreous floater for complete removal.

- For unlisted code 67299:
  - There is no stipulated reimbursement schedule for physicians.
  - Claims are evaluated and an appropriate payment rate is selected on a case-by-case basis.
  - There is no published global period.
  - Within Medicare, unlisted codes are ineligible for ASC facility fee reimbursement.
  - Each claim stands alone; reimbursement for one case does not set precedent for the next.
- The national Medicare Physician Fee Schedule amounts in 2020 for CPT 67031 are $399 for a physician in-office, $363 for a physician in a facility. Facility fees are $507 for a hospital outpatient department (HOPD) and $256 for an ASC.

CONCLUSION

Now with new technology, coupled with a better understanding of vitreous behavior and patient selection criteria, as well as new protocols, we do indeed have a safe and effective method to reduce the symptoms of floaters in certain groups of patients. In the past, surgeon's and physicians would often tell their patients, "Floaters are usually just a nuisance and often become less noticeable or more tolerable over time and can even disappear entirely. You need to just live with it." We would tell patients to ignore their floaters because we felt that vitrectomy was not worth the risk. As a result, we undermined and minimized the impact floaters have on a patient's quality of life. It is often easy to dismiss a condition when there is no good option to treat it. Now, when I merely ask a patient, even with a simple Weiss ring, I am amazed as to how many people feel the floaters are distracting to the point of interfering with vision and daily functioning. In my practice, this is the key to defining a CSVO. So now with a safer treatment option, a floater is "bad enough" when a patient states the floaters are interfering with their daily life, regardless of the number or size of the floater.

If one doesn't believe a condition is worth treating, then it is easy to find reasons not to address it and any adverse event is too many. But as with any disease state, it is a balance of safety and efficacy.

REFERENCES

1. Schulz-Key S, Carlsson JO, Crafoord S. Longterm follow-up of pars plana vitrectomy for vitreous floaters: complications, outcomes and patient satisfaction. *Acta Ophthalmol.* 2011;89(2):159–165.
2. Wagle AM, Lim WY, Yap TP, et al. Utility values associated with vitreous floaters. *Am J Ophthalmol.* 2011;152(1):60–65.
3. Webb BF, Webb JR, Schroeder MC, et al. Prevalence of vitreous floaters in a community sample of smartphone users. *Int J Ophthalmol.* 2013;6(3):402–405.
4. Garcia GA, Khoshnevis M, Yee KMP, Nguyen-Cuu J, Nguyen JH, Sebag J. Degradation of contrast sensitivity function following posterior vitreous detachment. *Am J Ophthalmol.* 2016;172:7–12. doi:10.1016/j.ajo.2016.09.005. Epub 2016 Sep 12. PMID: 27633841.

5. Delaney YM, Oyinloye A, Benjamin L. Nd:YAG vitreolysis and pars plana vitrectomy: surgical treatment for vitreous floaters. *Eye (Lond)*. 2002;16(1):21–26.
6. Singh IP. Real Time Ultrasound Evaluation of Vitreous Behavior during YAG Vitreolysis for the Treatment of Symptomatic Floaters. ASCRS 2019 Paper Presentation.
7. Shah CP, Heier JS. YAG laser vitreolysis vs sham YAG vitreolysis for symptomatic vitreous floaters: a randomized clinical trial. *JAMA Ophthalmol*. 2017;135(9):918–923.
8. Souza ES, Lima LH, Nascimento H, et al. Objective assessment of YAG laser vitreolysis in patients with symptomatic vitreous floaters. *Int J Retin Vitr*.2020;6.
9. Singh, IP. Treating Vitreous Floaters: Patient Satisfaction and Complications of Modern YAG Vitreolysis. ASCRS 2016. Paper Presentation.
10. Singh, IP. Neodymium: YAG Laser Vitreolytsis: Restrospective Safety Study: ASCRS 2017. Paper Presentation.
11. Singh, IP. Novel OCT application and optimized YAG laser enable visualization and treatment of mid-to posterior vitreous floaters. *Ophthalmic Surg Lasers Imaging Retina*. 2018;49(10):806–811.
12. Singh, IP. Pre-and Postoperative Objective Assessment of Quality of Vision in Patients Undergoing YAG Vitreolysis Using Wavefront Aberrometry, ASCRS 2017 Paper Presentation.

19 Panretinal Photocoagulation

Alan R. Hromas

Retinal ischemia is a common manifestation of a number of vascular diseases causing impairment of retinal circulation, including diabetic retinopathy, retinal arterial and venous occlusion, and inflammatory vasculitis. Ischemia and the resulting retinal tissue hypoxia upregulate the production of vascular endothelial growth factor (VEGF), which in turn may lead to deleterious effects on vision via increased vascular permeability or neovascularization. Neovascularization may manifest on the optic nerve head or elsewhere on the retina, leading to tractional elevation and detachment, or vitreous hemorrhage. Anterior segment neovascularization may produce a secondary angle closure, leading to neovascular glaucoma.

Diabetic retinopathy has long been recognized as a common cause of retinal ischemia via progressive hyperglycemia-mediated damage to the retinal microcirculation. The landmark Diabetic Retinopathy Study (DRS, 1979) demonstrated a significant reduction in the risk of severe vision loss in patients with proliferative diabetic retinopathy (PDR) treated with panretinal photocoagulation (PRP).[1-3] The subsequent Early Treatment of Diabetic Retinopathy Study (EDTRS, 1991) further refined the indications and thresholds for treatment.[4] Over the last 15 years, intravitreal injections of anti-VEGF drugs have gradually begun to emerge as an alternative treatment for many of the situations previously treated with PRP, and the Diabetic Retinopathy Clinical Research Network (DRCR.net) protocol S (2016) confirmed that intravitreal injections of the anti-VEGF drug ranibizumab was a viable, and sometimes superior, treatment option as compared to traditional laser.[5]

Though the research and data regarding PRP are most robust in the case of diabetic retinopathy, many of the findings have been extrapolated to other ischemic retinal diseases. The effectiveness of PRP in causing reduction or regression of neovascularization is believed to be related to its ability to improve oxygenation of the ischemic inner retina and downregulate the production of VEGF. The resulting reduction in circulating VEGF generally leads to stabilization or regression of existing neovascularization.[6,7]

Treatment generally involves the administration of multiple individual laser spots throughout the ischemic area, ideally using preoperative fluorescein angiography to delineate the areas of nonperfusion. PRP can be performed in-office with a slit-lamp-mounted laser or laser indirect ophthalmoscope (LIO), as well as in the operating room, with an endolaser, in conjunction with pars plana vitrectomy. Though the principles are similar regardless, this chapter will focus on in-office treatment.

INDICATIONS

Key Indications

- PDR
- Branch retinal vein occlusion (BRVO) or central retinal vein occlusion (CRVO), when associated with neovascularization[8,9]
- Branch retinal artery occlusion or central retinal artery occlusion (CRAO), when associated with neovascularization[10]
- Sickle cell retinopathy[11]
- Inflammatory retinal vasculitis with neovascularization
- Radiation retinopathy
- Inherited or genetic abnormalities causing retinal ischemia and neovascularization
  - Familial exudative vitreoretinopathy
  - Eales' disease
  - Incontinentia pigmenti

Though the most common indications for PRP are listed here, treatment may be indicated for any condition producing ischemia with neovascularization. Neovascularization may be found in multiple locations, including on the optic disc (NVD), elsewhere on the retina (NVE) (Figs. 19.1 and 19.2), on the iris (NVI), or within the iridocorneal angle (NVA).

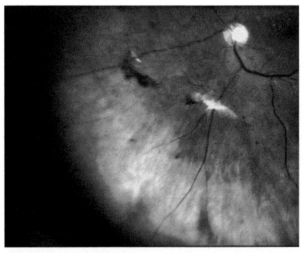

FIGURE 19-1 Fundus photograph showing neovascularization elsewhere.

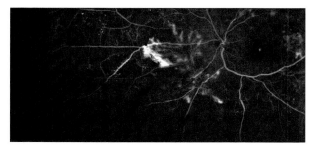

FIGURE 19-2 Fluorescein angiogram showing neovascularization elsewhere with peripheral ischemia.

Because of the potential for significant side effects resulting from PRP, extensive research has been undertaken to determine the optimal timing to perform treatment; that is, whether treatment should be performed at the first sign of neovascularization, only in more high-risk cases, or even prior to neovascularization developing (DRS, ETDRS). In brief, the authors concluded that PRP during the mild and moderate pre-proliferative stages tended to produce untoward side effects such as peripheral vision loss without significant benefit. In general, PRP can reasonably be performed in cases of severe non-PDR, particularly when the treating physician determines that there is high risk of progression to proliferative disease or if there are socioeconomic factors that may prevent the patient from following up on the recommended schedule for monitoring.[4,12]

When PDR is present (defined as the presence of NVD, NVE, NVI, or NVA), treatment is generally recommended. Some treating physicians may elect to delay treatment until "high-risk characteristics" develop, including neovascularization over one third of the optic disc, NVD associated with vitreous hemorrhage, or NVE greater than half of the disc area in size associated with vitreous hemorrhage.[13,14]

Note: Ablative laser to peripheral avascular retina is widely used for the treatment of advanced stages of retinopathy of prematurity. The principle is similar to that employed in acquired retinal vascular diseases, but there are important differences in the laser technique that are beyond the scope of this chapter.[15]

CONTRAINDICATIONS

Key Contraindications

- Media opacity preventing clear view of posterior segment
- Patient inability to cooperate

Performing safe PRP requires an adequate view of the posterior segment. By nature of the conditions being treated with PRP, the fundus view is often compromised by vitreous hemorrhage; other conditions such as corneal opacities, cataract, or inadequate mydriasis may be compounding factors. If the view is inadequate to safely aim the laser, treatment is best deferred until circumstances have improved spontaneously (i.e., via natural reabsorption of vitreous hemorrhage) or through other methods (cataract surgery or vitrectomy as indicated). Intravitreal injections of anti-VEGF medications can often be used to induce rapid regression of neovascularization and control neovascular complications in the meantime.

PRP is frequently employed in an in-office setting on patients who are awake and alert. For patients that are unable to cooperate with treatment due to age or mental status, treatment in an operating suite while under sedation administered by an anesthesiologist is an option. Patients who are awake during the procedure require some degree of cooperation to facilitate treatment and decrease the risk of inadvertent laser damage to the macula and optic nerve. This is particularly important when treatment is being administered via LIO, as compared to treatment via a slit-lamp-mounted laser with contact lens. In-office cooperation is facilitated by ensuring the patient receives adequate anesthesia preoperatively and ensuring that the patient is in a comfortable position, whether at the slit-lamp or in a reclining chair.

INFORMED CONSENT CONSIDERATIONS

Key Informed Consent Adverse Events

- Decrease in peripheral vision
- Nyctalopia
- Inadvertent laser damage to optic nerve or macular area with resulting scotoma
- Contraction of neovascular tissue with tractional elevation of the retina
- Vitreous hemorrhage
- Discomfort during the procedure
- Failure to adequately induce regression of the neovascularization
- Worsening cataract
- Worsening macular edema
- Transient choroidal effusion

Informed consent should include a description of the procedure to be performed, as well as the purpose, in plain language. For instance, "laser treatment to cause regression of abnormal blood vessels on the retina," which is intended to "decrease the risk of bleeding in the eye and retinal detachment" or "decrease the risk of glaucoma (high eye pressure)" as indicated.

In addition to the proposed benefits of the procedure, the risks listed previously should be addressed. In particular, some degree of peripheral vision loss and decreased low-light vision (nyctalopia) is very common among patients following PRP[16,17] and may be especially problematic for patients in certain professions (e.g., truck drivers). If the eye is being anesthetized with retrobulbar injection, the rare but potentially fatal complication of brainstem anesthesia should also be discussed.

As noted previously, the goal of treatment via PRP is to induce regression of neovascular tissue. It is important to discuss with patients preoperatively that, in the process of regression, neovascular tissue will sometimes contract, causing anterior traction on the retina and hemorrhage into the vitreous or progression of tractional retinal detachment. As patients are often asymptomatic or minimally symptomatic from a visual acuity perspective prior to treatment (despite having what may be heavy neovascularization), failure to adequately explain the risks of these outcomes beforehand may lead to them placing the blame on the surgeon or procedure itself.

The alternatives to treatment via PRP should be addressed as well; with consideration of the natural history of the condition should no treatment be performed at all. For instance, in a BRVO with neovascularization and vitreous hemorrhage, if the vitreous has spontaneously separated from the retina and neovascular tissue, the risk of future bleeding or retinal detachment may be low and thus observation may be very reasonable.

In recent years, particularly following the published results of the DRCR.net Protocol S ("Panretinal photocoagulation versus intravitreous ranibizumab for PDR"), intravitreal injection of anti-VEGF medications has been confirmed as a non-inferior alternative to PRP.[5] Though Protocol S specifically studied PDR, its findings could reasonably be extrapolated to other ischemic neovascular retinal diseases as well. As compared to PRP, anti-VEGF injections have multiple benefits: there is no destruction of the retinal tissue (and thus no peripheral vision, contrast sensitivity or low-light vision decrease), inadequate ocular media is less of a concern, treatment is quicker, and injections offer the added benefit of treating any concurrent diabetic macular edema, potentially leading to better vision outcomes. There are, however, also significant downsides to anti-VEGF treatment of neovascular retinal diseases; most significantly, anti-VEGF injections do not confer a long-lasting benefit and treatment generally must be repeated (potentially indefinitely) on a regular basis. Loss of patients to follow-up may find them returning years later with significant progression of disease, which is often not the case for patients who fail to follow up following PRP. Another potential downside to treatment with anti-VEGF is the remarkable ability of injections to induce rapid regression of neovascularization, which in some cases may precipitate rapid progression of tractional retinal detachment in a phenomenon often referred to as "crunch."[18] Though rare, intravitreal injections also confer a small risk of endophthalmitis, which is not a concern with PRP. In the author's anecdotal experience, when presented with both options, patients will often choose to undergo PRP rather than potentially ongoing intravitreal injections, regardless of the risks of peripheral vision loss and nyctalopia.

Informed consent should include a statement indicating that the risks, benefits, and alternative options were discussed, and the patient's questions were answered. It should also clearly state that the patient indicated they would like to proceed with the proposed procedure.

PREOPERATIVE CARE

Key Preoperative Considerations

- A complete eye examination should be done to ensure there is no media opacity that would preclude adequate treatment.
- The pupil should be widely dilated.
- Surgeon should verify the laser is functioning normally and be familiar with its operation.
- Topical anesthesia should be administered prior to the application of a contact treatment lens (and may be helpful even when the LIO is being used, to decrease the patient's need to blink during treatment).
- Consideration should be given to globe anesthesia.

Patients suffering from vascular diseases often have ocular comorbidities that could make adequate laser treatment difficult or dangerous. This may include vitreous hemorrhage, cataract, or miotic pupils. If the fundus view is inadequate, treatment may best be delayed until it can be performed adequately and safely. Anti-VEGF injections or vitrectomy surgery can be considered in patients with significant vitreous hemorrhage, and treatment can often be delayed until after cataract removal can be completed if necessary.

Depending on the laser wavelength and power required to achieve an acceptable burn, there may be significant discomfort associated with treatment. Yellow-wavelength lasers (577 nm) tend to be more comfortable than green-wavelength lasers (532 nm).[19] Pattern lasers (Iridex, Pascal, Navilas) generally apply several spots in rapid succession, with a shorter duration per spot, which seems to be more comfortable for many patients as compared to single-spot modes with longer duration. Discomfort may be mitigated by preoperative anesthesia. Topical anesthesia decreases the comfort associated with a contact treatment lens but does not adequately anesthetize the posterior segment for the actual laser treatment. Retrobulbar anesthesia is very effective but requires an awake patient to remain still while the retrobulbar needle is advanced into the orbit and carries the small but serious risk of brainstem anesthesia with resulting respiratory failure. This method also leads to transient loss of vision and lack of motility, requiring patching for the remainder of the day. Subconjunctival or sub-Tenon's anesthesia is not as effective as retrobulbar anesthesia, but it is often easier to perform and associated with less risk (primarily being the common subconjunctival hemorrhage and the very rare globe perforation).

SETTINGS AND PROCEDURE

Key Laser Settings

- Power: 100 to 450 mW
- Duration: 0.1 to 0.2 seconds (100–200 ms, 20–30 ms in pattern mode)
- Interval: 0.1 to 0.5 seconds
- Spot size: 400 to 500 μm, accounting for lens magnification
- Spot spacing: Approximately 1.0-spot width

The total energy applied per spot of laser is a product of the spot size, power, and duration of application. The energy needed to produce the appropriate burn (and thus the laser settings required) varies depending on laser characteristics (for instance, the wavelength), patient factors (ocular media opacity and fundus pigmentation), and focus. Although "ballpark" initial settings are discussed herein, appropriate settings may vary greatly in different situations.

At the slit lamp, the specific contact lens being used will produce some degree of laser spot magnification; this value varies between lenses. For instance, the Mainster 165 lens (Ocular) produces a laser spot magnification of 1.96x (Figs. 19.3–19.5). The Super Quad 160 (Volk) produces a magnification of 2.0x. The characteristics of the

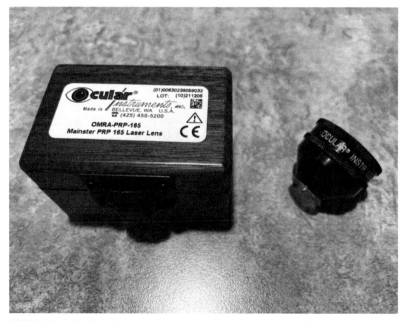

FIGURE 19-3 Ocular Mainster panretinal photocoagulation 165 Lens.

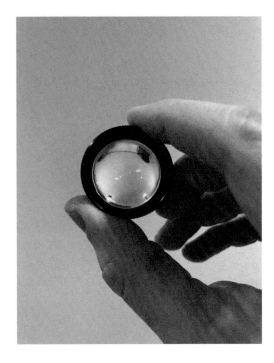

FIGURE 19-4 Physician view, Mainster panretinal photocoagulation 165 lens.

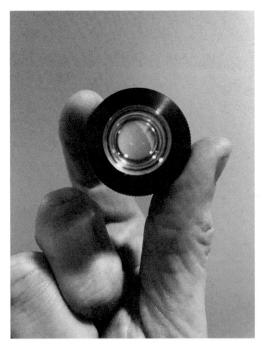

FIGURE 19-5 Patient view, Mainster panretinal photocoagulation 165 lens.

specific lens being used are clearly stated in the lens specifications documentation. When LIO is being used, lenses produce minification that must be considered; a 20D lens' laser spot magnification is approximately 0.32x, and for a 28D lens, 0.44x.[20–22]

The appropriate starting power is determined using a titration method. Aiming a single spot in a peripheral area of the retina, the laser is applied. Power is increased in increments to produce a slight greying of the tissue. Power and duration of the laser burn can be adjusted to increase or decrease the whitening effect. When treating at the slit lamp, the author generally begins with an approximately 400-μm spot size (200 μm selected on the reticule, 1.96x magnification using a Mainster 165 contact lens). Power is initially set at 150 mW with duration at 0.1 second (100 ms). Power is then adjusted to achieve the appropriate tissue effect.

If patient discomfort is present, this may at times be ameliorated by slightly decreasing the duration (i.e., to 70–80 ms) while increasing the power (10–20 mW increments) until an appropriate effect is again obtained.

The interval period refers to the time between applications of laser in single-spot mode when the pedal is held in the depressed position. The desired speed is based on surgeon preference and comfort; a shorter interval speeds treatment but also increases the risk of inadvertent laser damage should the patient move unexpectedly during treatment. An initial interval of 500 ms (0.5 s) is reasonable for beginning surgeon's, and this can be significantly shortened as confidence is gained.

All methods of treatment feature an aiming beam with adjustable brightness that is independent of the scope illumination. If the aiming beam is not visible, ensure the brightness is turned up and the laser is set to "ready"; often, the aiming beam is not visible until this is the case.

Once the chosen lens is positioned, laser spots are applied to the area to be treated, either in a "scatter" fashion (for single-spot mode) or using repeated patterns of spots (i.e., multiple 5 × 5 grids placed in a "patchwork" fashion) (Fig. 19.6).

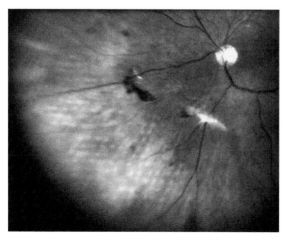

FIGURE 19-6 Immediate posttreatment photo showing grey-white burns.

The ultimate goal of treatment for panretinal cases is to fill the entire ischemic periphery with 1600 to 2000 individual spots, spaced approximately 1.0-spot width apart. While some surgeon's will elect to fully treat a given eye in one session of laser, many surgeon's elect to complete a full course of treatment across multiple sessions. The latter method may be less taxing on both the patient and surgeon, particularly when a "single-spot" mode is being used, as compared to a "pattern" mode.[23] Dividing treatment into multiple sessions may have the added benefit of decreasing the incidence of the "crunch" phenomenon that can sometimes occur with rapid regression of prominent neovascularization. When multiple sessions are performed, the goal may be to fully treat one half of the retina per session; another strategy may be to treat 360° with 2.0- to 3.0-width spot spacing, with the intention of adding denser spots at a later session.

PRP can be performed with the patient upright, using a slit-lamp-mounted laser unit, or via LIO. Both methods have relative advantages and disadvantages: Advantages of LIO treatment include potentially faster treatment in single-spot modes and a wider static field of view. Relative advantages of slit-lamp-mounted units include greater precision in treatment and a beneficial eye motion-stabilizing effect from the contact lens employed in treatment, in addition to the possibility of pattern-style treatment, which can significantly reduce treatment time. Patient comfort in terms of positioning may be better in LIO, as this method can be done with the patient reclining; however, the laser treatment itself is often more uncomfortable when LIO is used. With either option, taking time to ensure proper setup and patient positioning beforehand will often help make treatment go as smoothly as possible.

Considerations for Slit-Lamp-Mounted Laser Units

When a slit-lamp-mounted laser is being used, the position is similar to that used for a general exam. The patient is positioned at the slit lamp and advised to keep their forehead against the forehead support strap and their chin on the chin rest. Patients will often gradually drift out of position during the procedure, and it can be helpful to have an assistant help the patient maintain the proper position.

A coupling solution (i.e., carboxymethylcellulose [Celluvisc], hydroxypropyl methylcellulose [Gonak], or hypromellose [Genteal Gel]) is applied to the patient side of the contact lens to be utilized. The operative eye is anesthetized with topical tetracaine or proparacaine, and the contact lens is placed on the eye. This can be facilitated by asking the patient to look downward while the surgeon manually elevates the upper lid.

Once the lens is placed, titration and treatment can begin. The patient can be asked to direct their gaze in the direction of the pathology to facilitate visualization.

Considerations for Laser Indirect Ophthalmoscopy

When using LIO, reclining the patient back 45° or more can create a more comfortable situation for both the surgeon and patient. A drop of topical anesthetic is instilled in the operative eye; this can mitigate some of the involuntary eyelid clenching that often results if the ocular surface begins to dry during treatment. The lid can be manually elevated by the surgeon during treatment, or a wire lid speculum may be used; the latter is generally more uncomfortable for the patient. The patient is asked to look in various directions during the procedure to facilitate peripheral treatment.

Considerations for Pattern-Type or Navigated Lasers

When using a pattern-type laser (PASCAL, Iridex), the desired pattern must be selected. These units generally allow for the placement of a 2 × 2, 3 × 3, 4 × 4, or 5 × 5 grid of individual spots and feature the ability to adjust the spacing between the spots. The author generally uses a 3 × 3 to 5 × 5 square grid with spot spacing set to 2.0 to 3.0, and then places multiple overlapping grids to achieve good coverage through the ischemic areas and an effective spot spacing of about 1-spot width. Though smaller, 1.0-spot width grids can be used and applied in a patchwork fashion, the rapid placement of multiple spots within a smaller area anecdotally seems to produce more patient discomfort.

A navigated laser (Navilas) allows planned treatment by "painting" a grid of evenly spaced spots over the desired area in a preoperative fundus photo. The unit's software aligns the photo with a live view of the patient's fundus to ensure that spots are placed in the desired location. Again, spot spacing is adjustable.

When the pedal is depressed, the spots are applied in rapid succession; the pattern can be aborted partway through its application if the pedal is released. As the spots are applied rapidly, the duration for individual spots is shorter than what would usually be used in single-spot mode (0.02–0.03 seconds vs. 0.1 seconds). The initial power must therefore be correspondingly higher to achieve a similar effect as that obtained using the single-spot settings noted previously; this should be kept in mind while titrating.

Considering the relative advantages and disadvantages of each approach, the author generally treats via a slit-lamp–mounted laser when pattern or navigated modes are available, and via LIO when single-spot treatment is the only option (Fig. 19.7).

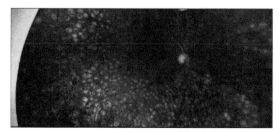

FIGURE 19-7 Several months post-panretinal photocoagulation, showing scars following treatment.

POSTOPERATIVE CARE/CO-MANAGEMENT (FOLLOW-UP SCHEDULE)

Key Postoperative Care Considerations

- Patient counseling
- Follow-up

As compared to anterior segment laser, intraocular inflammation and intraocular pressure rise are rare following posterior segment procedures, and thus no topical ocular antihypertensives or anti-inflammatories are prescribed. Patients are counseled to avoid touching or rubbing the eye to decrease the possibility of causing a corneal abrasion while the eye is anesthetized. If a preoperative retrobulbar block was performed, the ability to close the eyelid will be impaired, and temporarily patching the eyelid shut is advisable to decrease the risk of exposure keratopathy.

The patient should be counseled to call with any significant pain, decrease in vision, or increase in floaters postoperatively. As previously noted, vitreous hemorrhage or progression of tractional retinal detachment are possible following treatment; while mild-to-moderate vitreous hemorrhage will often resolve spontaneously with only observation, tractional or combined retinal detachment threatening the fovea often necessitates proceeding with pars plana vitrectomy.

Regression of neovascularization following PRP is generally significantly slower than that seen following intravitreal anti-VEGF injection. Following up on the patient four to six weeks post-treatment for a dilated exam is reasonable. Assuming neovascularization is regressing (as indicated by a "knuckled over" or by a whitish fibrotic appearance), patients can then be seen two to three months thereafter for a follow-up exam and fluorescein angiography to complete regression.

POTENTIAL COMPLICATIONS AND THEIR TREATMENT

Key Potential Complications

- Vitreous hemorrhage
- Progression of tractional retinal detachment
- Inadvertent central retinal laser damage
- Choroidal effusion
- Corneal abrasion

As stated previously, mild vitreous hemorrhage following laser often resolves spontaneously without the need for further treatment.[24] When hemorrhage is significant enough to preclude an adequate view of the retina and exclude the possibility of progressive retinal detachment, B-Scan ultrasound is indicated. Tractional detachment involving the macula is an indication for surgical repair via pars plana vitrectomy. Combined tractional and rhegmatogenous detachment is an indication for urgent surgical repair, regardless of the macular status. Vitreous hemorrhage without detachment noted on the B-Scan can be monitored with serial ultrasounds to allow for spontaneous clearing. Depending on the extent of the underlying neovascularization and the surgeon's estimated risk of "crunch," anti-VEGF may be used to help speed resolution.

Choroidal effusion can sometimes occur following heavy laser, particularly in hyperopic patients. Patients may remain asymptomatic if the effusion is small or develop significant discomfort and associated myopic shift in larger effusions. A short course of topical cycloplegics (i.e., Cyclopentolate 1% TID) can help with discomfort, and some have advocated for the use of topical or oral steroids.

Corneal abrasion can be related to trauma from multiple sources, including the contact lens used in treatment, a lid speculum when utilized, or by the patient rubbing the eye in the postoperative period. It is important to be aware that diabetics are at a higher risk for prolonged or poorly healing abrasions relative to the general population, and careful manipulation of the contact lens and good patient counseling may help to prevent a frustrating situation for the patient and surgeon.

EFFICACY

The DRS clearly demonstrated that PRP, applied in eyes with PDR when high-risk characteristics developed, reduced the rate of severe vision loss by over 50%. Later studies demonstrated the ability of PRP to induce regression of neovascularization in numerous other conditions associated with retinal ischemia. This method has been the recognized standard of care for such situations for much of the past 40 years.

As noted, anti-VEGF injections have emerged as an alternate option for patients with ischemia and neovascularization, with potential to produce better visual outcomes with fewer side effects in many patients. There have, however, been concerns raised about the high rate of diabetic patients who are lost to follow-up, only to return months or years later with significantly worsened disease. The persistent and long-lasting effect of PRP on the regression of neovascularization, as compared to the limited duration of effect from anti-VEGF injections, continues to maintain PRP as a relevant treatment.

CODING/BILLING

PRP is coded as CPT 67228 (treatment of extensive or progressive retinopathy (e.g., diabetic retinopathy), photocoagulation. The global period is ten days. If the contralateral eye is treated within the global period for a given eye, modifier-79 (distinct procedural service) is used.

The Centers for Medicare and Medicaid Services website (CMS.gov) maintains a list of ICD-10CM diagnosis codes that "support medical necessity" for CPT 67228. The list currently contains 200 separate codes, although some of the codes listed do not describe conditions where PRP is indicated, according to American Academy of Ophthalmology Preferred Practice Pattern guidelines (for instance, mild nonproliferative diabetic retinopathy). The codes listed in the following section are those where PRP is sometimes indicated, though this list is not comprehensive.

ICD-10CM

E08.341× to E08.359× (Range of diabetes due to an underlying condition, severe non-proliferative diabetic retinopathy [NPDR] to PDR

E09.341× to E10.359× (Range of drug- or chemical-induced diabetes with severe NPDR to PDR)

E10.341× to E10.359× (Range of Type 1 Diabetes with Severe NPDR to PDR)

E11.341× to E11.359× (Range of Type 2 Diabetes with Severe NPDR to PDR)

H21.1×× (Other vascular disorders of the iris and ciliary body [e.g., NVI])

H34.11 to H34.23 (Branch and CRAO)

H34.81× to H34.83× (Branch and CRVO)

H35.02× (Exudative retinopathy)

H35.05× (Retinal neovascularization)

H35.82 (Retinal ischemia)

H40.89 (Other specified glaucoma [e.g., neovascular glaucoma])

REFERENCES

1. Diabetic Retinopathy Study Research Group. Photocoagulation treatment of proliferative diabetic retinopathy: the second report of Diabetic Retinopathy Study findings. *Ophthalmology.* 1978;85(1): 82–106.
2. Photocoagulation treatment of proliferative diabetic retinopathy. Clinical application of Diabetic Retinopathy Study (DRS) findings, DRS Report Number 8. The Diabetic Retinopathy Study Research Group. *Ophthalmology.* 1981;88(7):583–600.
3. Preliminary report on effects of photocoagulation therapy. The Diabetic Retinopathy Study Research Group. *Am J Ophthalmol.* 1976;81(4):383–396. doi:10.1016/0002-9394(76)90292-0
4. Early Treatment Diabetic Retinopathy Study Research Group. Early photocoagulation for diabetic retinopathy: ETDRS report number 9. *Ophthalmology.* 1991;98(5 Suppl):766–785.
5. Writing Committee for the Diabetic Retinopathy Clinical Research Network, Gross JG, Glassman AR, et al. Panretinal photocoagulation vs intravitreous ranibizumab for proliferative diabetic retinopathy: a randomized clinical trial [published correction appears in JAMA. 2016 Mar 1;315(9):944] [published correction appears in JAMA. 2019 Mar 12;321(10):1008]. *JAMA.* 2015;314(20): 2137–2146. doi:10.1001/jama.2015.15217
6. Stefansson E. Oxygen and diabetic eye disease. *Graefes Arch Clin Exp Ophthalmol.* 1990;228(2): 120–123. doi:10.1007/BF00935719
7. Stefánsson E. The therapeutic effects of retinal laser treatment and vitrectomy. A theory based on oxygen and vascular physiology. *Acta Ophthalmol Scand.* 2001;79(5):435–440. doi:10.1034/j.1600-0420.2001.790502.x
8. Central Vein Occlusion Study Group. Natural history and clinical management of central retinal vein occlusion. *Arch Ophthalmol.* 1997;115(4):486–491.

9. Flaxel CJ, Adelman RA, Bailey ST, et al. Retinal Vein Occlusions Preferred Practice Pattern [published correction appears in Ophthalmology. 2020 Sep;127(9):1279]. *Ophthalmology*. 2020;127(2): P288–P320. doi:10.1016/j.ophtha.2019.09.029

10. Flaxel CJ, Adelman RA, Bailey ST, et al. Retinal and ophthalmic artery occlusions preferred practice pattern [published correction appears in Ophthalmology. 2020 Sep;127(9):1280]. *Ophthalmology*. 2020;127(2):P259–P287. doi:10.1016/j.ophtha.2019.09.028

11. Abdalla Elsayed MEA, Mura M, Al Dhibi H, et al. Sickle cell retinopathy. A focused review. *Graefes Arch Clin Exp Ophthalmol*. 2019;257(7):1353–1364. doi:10.1007/s00417-019-04294-2

12. Flaxel CJ, Adelman RA, Bailey ST, et al. Diabetic retinopathy preferred practice pattern [published correction appears in Ophthalmology. 2020 Sep;127(9):1279]. *Ophthalmology*. 2020;127(1): P66–P145. doi:10.1016/j.ophtha.2019.09.025

13. Davis MD, Fisher MR, Gangnon RE, et al. Risk factors for high-risk proliferative diabetic retinopathy and severe visual loss: Early Treatment Diabetic Retinopathy Study report number 18. *Invest Ophthalmol Vis Sci*. 1998;39(2):233–252.

14. Mohamed Q, Gillies MC, Wong TY. Management of diabetic retinopathy: a systematic review. *JAMA*. 2007;298(8):902–916.

15. Jalali S, Azad R, Trehan HS, Dogra MR, Gopal L, Narendran V. Technical aspects of laser treatment for acute retinopathy of prematurity under topical anesthesia. *Indian J Ophthalmol*. 2010;58(6): 509–515. doi:10.4103/0301-4738.71689

16. Fong DS, Girach A, Boney A. Visual side effects of successful scatter laser photocoagulation surgery for proliferative diabetic retinopathy: a literature review. *Retina*. 2007;27(7):816–824. doi:10.1097/IAE.0b013e318042d32c

17. Reddy SV, Husain D. Panretinal photocoagulation: a review of complications. *Semin Ophthalmol*. 2018;33(1):83–88. doi:10.1080/08820538.2017.1353820

18. Arevalo JF, Maia M, Flynn HW Jr, et al. Tractional retinal detachment following intravitreal bevacizumab (Avastin) in patients with severe proliferative diabetic retinopathy. *Br J Ophthalmol*. 2008;92(2):213–216. doi:10.1136/bjo.2007.127142

19. González-Saldivar G, Rojas-Juárez S, Espinosa-Soto I, Sánchez-Ramos J, Jaurieta-Hinojosa N, Ramírez-Estudillo A. Single-spot yellow laser versus conventional green laser on panretinal photocoagulation: patient pain scores and preferences. *Ophthalmic Surg Lasers Imaging Retina*. 2017;48(11): 902–905. doi:10.3928/23258160-20171030-05

20. Mainster MA, Crossman JL, Erickson PJ, Heacock GL. Retinal laser lenses: magnification, spot size, and field of view. *Br J Ophthalmol*. 1990;74(3):177–179. doi:10.1136/bjo.74.3.177

21. Ocular Instruments. Ocular Mainster PRP 165 Laser Lens Specifications. [Accessed Aug 21, 2020] Available at: https://ocularinc.com/media/wysiwyg/pdf/5805T-_OMRA-PRP_165_Rev_Q.pdf

22. Volk Instruments. Super Quad 160 Laser Lens Specifications. [Accessed Aug 21, 2020] Available at: https://www.volk.com/products/super-quad-160-indirect-contact-laser-lens

23. Nemcansky J, Stepanov A, Nemcanska S, Masek P, Langrova H, Studnicka J. Single session of pattern scanning laser versus multiple sessions of conventional laser for panretinal photocoagulation in diabetic retinopathy: efficacy, safety and painfulness. *PLoS One*. 2019;14(7):e0219282. Published 2019 Jul 16. doi:10.1371/journal.pone.0219282

24. Zweng HC, Little HL, Hammond AH. Complications of argon laser photocoagulation. *Trans Am Acad Ophthalmol Otolaryngol*. 1974;78(2):OP195–OP204.

20 Focal and Grid Macular Laser

James R. Singer

Focal and grid macular laser have been a cornerstone treatment of various retinal diseases for decades. The most common applications over the years have been diabetic macular edema (DME), macular edema due to branch retinal vein occlusions (BRVO), and central serous retinopathy (CSR). The first solar photocoagulator was developed by Meyer-Schwickerath in the 1940s. He and Littman later developed the xenon arc photocoagulator, which was used for both anterior and posterior segment applications.[1]

Since being described for the treatment of clinically significant DME (CSDME) in the Early Treatment of Diabetic Retinopathy Study (ETDRS) in 1985,[2] focal laser had been the first-line treatment modality for this condition until it was supplanted by intravitreal anti-vascular endothelial growth factor (anti-VEGF) therapy in the mid-2000s. That notwithstanding, focal laser still has a role as it remains the preferred treatment for non-center-involved DME (NCI-DME) and is sometimes used to augment anti-VEGF treatment in cases of center-involved DME (CI-DME). Recent clinical trials suggest that while anti-VEGF monotherapy for macular edema from diabetic retinopathy is effective for a large portion of patients, combination therapy with laser treatment is required to achieve the best possible outcome for many patients (approximately 50% of patients in the Diabetic Retinopathy Clinical Research Network [DRCR.net] protocol T study)[3] and may potentially reduce the frequency of anti-VEGF injections.

Macular laser treatment for BRVO was found to be effective for macular edema in the landmark Branch Vein Occlusion Study (BVOS) trial in 1984.[4] Treatment of this condition has also transitioned from macular grid laser to intravitreal anti-VEGF therapy much like DME, but laser still plays a useful role in some clinical scenarios (i.e., focal leakage from capillary breakdown, persistent and/or diffuse leakage despite anti-VEGF therapy, and treatment in patients who wish to forego or minimize injection therapy).

Macular focal laser also has a pertinent role in the treatment of CSR.[5] Additionally, focal laser has demonstrated efficacy in the treatment of several other retinal conditions such as retinal arterial macroaneurysms (RAM),[6] Coats' disease,[7] retinal capillary hemangiomas,[8] and optic disc pit maculopathy.[9]

The mechanism of action of laser photocoagulation involves light energy being absorbed and converted into a thermal burn at the level of the pigmented tissues of the retinal pigment epithelium (RPE) and choroid, triggering local protein denaturation. The mechanism by which this process leads to beneficial physiologic and anatomical effects in the macula is speculative, but there are numerous theories. The direct effect from destruction of the RPE and photoreceptors leading to reduced oxygen consumption and increased oxygenation of the inner retina is one proposed mechanism.[10] Another is the direct effect on retinal blood vessels, inducing closure and a corresponding reduction in leakage.[10] A third theory asserts that photocoagulation induces the release of transforming growth factor-beta 2 and other cytokines from RPE cells, which in turn suppresses the proliferation of vascular endothelial cells contributing to macular edema.[11] Other speculated mechanisms are that focal laser increases the RPE pump action[12] and/or induces recruitment of healthy RPE cells as a healing response.[13]

This chapter focuses on guidelines and treatment parameters for conventional macular lasers (532-nm argon green and 577-nm yellow), which are widely available and have been the standard for decades. It does bear mentioning that there are numerous other laser types (various multicolor lasers, subthreshold) and delivery systems (pattern scanning laser, camera-navigated contactless lasers with retinal landmark tracking), each of which has its own specific unique applications, benefits, and shortcomings. It is beyond the purview of this chapter to explore each of these laser technologies individually, but further discussion on the basic science of lasers can be found in Chapter 3. The treating clinician should have a comprehensive understanding of the laser unit itself (laser parameters, computerized algorithms if available), how the laser functions with the associated delivery device (slit lamp), and the properties of the selected laser wavelength prior to embarking on treatment.

INDICATIONS

Key Indications

- CSDME, including CI-DME and NCI-DME
- BRVO with macular edema
- CSR
- RAM
- Coats' disease
- Retinal capillary hemangioma
- Optic disc pit maculopathy

*Macular choroidal neovascularization is no longer an indication for focal laser treatment since the implementation of anti-VEGF therapies except in rare circumstances.

CONTRAINDICATIONS

Key Contraindications

- Dense media haze (i.e., corneal scarring, dense cataract, vitreous hemorrhage)
- Active ocular infection (i.e., conjunctivitis, corneal ulcer)
- Recent intraocular surgery
- Inability to fixate
- Patient tremor
- Inability to position patient at slit lamp

PREOPERATIVE PREPARATION

- Obtain written informed consent.
- Ensure adequate pupillary dilation.
- Apply topical anesthetic drops to the ocular surface (proparacaine, tetracaine, etc.).
- Identify and prepare the macular lens to be used, including application of methylcellulose gel if necessary.
- Review multimodal imaging studies (e.g., fundus photographs, fluorescein angiography, optical coherence tomography [OCT]) to formulate treatment plan and guide treatment.
- Position patient at laser slit lamp, make sure laser foot pedal and laser adjustment controls are within reach, and place laser lens against the patient's cornea.
- Have patient fixate forward with the fellow eye and focus the slit lamp into the treatment eye, taking note of ocular landmarks. (Moving the slit beam ~15° off-center will help to minimize glare.)

SETTINGS AND PROCEDURE

The following recommendations are for conventional green 532-nm or yellow 577-nm lasers:

Laser Parameter/Settings Ranges

- Power, duration, interval, and spot size are the standard adjustable laser parameters. Power, duration, and spot size (in conjunction with the type of lens being used) determine burn intensity, whereas the interval determines the time between laser applications when the laser foot pedal remains engaged. In general, the clinician should use the lowest settings possible initially and then titrate the laser settings to achieve the desired treatment effect. It is important to be mindful that various factors such as the ocular media (i.e., corneal haze, cataract, vitreous hemorrhage, etc.) and even the integrity of the fiber-optic laser cable can affect the laser intensity. Consequently, laser settings can vary significantly depending upon these factors in addition to the pathology being treated. As a general starting point for macular disease, the clinician could begin with the following laser parameters and adjust accordingly:

- Power: 50 to 80 mW
- Duration: 50 to 100 ms (much longer for intraretinal vascular lesions such as macroaneurysms)
- Spot size: 50 to 100 microns
- Interval: None (under this setting, laser will default to one laser application per foot pedal trigger)

Lenses

- Goldmann 3-mirror (0.93x image magnification, 1.08x laser spot magnification, mirrored lens can allow treatment of more peripheral lesions)
- Ocular NMR (no methylcellulose required) Fundus Laser (0.97x image magnification, 1.04x laser spot magnification, methylcellulose not required)
- Ocular Mainster Standard Focal/Grid (0.96x image magnification, 1.05x laser spot magnification, NMR version does not require methylcellulose)
- Ocular Mainster High Magnification (1.25x image magnification, 0.80x laser spot magnification, NMR version does not require methylcellulose)
- Ocular Reichel-Mainster 1x Retina (0.95x image magnification, 1.05x laser spot magnification)
- Ocular Yannuzzi Fundus Ocular (0.93x image magnification, 1.08x laser spot magnification, large scleral flange enhances manipulation of globe/eyelids)
- Volk Area centralis (1.06x image magnification, 0.94x laser spot magnification)
- Volk H-R Centralis (1.08x image magnification, 0.93x laser spot magnification)
- Volk Super Macula 2.2 (1.49x image magnification, 0.67x laser spot magnification)
- Volk Fundus Laser (1.25x image magnification, 0.80x laser spot magnification)

General Considerations

- For a given power and duration setting, decreasing the spot size will result in correspondingly higher relative energy delivery over a smaller area. Reducing the spot size without a corresponding adjustment in the power/duration can result in an overly intense burn, with the potential to produce rupture of Bruch's membrane resulting in hemorrhaging and/or secondary choroidal neovascularization.
- Laser applications should be placed more than 500 microns away from the foveal center and not within the foveal avascular zone with rare exceptions.
- Caution should be utilized during treatment in the papillomacular bundle to avoid inducing a cecocentral scotoma.

- Consider using small spot size (50 microns) and short-duration burns (50 ms) when treating close to the fovea or within the papillomacular bundle.
- Direct laser treatment of shunt vessels/collaterals should be avoided as well as areas of dense intraretinal hemorrhage (which can damage the inner-retinal layers leading to a scotoma).
- Several treatment sessions spaced several months apart may be required to achieve maximal resolution of edema from diabetic retinopathy and BRVO. CSR often responds well to a single laser treatment of focal hotspots but recurrences are not uncommon.

For Diabetic Macular Edema

- Treatment guidelines have evolved per recommendations of the DRCR.net (Modified-ETDRS technique)[14]:
- Directly treat all leaking microaneurysms in areas of retinal thickening between 500 and 3000 microns from the center of the macula (although treatment may be performed between 300 and 500 microns of macula if center-involved edema and visual acuity worse than 20/40 persist after initial focal photocoagulation).
- Treatment of microaneurysms does not require blanching of the lesion, but at least a mild gray-white burn should be evident beneath.
- The spot size for direct treatment should be 50 microns with a duration of 50 to 100 ms.
- Grid treatment is applied to all areas with edema not associated with microaneurysms. If fluorescein angiography is obtained, grid laser is applied to areas of edema with angiographic non-perfusion.
- When indicated, grid laser should be applied 500 to 3000 microns superiorly, nasally, and inferiorly from center of macula, 500 to 3500 microns temporally from macular center, with no burns placed within 500 microns of disc.
- The burn intensity for grid treatment should be a barely visible light gray with a burn separation of 2 burn widths.
- The laser wavelength should be in the green–yellow spectrum.
- Lenses used for laser treatment should not increase or reduce the burn size by more than 10%.
- See Figure 20.1 for example of focal laser treatment for DME.

For Macular Edema Secondary to Branch Retinal Vein Occlusions

- Apply laser treatment to regions of retinal edema/thickening in a grid pattern with laser spots spaced one to two burn widths apart.
- Burns should achieve a light grayish whitening of the RPE.
- Treatment may extend from the edge of the foveal avascular zone to the arcades.
- See Figure 20.2 for example of focal laser treatment for BRVO with macular edema.

For Central Serous Retinopathy

- Apply laser treatment to focal leaking "hot spots" noted on angiography (usually noted on examination as focal RPE alterations/detachments) until a very subtle blanching of the RPE is achieved.
- Treatment should be at least 375 microns or more from the fovea (and not within the foveal avascular zone) with a small spot size of 50 to 200 microns and short duration of 50 to 100 ms, favoring smaller and shorter duration burns when in close proximity to the fovea.
- See Figure 20.3 for example of focal laser treatment for CSR.

For Coats' Disease, Retinal Capillary Hemangiomas, and Macroaneurysms

- Laser can be used to reduce leakage or induce closure of an anomalous vessel.
- The clinician should be familiar with the latest published reports and clinical studies for treatment of these conditions as there are no established guidelines for laser.
- In general, the entire vascular lesion (and sometimes the immediate surrounding area) is treated directly, using low-power and long-duration (200–500 ms) burns.
- A gentle and slow-forming grayish whitening of the lesion/vessel should be noted with each burn.
- See Figure 20.4 for example of focal laser treatment for RAM with macular edema and exudation.

POSTOPERATIVE CARE/CO-MANAGEMENT (FOLLOW-UP SCHEDULE)

- Patients should be followed closely with a repeat exam within one to two months to gauge treatment response. Examinations typically include a dilated funduscopic exam, OCT, and possibly a fluorescein angiogram to assess for persistent areas of leakage and/or non-perfusion. Those requiring combination therapy (intravitreal anti-VEGF and/or corticosteroids) should remain on an appropriate follow-up schedule depending upon disease severity and timing of prior treatments. Typically, a response to laser can be seen within a few weeks but anatomical and functional improvements can continue over months. Continued management decisions should be based on disease type, activity, severity, and patient-specific factors such as unique treatment preferences, ability to follow up, and treatment burden.

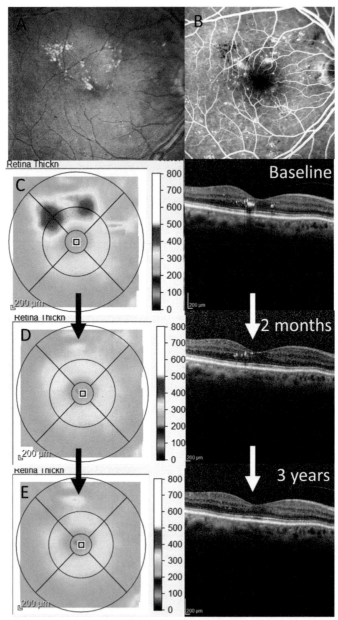

FIGURE 20-1 Diabetic macular edema pre- and post-focal laser treatment. Baseline multicolor scanning laser image **(A)** demonstrates scattered microaneurysms with lipid exudates extending into the fovea from two foci of leakage superonasally and superotemporally. Pretreatment fluorescein angiography **(B)** reveals scattered pinpoint foci of hyperfluorescence consistent with microaneurysms and blockage correlating to the lipid exudates. There is angiographic leakage superotemporal and superonasal to the fovea. Baseline **(C)** and post-laser **(D,E)** optical coherence tomography images at 2 months and 3 years reveal subfoveal hyperreflective debris consistent with lipid and juxtafoveal thickening in the regions of angiographic leakage. The edema and lipid resolved with focal laser treatment alone. A single application of modified ETDRS-style focal/grid laser was delivered to the area of leakage noted on fluorescein angiography just superonasal and superotemporal to the fovea.

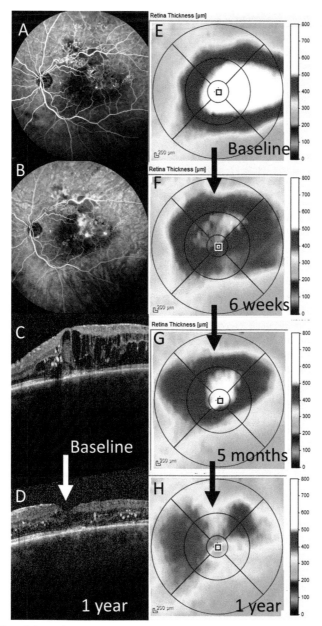

FIGURE 20-2 Chronic branch retinal vein occlusion with macular edema pre-and post-focal laser treatment. Patient had history of recalcitrant edema and lipid exudation despite prior treatment with bevacizumab, aflibercept, ranibizumab, and dexamethasone intravitreal implants. Baseline fluorescein angiography **(A,B)** demonstrates scattered areas of blockage from lipid exudates, capillary non-perfusion, and late leakage in the superior/superotemporal macula. Baseline **(C,E)** and post-laser **(D, F–H)** optical coherence tomography images reveal significant improvement 6 weeks after laser treatment with continued anatomical gains over the following year. The patient only received two intravitreal injections after laser treatment in the following year, whereas monthly treatment had been required previously with little change noted on OCT. A single application of macular grid laser was delivered to the areas of leakage and non-perfusion that were noted on fluorescein angiography.

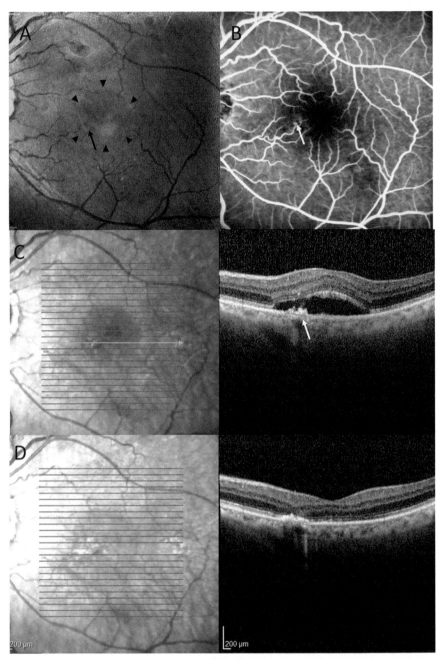

FIGURE 20-3 Central serous retinopathy pre-focal and 6-week post-focal laser treatment. Baseline multicolor scanning laser image **(A)** demonstrates a focal area of RPE disruption adjacent to the fovea (black arrow) with surrounding subretinal fluid (arrowheads). Pretreatment fluorescein angiography **(B)** reveals focal leakage (white arrow) corresponding to the RPE alterations noted clinically. Baseline **(C)** and post-laser **(D)** optical coherence tomography images exhibit subfoveal/subretinal fluid, which regressed entirely after treatment. A single-light application of focal laser was delivered to the area of leakage noted on fluorescein angiography.

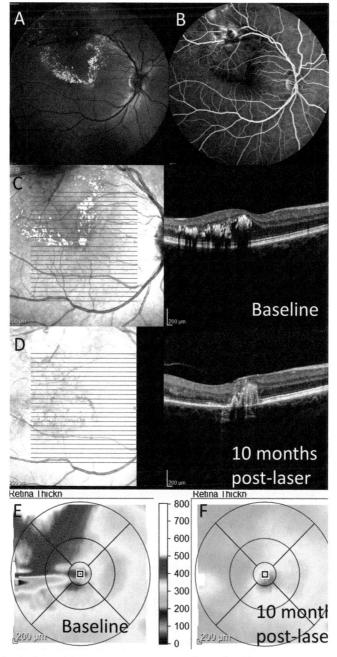

FIGURE 20-4 Retinal arterial macroaneurysm pre- and post-focal laser treatment. Chronic macular edema and lipid exudation resulted in severe vision loss. Initial treatment with bevacizumab had negligible effects on the leakage, which prompted treatment with focal laser. Baseline multicolor scanning laser and fluorescein angiography images **(A,B)** demonstrate fusiform dilatation and leakage from the superotemporal arterial lesion. Baseline **(C,E)** and post-laser **(D,F)** optical coherence tomography images reveal significant improvement 10 weeks after laser treatment but with persistent subfoveal hyperreflective retinal debris from the chronic lipid exudate. Several long-duration applications of laser (200–400 ms) with varying spot sizes (200–500 microns) were delivered to the macroaneurysm until a light blanching was noted.

POTENTIAL COMPLICATIONS AND THEIR TREATMENT

Overly Intense Laser Burns

- Can result in a variety of deleterious effects such as a central/paracentral scotoma, subretinal fibrosis, subretinal hemorrhage, and rupture of Bruch's membrane with secondary choroidal neovascularization. In most cases, close observation alone is appropriate. If choroidal neovascularization develops, anti-VEGF injections should be promptly initiated. It is also important for the clinician to be mindful of the concept colloquially known as "laser creep," a phenomenon in which a slowly progressive zone of RPE atrophy develops immediately adjacent to prior laser burns, particularly those large in size associated with higher-power and longer-duration burns. The atrophy can progress for months to years after laser treatment, possibly enlarging up to 300% of the original burn size,[15] and lead to irreversible vision loss. Hence, avoidance of intense burns, particularly those close to the foveal avascular zone, is of paramount importance. Using a small spot size (50 microns) and low power and duration can reduce the likelihood of this complication.

Foveal Burns

- Lead to permanent central vision loss. No treatment is available.

Vascular Occlusion/Rupture

- Direct laser treatment to a retinal blood vessel can result in an occlusion or rupture, resulting in retinal ischemia distal to the occlusion or hemorrhage, respectively. Treatment would be directed at minimizing the resulting retinal vascular complications and/or mitigating the effects of the intraocular hemorrhage (e.g., injection therapy, sectoral scatter laser, vitrectomy).

Exudative Retinal Detachment

- Rarely, treatment of retinal vascular lesions such as a retinal arterial macroaneurysm can trigger an inflammatory response that leads to exudation. This may in turn cause an exudative retinal and/or choroidal detachment. Treatment options generally include corticosteroids (topical, periocular or intraocular, and/or oral) and observation alone.

VIDEO OF PROCEDURE

Video 20.1—Focal laser treatment for diabetic macular edema using a 532 nm Argon green laser. Laser settings: laser power 50 to 100 mW, laser duration 50 ms, spot size 50 μm, lens: Volk HR-centralis. Video courtesy of James Singer.

EFFICACY

Diabetic Macular Edema

- The ETDRS clinical trial confirmed the benefits of focal/grid macular laser treatment for clinically significant macular edema in 1985. This treatment modality remained the primary therapy until the mid-2000s when anti-VEGF treatment became the standard of care for CI-DME. The ETDRS demonstrated that macular laser decreased the risk of moderate vision loss in patients with CSDME by 50% at 3 years, while a significant vision gain (15+ letters) was only experienced by approximately 3% of study patients.[2]
- A major review of macular laser photocoagulation monotherapy for DME in 2018 showed that laser reduced the chance of visual loss and increased the likelihood of DME resolution compared to no intervention at 1 to 3 years.[16] This Cochrane review analyzed 24 randomized controlled trials and the outcomes of 4422 eyes.
- The Diabetic Retinopathy Clinical Research Network (DRCR.net) published numerous studies demonstrating the benefit of focal/grid macular laser treatment for CI-DME, including protocols B, I, K, and T. Since anti-VEGF therapy is now first-line therapy and has been shown to be superior to laser monotherapy, it is difficult to independently assess the efficacy of macular focal laser in the setting of concurrent anti-VEGF treatments. Nonetheless, it has been shown that many patients still require macular focal laser despite anti-VEGF therapy. DRCR.net protocol T, a landmark clinical trial that focused on treatment of patients with vision impairment from CI-DME, revealed that a large percentage of patients undergoing anti-VEGF treatment still had persistent DME and needed macular laser.[3] Patients were randomized to receive intravitreal injections of 2 mg of Eylea (aflibercept, Regeneron), 1.25 mg of compounded Avastin (bevacizumab, Genentech), or 0.3 mg of Lucentis (ranibizumab, Genentech) and were followed over two years. If DME persisted at six months despite injection therapy per study parameters, focal macular laser was administered according to the modified ETDRS protocol. The number of patients who underwent at least one session of macular laser during the two years comprised 41%, 64%, and 52% of the aflibercept, bevacizumab, and ranibizumab groups, respectively. Anti-VEGF therapy, and focal laser in cases of persistent DME, resulted in mean visual acuity improvements of 12.8 letters in the aflibercept group, 10 letters in the bevacizumab group, and 12.3 letters in the ranibizumab group at 2 years.
- Treatment of NCI-DME with anti-VEGF has not been rigorously studied. Consequently, focal/grid laser treatment is the recommended treatment for this condition.

Branch Retinal Vein Occlusion

- Grid laser for macular edema due to BRVO has been shown to be beneficial since the BVOS study of 1984.[4] Eyes with visual acuity of 20/40 or worse due to perfused BRVO with macular edema were randomized to grid-pattern laser photocoagulation or observation. Treated eyes were much more likely to gain at least 2 lines of vision versus the observation group (65% vs. 37%). Treated eyes were almost twice as likely to have 20/40 or better vision than those in the observation group.

- The utility of grid laser for treatment of macular edema due to BRVO was further confirmed after the Standard Care versus Corticosteroid for Retinal Vein Occlusion study in 2009, which concluded that grid laser photocoagulation should be recommended for macular edema secondary to BRVO over intravitreal triamcinolone.[17] This study showed that 29% of eyes treated with macular laser gained 3 or more lines of vision at 1 year compared with 26% of eyes treated with 1-mg intravitreal triamcinolone and 27% of eyes treated with 4-mg intravitreal triamcinolone. Despite all three groups experiencing similar vision gains, the groups treated with corticosteroids had higher rates of side effects, leading to the recommendation of macular laser over corticosteroid therapy.

- Once the BRAVO[18] trial results were published demonstrating excellent vision gains and minimal side effects with anti-VEGF therapy, macular grid laser became the second-line treatment for macular edema due to BRVO. Nonetheless, many patients who underwent ranibizumab therapy still required macular laser treatment during the BRAVO study (36%–43%) and eventually around 50% of those patients underwent macular laser treatment by the conclusion of the HORIZON[19] trial, which was an open-label extension trial of the BRAVO study.

- Recent publications have actually brought into question the utility of adding laser in the setting of ongoing anti-VEGF treatment for macular edema due to BRVO. Neither the BRIGHTER[20] trial nor the RETAIN[21] trial revealed that adding laser to ranibizumab intravitreal therapy improved vision or decreased treatment burden.

Retinal Arterial Macroaneurysm

- It is important to note that there are no treatment guidelines for RAM. The majority of macroaneurysms spontaneously involute and will therefore not require laser treatment. There are few studies regarding the efficacy of focal laser treatment for macroaneurysms due to their significant clinical variability. Hence, data from well-designed clinical trials are lacking. Nonetheless, information regarding the efficacy of focal laser for macroaneurysms dates back to 1976 when Gass and colleagues published a case series showing that it obliterated the macroaneurysms and reduced leakage in several patients.[22] It should also be noted that anti-VEGF therapy can be beneficial without the risk of hemorrhage, exudation, and vessel occlusion that can accompany laser treatment.[23]

Central Serous Retinopathy

- There are no well-defined treatment guidelines for CSR. However, in select cases, thermal laser can be used and has been shown to be effective. The mechanism of thermal laser for CSR is unknown. It has been speculated that photocoagulation may seal focal RPE defects, trigger a healing response and recruitment of healthy RPE cells, or stimulate the RPE cellular "pump" near the leak.[5]

- Two small randomized, controlled trials[24,25] suggested more rapid resolution of subretinal fluid with focal laser treatment in CSR but these studies included relatively few patients and preceded the advent of OCT. Several other trials reported quicker resolution of subretinal fluid in CSR, but some studies have suggested no significant long-term differences in outcomes between treated and untreated eyes.[26]

CODING/BILLING AND MODIFIERS

- Focal/grid laser procedures are billed with CPT code 67210 (Destruction of localized lesion of retina [e.g., macular edema, tumors], 1 or more sessions; photocoagulation), which at the time of this publication has a 90-day global period.
- Common ICD-10 diagnoses codes that support this procedure are:
  - E10.3211, E10.3212, E10.3213-Type 1 Diabetes Mellitus with Mild Nonproliferative Diabetic Retinopathy with Macular Edema
  - E10.3311, E10.3312, E10.3313-Type 1 Diabetes Mellitus with Moderate Nonproliferative Diabetic Retinopathy with Macular Edema
  - E10.3411, E10.3412, E10.343-Type 1 Diabetes Mellitus with Severe Nonproliferative Diabetic Retinopathy with Macular Edema
  - E10.3511, E10.3512, E10.3513-Type 1 Diabetes Mellitus with Proliferative Diabetic Retinopathy with Macular Edema
  - E11.3211, E11.3212, E11.3213-Type 2 Diabetes Mellitus with Mild Nonproliferative Diabetic Retinopathy with Macular Edema
  - E11.3311, E11.3312, E11.3313-Type 2 Diabetes Mellitus with Moderate Nonproliferative Diabetic Retinopathy with Macular Edema
  - E11.3411, E11.3412, E11.3413-Type 2 Diabetes Mellitus with Severe Nonproliferative Diabetic Retinopathy with Macular Edema
  - E11.3511, E11.3512, E11.3513-Type 2 Diabetes Mellitus with Proliferative Diabetic Retinopathy with Macular Edema
  - H34.8310, H34.8320, H34.8330-Tributary (branch) Retinal Vein Occlusion with Macular Edema
  - H35.711, H35.712, H35.713-Central serous chorioretinopathy
  - H35.09-RAM

REFERENCES

1. Meyer-Schwickerath GRE. The history of photocoagulation. *Aust N Z J Ophthalmol.* 1989;17: 427–434.
2. Photocoagulation for Diabetic Macular Edema: Early Treatment Diabetic Retinopathy Study Report Number 1 Early Treatment Diabetic Retinopathy Study Research Group. 11.
3. Wells JA, et al. Aflibercept, bevacizumab, or ranibizumab for diabetic macular edema. *Ophthalmology.* 2016;123:1351–1359.

4. The Branch Vein Occlusion Study Group. Argon laser photocoagulation for macular edema in branch vein occlusion. *Am J Ophthalmol*. 1984;98:271–282.

5. Nicholson B, Noble J, Forooghian F, et al. Central serous chorioretinopathy: update on pathophysiology and treatment. *Surv Ophthalmol*. 2013;58:103–126.

6. Rabb F. Retinal arterial macroaneurysms. *Surv Ophthalmol*. 1988;33:73–96.

7. Kodama A, Sugioka K, Kusaka S, et al. Combined treatment for Coats' disease: retinal laser photocoagulation combined with intravitreal bevacizumab injection was effective in two cases. *BMC Ophthalmol*. 2014;14:36.

8. Singh AD, Nouri M, Shields CL, et al. Treatment of retinal capillary hemangioma. *Ophthalmology*. 2002;109:1799–1806.

9. Moisseiev E, Moisseiev J, Loewenstein A. Optic disc pit maculopathy: when and how to treat? A review of the pathogenesis and treatment options. *Int J Retina Vitr*. 2015;1:13.

10. Stefansson E. The therapeutic effects of retinal laser treatment and vitrectomy. A theory based on oxygen and vascular physiology. *Acta Ophthalmol Scand*. 2001;79:435–440.

11. Matsumoto M, Yoshimura N, Honda Y. Increased production of transforming growth factor-beta 2 from cultured human retinal pigment epithelial cells by photocoagulation. *Invest Ophthalmol Vis Sci*. 1994 Dec;35(13):4245–4252.

12. Ogata N, Tombran-Tink J, Jo N, et al. Upregulation of pigment epithelium-derived factor after laser photocoagulation. *Am J Ophthalmol*. 2001;132:427–429.

13. Colome J, Ruiz-Moreno JM, Montero JA. Diode laser-induced mitosis in the rabbit retinal pigment epithelium. *Ophthalmic Surg Lasers Imaging* Retina. 2007;38:484–490.

14. Diabet. Retin. Clin. Res. Netw. Internet Cited 2020 Sept 3 Modif.-ETDRS Focal Photocoagul. Tech. Available HttppublicfilesjaeborgdrcrnetMiscFocalGridProcedure42711pdf.

15. Schatz H. Progressive enlargement of laser scars following grid laser photocoagulation for diffuse diabetic macular edema. *Arch Ophthalmol*. 1991;109:1549.

16. Jorge EC. et al. Monotherapy laser photocoagulation for diabetic macular oedema. *Cochrane Database Syst Rev*. 2018. doi:10.1002/14651858.CD010859.pub2

17. A randomized trial comparing the efficacy and safety of intravitreal triamcinolone with standard care to treat vision loss associated with macular edema secondary to branch retinal vein occlusion: the Standard Care vs Corticosteroid for Retinal Vein Occlusion (SCORE) Study Report 6. *Arch. Ophthalmol*. 2009;127:1115.

18. Brown DM, et al. Sustained benefits from ranibizumab for macular edema following branch retinal vein occlusion: 12-month outcomes of a phase III study. *Ophthalmology*. 2011;118:1594–1602.

19. Heier JS, et al. Ranibizumab for macular edema due to retinal vein occlusions. *Ophthalmology*. 2012;119:802–809.

20. Tadayoni R, et al. Sustained benefits of ranibizumab with or without laser in branch retinal vein occlusion. *Ophthalmology*. 2017;124:1778–1787.

21. Campochiaro PA, et al. Long-term outcomes in patients with retinal vein occlusion treated with ranibizumab. *Ophthalmology*. 2014;121:209–219.

22. Lewis RA, Norton EW, Gass JD. Acquired arterial macroaneurysms of the retina. *Br J Ophthalmol*. 1976;60:21–30.

23. Mansour AM, et al. Intravitreal anti-vascular endothelial growth factor injections for exudative retinal arterial macroaneurysms. *Retina*. 2019;39:1133–1141.

24. Leaver P, Williams C. Argon laser photocoagulation in the treatment of central serous retinopathy. *Br J Ophthalmol*. 1979;63:674–677.

25. Robertson DM, Ilstrup D. Direct, indirect, and sham laser photocoagulation in the management of central serous chorioretinopathy. *Am J Ophthalmol*. 1983;95:457–466.

26. Gilbert CM, Owens SL, Smith PD, et al. Long-term follow-up of central serous chorioretinopathy. *Br J Ophthalmol*. 1984;68:815–820.

Laser Retinopexy

Alan R. Hromas

Laser retinopexy refers to the use of photocoagulative laser in an attempt to halt the progression of retinal pathology threatening symptomatic retinal detachment. Treatment involves the application of confluent individual laser burns to demarcate an area of concern, with the goal of inducing a chorioretinal adhesion and thus preventing the start or progression of retinal detachment. This may include treatment of retinal flap tears ("horseshoe tears"), atrophic retinal holes, degenerative peripheral changes such as lattice degeneration, or subclinical peripheral retinal detachments.

The causative role of retinal breaks in retinal detachment was first asserted by Jules Gonin in 1918[1] and led to the treatment of retinal detachments with igni-puncture. Nearly 30 years later, Gerhard R.E. Meyer-Schwickerath introduced the concept of photocoagulation for therapeutic purposes within the eye. As applied to retinal breaks, he hypothesized that the chorioretinal scarring produced by focused light damage to the retina could prevent the accumulation or spread of subretinal fluid by effectively "tacking the retina down." After initially performing treatment using focused rays from the sun, he worked with Zeiss to develop the powerful xenon-arc coagulator. In the ensuing 30 years, the xenon-arc coagulator was gradually replaced with the laser technology that remains the most common mode of treatment today.[2] While trans-scleral cryotherapy remains commonly used for certain situations, for many surgeon's, the associated discomfort, inflammation, and increased rate of proliferative vitreoretinopathy[3] limit its use relative to laser.

There are many types of lasers employed in retinal applications. Currently, the most popular are green argon (514 nm) and frequency doubled neodymium yttrium aluminum garnet (Nd:YAG) (532 nm), and yellow krypton (568 nm) and dye (577 nm) lasers. These wavelengths lie within the peak absorption range for the tissues being treated, namely the pigmented and vascular structures of the retinal pigment epithelium and choroid.[4] Yellow wavelengths are believed to penetrate more effectively through nuclear sclerotic lenses.

Laser spots generate a controlled thermal effect ultimately resulting in chorioretinal scarring and adherence of the neurosensory retina to the underlying tissues, thus its usefulness in decreasing the risk of retinal detachment in patients with retinal breaks.

INDICATIONS

Key Indications

- Acute symptomatic retinal tear ("horseshoe tear")
- Retinal dialysis
- Traumatic retinal breaks
- Peripheral or asymptomatic retinal detachment
- Lattice degeneration, atrophic holes, or other peripheral pathology that has significant risk of progression to retinal detachment in the surgeon's opinion

Studies of the natural history of peripheral retinal defects have refined our knowledge regarding which retinal lesions confer the greatest risk of retinal detachment and thus require treatment.[5,6] Most acute, symptomatic flap or horseshoe tears are a consequence of posterior vitreous detachment (PVD) (Figure 21.1). A PVD is a natural, degenerative consequence of aging; complete PVD is defined as the separation of the posterior hyaloid from the optic nerve head. The process of PVD often produces patient symptoms of "flashes and floaters," and it has been estimated that retinal breaks occur in up to 10%–15% of patients with symptomatic PVD. Untreated breaks have been estimated to progress to clinical retinal detachment in up to 50% of cases, and thus an acutely symptomatic horseshoe tear is a clear indication for prophylactic treatment.[7]

Although acute flap tears are the classic cause of rhegmatogenous detachment, other retinal defects may also lead to detachment. Atrophic retinal holes are a degenerative thinning of the peripheral retina and often occur in conjunction with lattice degeneration. Operculated retinal breaks represent flap tears wherein the flap has been avulsed, thus reducing active traction on the retina. Observations with regard to the natural history of such lesions have shown that many never progress to detachment over a lifetime of monitoring, and thus the routine treatment of such lesions is generally not performed. Treatment can be considered on a case-by-case basis; for instance, documented accumulation of subretinal fluid around an atrophic hole is a reasonable situation to treat.

FIGURE 21-1 Retinal tear.

Retinal dialysis (separation of the neurosensory retina at the ora serrata) generally occurs as a result of significant blunt trauma to the eye. In some cases, dialysis may not lead to detachment for several years following the initial injury, but treatment of this and other traumatic retinal breaks is generally recommended due to the relatively high risk of progression.

Asymptomatic retinal defects are commonly found on routine dilated exam and may include the aforementioned flap tears, atrophic holes, operculated breaks, or even subclinical peripheral detachments. Signs of chronicity, such as pigment demarcation, indicate that a particular lesion has remained stationary for months; however, the presence of such pigment does not ensure the lesion will not progress in the future. The presence of subretinal fluid adjacent to a hole or a break (operculated or not) increases the chance of progression.

Lattice degeneration represents defined areas of thinning in the peripheral retina. Patches of lattice are generally roughly oval shaped and characterized by an overlying pocket of liquified vitreous, with especially adherent vitreous at the border of the lesion. Due to the abnormal vitreoretinal adherence, lattice is prone to tearing along its border, usually during the process of PVD. These lesions thus increase the risk of retinal detachment. There is no clear consensus with regard to whether prophylactic treatment of lattice is warranted.[8] The author generally only prophylactically treats lattice in cases that are especially high risk: Those patients with a personal history of retinal detachment in the contralateral eye or those with a strong family history of detachment.

CONTRAINDICATIONS

Key Contraindications

- Media opacity preventing clear view of posterior segment
- Patient inability to cooperate with treatment

Performing in-office laser retinopexy involves some degree of patient cooperation. Though the procedure is relatively safe with an adequate view and a stationary patient, sudden eye or bodily movements during the process of treatment can risk inadvertent laser to important structures (e.g., the macula and optic nerve). In patients who are too young, invalid, intoxicated, or exhibiting dementia, treatment may best be performed with laser indirect ophthalmoscopy (LIO) in the operating room under sedation. Ensuring adequate anesthesia helps with cooperation.

Performing safe laser retinopexy requires an adequate view of the posterior segment. In acute retinal breaks associated with PVD, vitreous hemorrhage is often present, which can make the view difficult. Other conditions such as corneal opacities, cataract, or inadequate mydriasis may be compounding factors.

It should be noted that in cases of acute PVD associated with vitreous hemorrhage, the risk of an underlying retinal break is high.[9] If the view is inadequate to exclude the presence of an underlying break, B-Scan ultrasound should be performed to exclude any clear tear or detachment. The presence of a clear retinal detachment or a break that is untreatable due to media opacity is an indication for urgent pars plana vitrectomy,[10] with the goal of treating or halting any concerning lesion prior to it progressing to a "macula off" status and irreversible vision decrease. If B-Scan does not demonstrate a break or detachment, options include close monitoring (every two to three days) with repeat B-Scans as necessary to allow for some clearing or proceeding with pars plana vitrectomy to clear the visual axis and treat any underlying pathology.

INFORMED CONSENT CONSIDERATIONS

Key Informed Consent Adverse Events

- Inadvertent laser damage to optic nerve or macular area with resulting scotoma
- Symptomatic visual field defect
- Discomfort during the procedure
- Progression of retinal detachment despite treatment
- Subsequent development of symptomatic epiretinal membrane

Informed consent should include a description of the procedure to be performed, as well as the purpose, in plain language. For instance, "laser treatment to minimize or decrease the risk of progression of retinal detachment." In addition to the proposed benefits of the procedure, the risks listed previously should be addressed.

For more posteriorly located breaks, or detachments associated with fluid posterior to the equator, there is significant risk of the patient noticing a posttreatment visual field abnormality. It should be noted that laser can only be applied to nondetached retina along the edge of the area being demarcated, and the risk of causing a symptomatic visual field defect must be considered when deciding whether a patient is a good candidate for this mode of treatment. For patients with borderline detachments, definitive surgical repair via pars plana vitrectomy, scleral buckling, or pneumatic retinopexy may be a better option.

Depending on a number of factors, including the amount of laser to be applied, the location of application, and the tolerance of the patient, treatment may be uncomfortable. Discomfort is greater when scleral depression is required. The horizontal meridians (3:00 and 9:00) are generally more uncomfortable due to the underlying long posterior ciliary nerves, though often the location of the pathology may necessitate treatment through these areas. Anesthesia in addition to topical drops can be considered, but subconjunctival, peribulbar, and retrobulbar anesthesia each confer additional risk, which should be discussed as part of informed consent. All methods may lead to subconjunctival hemorrhage, or the more serious globe perforation. If the eye is being anesthetized with retrobulbar injection, the rare but potentially fatal complication of brainstem anesthesia should also be discussed.

Though not technically an "adverse event," it should be discussed with the patient that no treatment can guarantee progression of retinal detachment will not occur. For an acute horseshoe tear, the risk of detachment may be reduced from 30%–50% to 5% or less with treatment.[3]

Patients should be advised that the intended effect of the laser is not immediate; that is, it takes two to four weeks before the chorioretinal adhesion is at full strength. Therefore, following laser, it is recommended that patients refrain from unnecessary strenuous or "jarring" activities. The author generally advises patients to avoid heavy reading for a few days after treatment, due to the potential for repetitive "back and forth" eye movements to cause progression of detachment before an adequate adhesion can form. Potentially "jarring" activities may include operating a riding lawn mower, waterskiing, or use of a firearm with recoil. High-impact sports should be avoided, though weightlifting seemingly does not confer the forces needed to promote further vitreoretinal traction.

It is also advisable to clearly inform the patient that laser treatment is not able nor intended to "improve their vision"; many patients are initially diagnosed with a retinal tear after experiencing flashes and floaters. Some patients mistakenly assume treatment with the laser will remove their floaters, if not clearly advised to the contrary.

Informed consent should include a statement indicating that the risks, benefits, and alternative options were discussed, and the patient's questions were answered. It should also clearly state that the patient indicated they would like to proceed with the proposed procedure.

PREOPERATIVE CARE

Key Preoperative Considerations

- A complete eye examination should be done to ensure there is no media opacity that would preclude adequate treatment.
- A detailed exam of the contralateral eye should be documented. If one is not carried out, the reason should be noted.
- The pupil should be widely dilated.
- Surgeon should verify the laser is functioning normally and be familiar with its operation.
- Topical anesthesia should be administered prior to the application of a contact treatment lens (and may be helpful even when the LIO is being used, to decrease the patient's need to blink during treatment).
- Consideration should be given to globe anesthesia.

In addition to ensuring that the view is adequate to treat the area of concern (accounting for vitreous hemorrhage, cortical spoke cataracts, poor dilation, etc.), the preoperative exam should carefully determine the extent of any subretinal fluid. For peripheral breaks, subretinal fluid may be shallow and often the extent of the detached area may be difficult to ascertain. As laser can only be applied to attached retina, an underestimation of the extent of subretinal fluid that can lead to a more extensive procedure than initially planned.

Depending on the laser wavelength and power required to achieve an acceptable burn, there may be significant discomfort associated with treatment. Newer yellow-wavelength lasers (577 nm) tend to be more comfortable than green-wavelength lasers (532 nm). Pattern lasers (Iridex, Pascal, Navilas) generally apply several spots in rapid succession, with a shorter duration per spot, which seems to be more comfortable for many patients as compared to single-spot modes with longer duration. In cases where comfort is a concern, symptoms may be mitigated by preoperative anesthesia. Topical anesthesia decreases the comfort associated with a contact treatment lens but does not adequately anesthetize the posterior segment for the actual laser treatment. Retrobulbar anesthesia is very effective but requires an awake patient to remain still while the retrobulbar needle is advanced into the orbit and carries the small but serious risk of brainstem anesthesia with resulting respiratory failure. Subconjunctival or sub-Tenon's anesthesia is not as effective as retrobulbar anesthesia, but it is often easier to perform and associated with less risk (primarily being the common subconjunctival hemorrhage and the very rare globe perforation).

SETTINGS AND PROCEDURE

Key Laser Settings

- Power: 100 to 450 mW
- Duration: 0.1 to 0.2 s (100–200 ms, 20–30 ms in pattern mode)
- Interval: 0.1 to 0.5 s
- Spot size: 400 to 500 μm, accounting for lens magnification
- Spot spacing: Confluent

The total energy applied per spot of laser is a product of the spot size, power, and duration of application. The energy needed to produce the appropriate burn (and thus the laser settings required) varies depending on laser characteristics (for instance, the wavelength), patient factors (ocular media opacity and fundus pigmentation), and focus. Although ballpark initial settings are discussed herein, appropriate settings may vary greatly in different situations.

At the slit-lamp, the specific contact lens being used produces magnification of the laser spot, and this should be taken into account when selecting the spot size on the

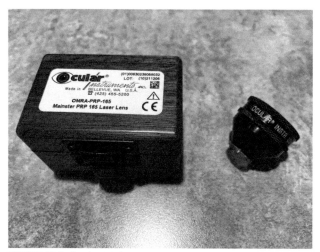

FIGURE 21-2 Ocular Mainster PRP 165 Lens.

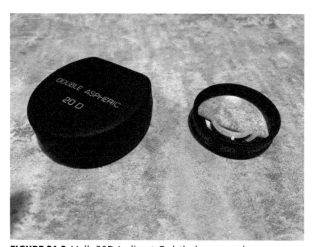

FIGURE 21-3 Volk 20D Indirect Ophthalmoscopy lens.

laser unit. For instance, the Mainster 165 lens (Ocular) produces a laser spot magnification of 1.96× (Figure 21.2). The Super Quad 160 (Volk) produces a magnification of 2.0×. When LIO is being used, lenses produce minification that must be considered; a 20D lens' laser spot magnification is approximately 0.32×, and for a 28D lens, 0.44× (Figure 21.3).[11,12] The characteristics of the specific lens being used are clearly stated in the lens specifications documentation and are also available on the manufacturer's website.

Prior to commencing treatment, the appropriate power is determined using a titration method. Aiming a single spot in a peripheral area of the retina, the laser is applied. Power is gradually increased to produce a slight greying of the tissue. Total energy released is a product of power and duration of the laser burn, and either variable can be changed to increase or decrease the whitening effect. When treating at the slit lamp, the author generally begins with an approximately 400-μm spot size (200 μm selected on the reticule, 1.96× magnification using a Mainster 165 contact lens). Power is initially set at 150 mW with duration at 0.1 s (100 ms). Power is gradually increased or decreased to achieve the appropriate tissue effect. Care must be taken to avoid overly hot, white burns; such spots applied in a confluent pattern may cause significant localized retinal thinning, necrosis, and new retinal breaks.

If patient discomfort is present once the appropriate power is found, occasionally this can be ameliorated by slightly decreasing the duration (i.e., to 70–80 ms) while increasing the power (10–20 mW increments) until an appropriate effect is again obtained.

The interval period refers to the time between applications of laser in single-spot mode when the pedal is held in the depressed position. The desired speed is based on surgeon preference and comfort; a shorter interval speeds treatment but also increases the risk of inadvertent laser damage should the patient move unexpectedly during treatment. An initial interval of 500 ms (0.5 s) is reasonable for beginning surgeon's, and this can be significantly shortened as confidence is gained.

All methods of treatment feature an aiming beam with adjustable brightness that is independent of the scope illumination. If the aiming beam is not visible, ensure the brightness is turned up and the laser is set to "ready"; often, the aiming beam is not visible until this is the case.

Once the appropriate settings are determined, treatment can commence. Laser spots are applied to the area to be treated in a confluent manner, with the goal of placing 3 to 5 rows of laser around the area of concern. Three rows are generally adequate for smaller breaks; larger breaks and detachments may benefit from five rows.

Ideally, any pathology being treated should be entirely encircled by confluent laser spots; in practice, however, it is often difficult to adequately encircle the anterior portion of lesions in the far periphery. If a break cannot be fully encircled, it is important that the "horns" of laser on either side of the lesion be extended up to the ora serrata. Subretinal fluid extending around the anterior extent of inadequate laser is a common cause of treatment failure and progression to retinal detachment.[7] If the laser cannot be extended to the equator as planned, occasionally widening the horns to an area that is more easily treated is helpful. In situations where inadequate visualization precludes anterior laser, trans-scleral cryotherapy can be used to treat the anterior portion on either side of the lesion.

Laser retinopexy can be performed with the patient upright, using a slit-lamp–mounted laser unit, or via LIO. Both methods have relative advantages and disadvantages: Advantages of LIO treatment include potentially faster treatment in single-spot modes and a wider static field of view, and the ability to perform scleral depression while treating and thus facilitate treatment of anterior lesions. Relative advantages of slit-lamp–mounted units include greater precision in treatment and a beneficial eye motion-stabilizing effect from the contact lens employed in treatment, in addition to the possibility of pattern-style treatment, which can significantly reduce treatment time. Patient comfort in terms of positioning may be better in LIO, as this method can be done with the patient reclining; however, the laser treatment itself is often more uncomfortable when LIO is used, particularly when it is used in combination with scleral depression. Regardless of the method of administration, taking time to ensure proper setup and patient positioning beforehand will often help make treatment go as smoothly as possible.

Considerations for Slit-Lamp–Mounted Laser Units

When a slit-lamp–mounted laser is being used, the position is similar to that used for a general exam. The patient is positioned at the slit lamp and advised to keep their forehead against the forehead support strap and their chin on the chin rest. Patients will often gradually drift out of position during the procedure, and it can be helpful to have an assistant help the patient maintain the proper position.

A coupling solution (i.e., carboxymethylcellulose [Celluvisc], hydroxypropyl methylcellulose [Gonak], or hypromellose [Genteal Gel]) is applied to the patient side of the contact lens to be utilized. The operative eye is anesthetized with topical tetracaine or proparacaine, and the contact lens is placed on the eye. This can be facilitated by asking the patient to look downward while the surgeon manually elevates the upper lid.

Once the lens is placed, titration and treatment can begin. The patient can be asked to direct their gaze in the direction of the pathology to facilitate visualization.

Considerations for Laser Indirect Ophthalmoscopy

When using LIO, reclining the patient back 45° or more can create a more comfortable situation for both the surgeon and patient. A drop of topical anesthetic is instilled in the operative eye; this can mitigate some of the involuntary eyelid clenching that often results if the ocular surface begins to dry during treatment. The lid can be manually elevated by the surgeon during treatment, or a wire lid speculum may be used; the latter is generally more uncomfortable for the patient. The patient is asked to look in various directions during the procedure to facilitate peripheral treatment.

Considerations for Pattern-Type Lasers

When using a pattern-type laser, the desired pattern must be selected. In laser retinopexy, the goal is generally to surround breaks or demarcate detached areas with 3 to 5 rows of confluent laser (Figure 21.4). Units generally offer a number of patterns, which can be useful for treating retinal breaks, including circular or hemi-circular arcs that can be resized and positioned to surround a given break. The author generally uses a 3 × 3 to 5 × 5 square grid with spot spacing set to zero, surrounding or demarcating the area of concern with confluent squares.

When the pedal is depressed, the spots are applied in rapid succession; the pattern can be aborted partway through its application if the pedal is released. As the spots are applied rapidly, the duration for individual spots is shorter than what

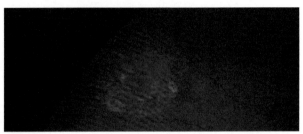

FIGURE 21-4 Retinal tear, several weeks posttreatment.

would usually be used in single-spot mode (0.02–0.03 s vs. 0.1 s). The initial power must therefore be correspondingly higher to achieve a similar effect as that obtained using the single-spot settings noted previously; this should be kept in mind while titrating.

Considering the relative advantages and disadvantages of each approach, the author generally treats via a slit-lamp–mounted laser when pattern or navigated modes are available and via LIO when single-spot treatment is the only option.

POSTOPERATIVE CARE/CO-MANAGEMENT (FOLLOW-UP SCHEDULE)

Key Postoperative Care Considerations

- Patient counseling
- Follow-up

As compared to anterior segment laser, intraocular inflammation and intraocular pressure rise are rare following posterior segment procedures, and thus no topical ocular antihypertensives or antiinflammatories are typically prescribed. Patients are counseled to avoid touching or rubbing the eye to decrease the possibility of corneal abrasion while the eye is anesthetized. If a preoperative retrobulbar block was performed, the ability to close the eyelid will be impaired, and temporarily patching the eyelid shut is advisable to decrease the risk of exposure keratopathy.

The patient should be counseled to monitor for any concerning symptoms (increase in floaters, change in flashes, or visual field loss) during the follow-up period. Studies have shown that up to 20% of patients may form subsequent breaks following treatment of the breaks initially found,[13] and a clear increase in floaters warrants a repeat exam to exclude this possibility. Patients will often continue to see brief, arc-like flashes in the temporal periphery, sometimes occurring for weeks after the initial onset; this tends to be noticeable in low-light levels and tends to accompany head movements, and presumably this is due to the detached vitreous contacting or placing mild traction on the peripheral retina. Patients can be informed that this type of photopsia is to be expected, but any changes outside of this typical pattern should be investigated.

As noted previously, it may take over two weeks to form a firm chorioretinal adhesion. Patients should be reexamined approximately two weeks following the laser to ensure there is no extension of subretinal fluid outside of the lasered area. Follow-up can be extended thereafter assuming stability. If vitreous hemorrhage is significant enough that additional breaks cannot be excluded at the time the initial break is found, it is probably prudent to reexamine in one week or less.

POTENTIAL COMPLICATIONS AND THEIR TREATMENT

Key Potential Complications

- Inadvertent damage to central retina or optic nerve
- Corneal abrasion

Complications are rare in laser retinopexy, with the most significant being the risk for damage to critical structures. Sudden, unexpected patient movement risks damage to the retina corresponding to the useful visual field (e.g., the macula) or the optic nerve. Unfortunately, such damage is irreversible and thus the best strategy is minimizing the risk of sudden patient movement by good preoperative patient counseling, adequate anesthesia, and use of a slow repeat speed with unreliable patients.

EFFICACY

With treatment, the risk of a horseshoe tear progressing to retinal detachment is decreased from 30%–50% to 5% or less.[7] The risk of posttreatment retinal detachment in atrophic holes, operculated breaks, and lattice degeneration is low regardless of treatment. For detachments, as a general rule, the greater the extent of subretinal fluid, the higher the chance of retinal detachment.

CODING/BILLING

Laser retinopexy for a retinal tear, hole, or lattice degeneration with no associated retinal detachment is coded as current procedural terminology (CPT) 67145 (prophylaxis of retinal detachment [e.g., retinal tear, lattice degeneration] without drainage, one or more sessions, photocoagulation). The global period for this code is 90 days.

When a retinal detachment is present, generally defined as one or more disc diameter of subretinal fluid surrounding the retinal break, retinopexy is coded as CPT

67105 (repair of retinal detachment, including drainage of subretinal fluid when performed, photocoagulation). The global period is ten days.
(ICD)-10CM

H33.00-H33.03 (Rhegmatogenous retinal detachment)
H33.04 (Retinal dialysis)
H33.30-H33.33 (Retinal break without detachment)
H35.41 (Lattice degeneration of retina)

REFERENCES

1. Schwartz SG, Garoon R, Smiddy WE, et al. The legacy of Jules Gonin: one hundred years of identifying and treating retinal breaks. *Graefes Arch Clin Exp Ophthalmol.* 2018;256(6):1051–1052. doi:10.1007/s00417-018-3999-4
2. Meyer-Schwickerath GR. The history of photocoagulation. *Aust N Z J Ophthalmol.* 1989;17(4): 427–434. doi:10.1111/j.1442-9071.1989.tb00566.x
3. Nagasaki H, Shinagawa K, Mochizuki M. Risk factors for proliferative vitreoretinopathy. *Prog Retin Eye Res.* 1998;17(1):77–98. doi:10.1016/s1350-9462(97)00007-4
4. Cordero I. Understanding and safely using ophthalmic lasers. *Community Eye Health.* 2015;28(92): 76–77.
5. Blindbaek S, Grauslund J. Prophylactic treatment of retinal breaks—a systematic review. *Acta Ophthalmol.* 2015;93(1):3–8. doi:10.1111/aos.12447
6. Byer NE. Long-term natural history of lattice degeneration of the retina. *Ophthalmology.* 1989; 96(9):1396–1401; discussion 1401–1392.
7. American Academy of Ophthalmology Retina/Vitreous Panel. Posterior vitreous detachment, retinal breaks, and lattice degeneration. San Francisco, CA: American Academy of Ophthalmology; 2014. [accessed July 10, 2020]. Preferred Practice Pattern Guidelines. 2014. Available at: www.aao.org/ppp
8. Wilkinson CP. Interventions for asymptomatic retinal breaks and lattice degeneration for preventing retinal detachment. *Cochrane Database Syst Rev.* 2014(9):CD003170.
9. Sarrafizadeh R, Hassan TS, Ruby AJ, et al. Incidence of retinal detachment and visual outcome in eyes presenting with posterior vitreous separation and dense fundus-obscuring vitreous hemorrhage. *Ophthalmology.* 2001;108(12):2273–2278.
10. Tan HS, Mura M, Bijl HM. Early vitrectomy for vitreous hemorrhage associated with retinal tears. *Am J Ophthalmol.* 2010;150(4):529–533.
11. Volk Instruments. Super Quad 160 Laser Lens Specifications. [Accessed Aug 21, 2020) Available at: https://www.volk.com/products/super-quad-160-indirect-contact-laser-lens
12. Ocular Instruments. Ocular Mainster PRP 165 Laser Lens Specifications. [Accessed Aug 21, 2020) Available at: https://ocularinc.com/media/wysiwyg/pdf/5805T-_OMRA-PRP_165_Rev_Q.pdf
13. Goldberg RE, Boyer DS. Sequential retinal breaks following a spontaneous initial retinal break. *Ophthalmology.* 1981;88(1):10–12.

SECTION 6

Oculoplastics

22 Intense Pulsed Light Therapy

Selina R. McGee • Karl Stonecipher

Intense pulsed light (IPL) therapy was initially developed for the treatment of leg telangiectasias and has become the standard treatment for rosacea, flushing, and facial redness, as well as manifestations of photodamage, including pigmented lesions.[1] IPL therapy is utilized by eye care professionals to treat aging changes due to photodamage, ocular rosacea, and most recently meibomian gland dysfunction (MGD) in dry eye disease (DED). In the Tear Film and Ocular Surface Society (TFOS) International Dry Eye Workshop II (DEWS II) treatment algorithm, the management and therapy subcommittee placed IPL as a step 2 treatment for dry eye and MGD.[2]

MGD is a chronic diffuse disease, commonly characterized by terminal duct obstruction with qualitative or quantitative changes in the glandular secretion. It can result in alteration of the tear film, symptoms of eye irritation, clinically apparent inflammation, and ocular surface disease.[3] Increased tear evaporation, tear hyperosmolarity, increased ocular surface staining, increased inflammation, symptomatic irritation of the eyelid and globes, as well as decreased visual acuity have all been observed with MGD.[4] MGD can be accompanied by ocular rosacea. One study reported that 80% of facial rosacea patients suffer from MGD and in 20% of patients, ocular rosacea precedes facial rosacea.[5] IPL therapy is very effective in managing rosacea and is thought to minimize the blood vessels that are responsible for leaking inflammatory mediators onto the ocular surface.[6]

It is thought that there are many factors that contribute to MGD. Inflammation, microbial/*Demodex* infestation, enzyme changes, stasis, hyperkeratinization, temperature changes, and obstruction are thought to contribute whether individually or in conjunction with one another.[7] IPL is still being studied on how it specifically improves MGD, but there are many retrospective and prospective studies in the literature that support the improvement in both signs and symptoms of MGD.[8-18]

MECHANISM OF ACTION, EFFICACY, AND SAFETY

An IPL unit consists of a flashlamp internally filtered to emit noncoherent light of wavelengths ranging from 500 to 1,200 nm, thereby targeting specific chromophores. Melanin absorption is in the range 400 to 700 nm and oxyhemaglobin absorption is in the range 900 to 1,200 nm. Of interest, the pigmented exoskeleton of *Demodex*

371

contains a chromophore that absorbs IPL energy. In fact, histologic analysis demonstrated that IPL induces coagulation and necrosis of *Demodex*.[19]

IPL is NOT a laser, as a laser emits coherent light. Quartz filters are available to remove wavelengths below 515, 550, 560, 570, 590, 615, 645, 690, and 755 nm depending on target, skin type, and desired outcome.

Modern IPL systems achieve efficacy and safety by selective photothermolysis, in which (1) target chromophores such as blood vessels (red's), pigment (brown's, including melanin in hair follicles) absorb more light energy than the surrounding tissue and (2) the energy is delivered and absorbed within the chromophore's thermal relaxation time. The thermal relaxation time is the time for the structure to lose half of the delivered energy (i.e., to cool).[20]

During IPL treatment, energy is delivered in one to three synchronized pulses rather than continuously. This allows the epidermis to cool between pulses while the target continues to heat. Safety is further enhanced through appropriate wavelength selection and aggressive contact cooling (e.g., sapphire chill plate). Advantages of this technique are that posttreatment purpura, a common adverse effect of pulsed dye laser treatment utilized in dermatology, occurs only infrequently with IPL treatment.[20]

Bitter and a host of other researchers have confirmed the efficacy and safety of full-face IPL treatment for photodamaged skin since IPL was introduced more than 20 years ago.[1] IPL has also been found to be a safe and successful treatment of ocular rosacea and MGD.[8-19]

INDICATIONS

Common indications for IPL treatment include rosacea, melasma, and photodamage including poikiloderma, telangiectasias, and dyschromia. In addition, IPL has been used to treat port wine stains, rough skin texture, freckles, lentigines, superficial wrinkling, large pores, unwanted hair, MGD, hordeola, and chronic chalazia.[21]

PATIENT SELECTION

The easiest patients to treat with IPL have fair skin (Fitzpatrick skin types I–III) with telangiectasia of the eyelid and/or face or pigmentary abnormalities of the periocular region. Darker skin types can also be treated (Fitzpatrick skin type IV)—with caution—by using lower energies, longer pulse durations, longer delay times, and higher-wavelength filters (e.g., 590, 615, and 640 nm). Fitzpatrick skin types V could be treated with extreme caution and skin type VI should never be treated with IPL.[21]

Patients must be willing to undergo multiple treatments at two- to four-week intervals. Most patients need a series of four to five treatments and then will continue to need a maintenance treatment every four to six months. Since IPL treatments are currently not covered by private insurance, patients must be willing to assume responsibility for the cost of treatment. Patients' medical history, medications, and previous cosmetic treatments must also be discussed.

FITZPATRICK SKIN TYPING SCALE

The Fitzpatrick skin phototypes were constructed based on an individual's skin color and their tendency to burn or tan when exposed to sunlight. There are six skin types characterized by the following as shown in Table 22.1[22]:

TABLE 22-1 FITZPATRICK SKIN TYPE SCALE

FITZPATRICK SKIN TYPE	SKIN COLOR BEFORE SUN EXPOSURE	EYE COLOR	HAIR COLOR	SUN REACTION
Skin type I	Ivory	Light blue, light gray, or light green	Red or light blonde	Skin always freckles, always burns and peels, and never tans
Skin type II	Fair or pale	Blue, gray, or green	Blonde	Skin usually freckles, burns and peels often, and rarely tans
Skin type III	Fair to beige, with golden undertones	Hazel or light brown	Dark blonde or light brown	Skin usually freckles, burns and peels often, and rarely tans
Skin type IV	Olive or light brown	Dark brown	Dark brown	Doesn't really freckle, burns rarely, and tans often
Skin type V	Dark brown	Dark brown to black	Dark brown to black	Rarely freckles, almost never burns, and always tans
Skin type VI	Deeply pigmented dark brown to darkest brown	Brownish black	Black	Never freckles, never burns, and always tans darkly

CONTRAINDICATIONS

Contraindications for IPL Treatment Include the Following:

- Active herpes simplex virus (HSV) infection
- Exposure to sun, remaining suntan or artificial tanning in the three to four weeks preoperatively
- Active lupus erythematosus
- A history of seizures induced by bright lights
- Dysplastic nevi
- Significant concurrent skin conditions or any inflammatory skin conditions

- Open lacerations or abrasions
- Chronic or cutaneous viral, fungal, or bacterial diseases
- Tattoos
- Unreasonable expectations
- Skin type VI

To the best of the authors' knowledge, IPL has not been studied in human pregnancy and therefore is not advised.

PRETREATMENT PATIENT EDUCATION

The following should be discussed with patients prior to performing IPL treatment:

- Results are not guaranteed.
- MGD and DED are multifactorial diseases in nature.
- Adjunctive treatments may still be needed such as artificial tears, warm compresses, lid hygiene, antiinflammatories, immunomodulators, oral antibiotics, or thermal pulsation therapies. (This list is not meant to be all-inclusive.)
- Not all red and brown areas will disappear. Red and brown spots removed by treatment may recur, especially with excessive sun exposure.
- Deep wrinkle lines will not be removed by the treatment.
- Adverse effects include redness, swelling, burning, pain, crust formation, bruising, hyperpigmentation and hypopigmentation, and scar formation.
- Multiple treatment sessions (typically three to five) are required for optimal results.
- Maintenance treatments are often recommended four to six months after the initial series. In addition, patients should be quoted a price for the treatment course.

PRETREATMENT PATIENT INSTRUCTIONS

Patients are given the following instructions prior to treatment:

- Do not take isotretinoin (Accutane) for one month before your treatment. Of note, because Accutane targets sebaceous glands and meibomian glands are sebaceous glands, imaging and close monitoring should be performed while on isotretinoin as they can be entirely decimated with continued use of the medication.
- Discontinue doxycycline medication two weeks before your treatment. The medication can be resumed post treatment if needed.
- If you are tanned, please reschedule your appointment.
- Do not apply makeup or lotions on your day of treatment, or be prepared to remove them at the clinic.

- If you have a history of cold sores, take your prescribed medication (e.g., valacyclovir [Valtrex], famciclovir [Famvir], acyclovir [Zovirax]) on the day before, day of, and day after treatment. If any active lesions are present the appointment will need to be rescheduled.
- Inform the technician before each appointment if you (1) are taking new medications or (2) have tattoos or beauty marks you do not want treated.
- Inform the clinician immediately if the area being treated feels "too hot."

INFORMED CONSENT CONSIDERATIONS

Informed consent should include a description of the procedure in plain language, for example, "IPL will be used to treat MGD related to keratoconjunctivitis sicca and/or ocular rosacea. This will help decrease inflammation and may help eye irritation related to ocular surface disease."

Potential alternative treatments, such as prescription eye drops, oral medications, monitoring, or other in office procedures, should be listed. Risks and complications inherent to any IPL procedure include but are not limited to redness, swelling, burning, pain, crust formation, bruising, hyperpigmentation and hypopigmentation, and scar formation.

A note from the counseling practitioner should be included and phrased similar to "I have counseled this patient as to the nature of the proposed procedure, the attendant risks involved, and the expected results." The patient's and doctor's name should be printed and signed with the date as well as a witness (typically a staff member).

As part of the informed consent, the patient needs to determine their skin typing with the assistance of the clinician. This should be in writing, and both patient and clinician should sign and date.

PROCEDURE PROTOCOL

Tray Setup

The setup tray may include IPL grade eye shields, cooled gel (clear only), tongue blade, washcloth, hair band, and nonsterile gloves. In addition, cleanser and sunscreen lotion may be available for use by the patient. See Figure 22.1.

Anesthesia

Topical anesthetic cream should not be used prior to treatment.[21] Formulations of anesthesia typically contain a combination of benzocaine, tetracaine, and lidocaine, which can vasoconstrict blood vessels. When the blood vessels are constricted, there

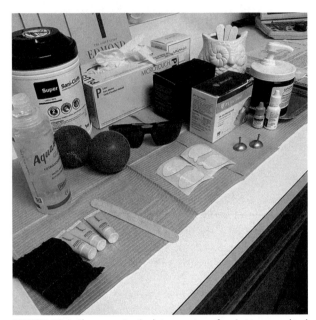

FIGURE 22-1 Shows a typical tray setup for intense pulsed light procedure including hair band, makeup remover wipes, tongue blade, clear ultrasound gel, comfort squeeze devices, intense pulsed light/laser grade pasties, laser grade corneal shields, corneal anesthetic, safety goggles, sunscreen, and postoperative skin care kit.

are less chromophores to target, and the patient may be undertreated. Coach patients through the procedure and utilize frequent breaks to help with patient comfort if the need arises.

Medications

Antiviral medications (valacyclovir, famciclovir, or acyclovir) may be prescribed prophylactically in patients with a history of HSV.

Safety Concerns

Patients, IPL operators, and assistants in the room should **ALWAYS** wear protective eye shields appropriate for the wavelengths used in treatment. In Dr. Selina McGee's office, each patient contemplating IPL treatment that is high risk such as a skin type IV must undergo a test site treatment at least 48 hours before the initial treatment session. This is to check for a delayed reaction to treatment and to determine the appropriate treatment settings.

PROCEDURE

The first treatment begins after pretreatment photographs have been obtained, the test site has been evaluated, and appropriate treatment parameters have been selected. Treatment settings vary by device; an operator's manual specific to the IPL unit should be consulted. A discussion of treatment parameters is presented here. As an example, Tables 22.2 to 22.7 show treatment variables for a specific IPL device[21] as well as the Protocol settings of pioneers Rolando Toyos[15] and Laura Periman.[23]

TABLE 22-2 SETTINGS FOR THE TREATMENT OF MEIBOMIAN GLAND DYSFUNCTION[10,21,23]

FITZPATRICK SKIN TYPE	LIGHT GUIDE	FILTER (NM)	NUMBER OF PULSES	PULSE DURATION (MS)	DELAY (MS)	FLUENCE (J/CM²)
Skin type I	Large	590	3	6.0	50	16
Skin type II	Large	590	3	6.0	50	14
Skin type III	Large	590	3	6.0	50	12
Skin type IV	Large	590	3	6.0	50	10

TABLE 22-3 SETTINGS FOR THE TREATMENT OF HORDEOLA/CHALAZIA

FITZPATRICK SKIN TYPE	LIGHT GUIDE	FILTER (NM)	NUMBER OF PULSES	PULSE DURATION (MS)	DELAY (MS)	FLUENCE (J/CM²)
Skin type I	8 × 15	560	3	3.0	15.0	20.0
Skin type II	8 × 15	560	3	3.5	20.0	19.0
Skin type III	8 × 15	560	3	3.0	25.0	18.0

TABLE 22-4 SETTINGS FOR THE TREATMENT OF HYPERPIGMENTATION (PHOTOFACIAL)

FITZPATRICK SKIN TYPE	LIGHT GUIDE	FILTER (NM)	NUMBER OF PULSES	PULSE DURATION (MS)	DELAY (MS)	FLUENCE (J/CM²)
Skin type I	8 × 35	560	Double	3.5	10	17.0
Skin type II	8 × 35	560	Double	3.5	15	17.0
Skin type III	8 × 35	560	Double	4.0	20	16.0

TABLE 22-5 SETTINGS FOR THE SPOT TREATMENT OF PIGMENT (LENTIGINES) USING 6 MM CIRCLE CRYSTAL

FITZPATRICK SKIN TYPE	LIGHT GUIDE (MM)	FILTER (NM)	NUMBER OF PULSES	PULSE DURATION (MS)	DELAY (MS)	FLUENCE (J/CM^2)
Skin type I	6	515	Single	4.0	—	19.0
Skin type II	6	515	Single	4.0	—	19.0
Skin type III	6	560	Single	4.0	—	20.0

TABLE 22-6 SETTINGS FOR THE TREATMENT OF ERYTHEMA (FLUSHING SKIN)

FITZPATRICK SKIN TYPE	LIGHT GUIDE (MM)	FILTER (NM)	NUMBER OF PULSES	PULSE DURATION (MS)	DELAY (MS)	FLUENCE (J/CM^2)
Skin type I	8 × 35	560	Double	4.5	10	17.0
Skin type II	8 × 35	560	Double	4.5	15.0	16.0
Skin type III	8 × 35	560	Double	5.0	20.0	15.0

TABLE 22-7A SETTINGS FOR THE TREATMENT OF TELANGIECTASIAS (BROKEN CAPILLARIES) MEDIUM DEPTH

FITZPATRICK SKIN TYPE	LIGHT GUIDE	FILTER (NM)	NUMBER OF PULSES	PULSE DURATION (MS)	DELAY (MS)	FLUENCE (J/CM^2)
Skin type I		590	Triple	3.5	20.0	22.0
Skin type II		590	Triple	3.5	25.0	21.0
Skin type III		590	Triple	3.5	30.0	20.0

TABLE 22-7B SETTINGS FOR THE TREATMENT OF TELANGIECTASIAS (BROKEN CAPILLARIES) SHALLOW DEPTH

FITZPATRICK SKIN TYPE	LIGHT GUIDE	FILTER (NM)	NUMBER OF PULSES	PULSE DURATION (MS)	DELAY (MS)	FLUENCE (J/CM^2)
Skin type I		560	Triple	3.0	15.0	20.0
Skin type II		560	Triple	3.5	20.0	19.0
Skin type III		560	Triple	3.0	25.0	18.0

TABLE 22-7C SETTINGS FOR THE SPOT TREATMENT OF TELANGIECTASIAS

FITZPATRICK SKIN TYPE	LIGHT GUIDE (MM)	FILTER (NM)	NUMBER OF PULSES	PULSE DURATION (MS)	DELAY (MS)	FLUENCE (J/CM²)
Skin type I	6	Vascular	Double	3.5	10	28.0
Skin type II	6	Vascular	Double	3.5	15	28.0
Skin type III	6	Vascular	Double	3.5	20	27.0

The patient needs to remove all products from the skin including moisturizer. Clean skin is essential to proper treatment. The IPL operator should remove all stray hair from the procedure field; the use of a disposable hair band pushes hair out of the treatment area very effectively as shown in Figure 22.2.

Utilize a white makeup pencil to cover pigment that patients want to keep, as shown in Figure 22.3.

The IPL operator places protective eye shields on the patient. These can be IPL-specific adhesive shields or similar to the laser grade eye adhesive shields shown in Figure 22.4.

Exposed lashes will be singed with the IPL application and should be avoided.

Adhesive shields should be avoided in patients with lash extensions, as they can be difficult to remove post-procedure without affecting the lashes. Laser grade shields

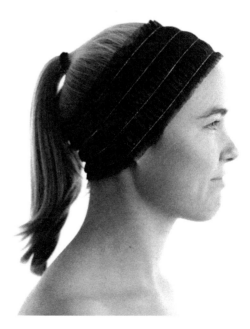

FIGURE 22-2 Disposable hair band to effectively remove hair from the treatment field. This will be discarded at the end of the treatment.

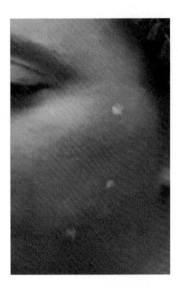

FIGURE 22-3 A white waterproof eyeliner pencil that safely shields pigmented lesions so they cannot absorb light. Utilize this when patients have pigmented beauty marks that are desirable and the practitioner does not want affected.

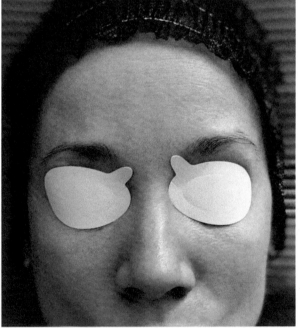

FIGURE 22-4 Intense pulsed light/laser grade pasties. For proper placement, have the patient look down and capture their eyelashes as you apply the adhesive from the bottom to the top of the lid. The bottom of the adhesive should be as close to the lash line as possible without lash exposure. Exposed lashes will be signed with the intense pulsed light application and should be avoided.

as shown in Figure 22.5 are optimal as the nose piece can be moved up and down to facilitate maximum treatment area.

Once shields are in place, the operator applies a thin (1–2 mm) layer of cold, clear, ultrasonic gel to cool the skin and allow the sapphire crystal to glide easily. The crystal (cut-off filter) is placed perpendicular to the area to be treated (Fig. 22.7).

After three pulses, the operator evaluates the treated area for severe erythema, welts, purpura, blisters, or any other adverse reaction. If no reactions are evident, the operator resumes treatment. The pattern follows along V2 of the trigeminal area or tragus to tragus with no more than 1 mm of overlapping treatment sites (Fig. 22.8).

Be mindful of areas with hair (eyebrows, hairline, and beard), particularly if the patient wants to retain facial hair growth. Two passes are made along the same distribution as long as no adverse effects occur.

Treatment of the eyelids may also be performed. Laser grade corneal shields must be in place before treatment of the eyelids (Fig. 22.9).

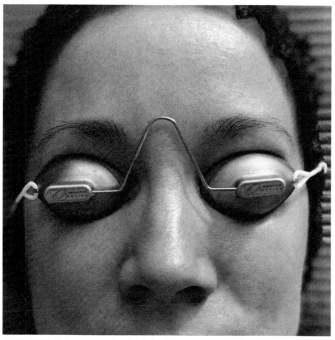

FIGURE 22-5 Laser grade shields that are optimal as the nose piece can be moved up and down to facilitate maximum treatment area. More aggressive therapy for the seasoned practitioner involves treating eyelids as well. When treating the eyelids, laser grade corneal shields should be in place as shown in Figure 22.6.

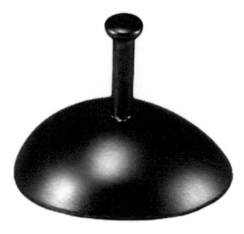

FIGURE 22-6 26 mm laser grade metal corneal shields. These shields can be cleaned in an autoclave or with alcohol between treatments.

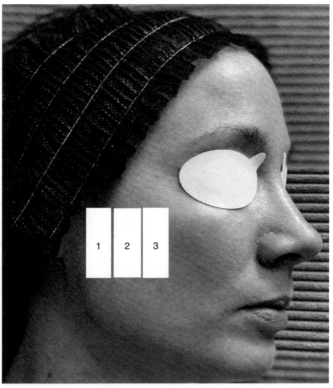

FIGURE 22-7 Proper placement of the first 3 pulses. Observe the skin reaction before moving on to ensure proper clinical end points. If appropriate then perform the rest of the treatment area.

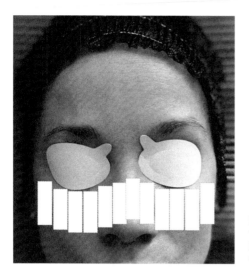

FIGURE 22-8 Proper alignment and treatment pattern with handpiece held perpendicular to maximize the target tissue treatment area.

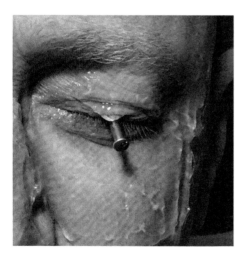

FIGURE 22-9 Proper placement of corneal metal shield of patient's left eye with clear ultrasound gel in place for treatment.

If using laser grade shields, instill one drop of proparacaine and one drop of a higher viscosity artificial tear or small ribbon of bland ophthalmic ointment prior to inserting shields. The author's preference is the 26-mm laser grade shield (largest). Gel is also applied to lids and the 15×35 mm^2 crystal is exchanged for the smaller 8×15 mm^2 crystal. Three pulses are applied to the upper eyelid and then 3 pulses to the lower eyelid, staying 2 mm away from the lash line. Treat the right eyelids and then left eyelids with one pass and then perform a second pass for a total of 24 pulses.[23]

After the second pass, the gel is removed with the tongue blade followed by a washcloth, and the patient is instructed to apply sunscreen before leaving the office and to wear sunglasses. If the patient experiences swelling and edema immediately after treatment, an ice pack may be provided.

PROCEDURE CHECKLIST

- Patient education form read and understood
- Pretreatment instructions reviewed and understood
- Informed consent signed
- Skin type identified
- Confirm that patient has taken prophylactic antiviral medication (if positive history of HSV) and has no contraindications for treatment
- Pretreatment photograph taken
- Set up procedure tray including eye shields/safety goggles
- Select treatment parameters
- Pretreatment test site confirmed with no adverse reaction
- Perform IPL treatment
- Provide verbal and written posttreatment instructions to patient
- Complete procedure note including device settings
- Subsequent treatment scheduled

Key Procedural Points

- Educate the patient that the tip is very cool at first, and the bright light may be surprising. Use of handheld stress balls can be effective for patients to remain calm. Educate patients that it feels like a hot rubber band or pin prick to the skin. Count 1, 2, 3 and pulse so the patient isn't surprised. Take breaks as needed for the patient to tolerate the procedure.
- The handpiece and crystal should be held perpendicular to the eyelid to maximize the amount of energy delivered to the area.
- Do not press down hard with handpiece as this will blanch the blood vessels therefore minimizing the target tissues and the patient may be undertreated.
- A good rule of thumb is to use mild to moderate erythema as a treatment endpoint as shown in Figure 22.10.
- Darkening of target pigment also represents a treatment endpoint if removing pigment is target treatment goal.
- Always double-check that the settings you want to use are the settings you are using.
- As a rule, darker skin types require cautious treatment with lower energies, longer pulse durations, longer delay times, and higher-wavelength filters (e.g., 590, 615, and 640 nm).

- Utilize a white makeup pencil to cover pigment that patients want to keep.
- Tanning of all forms (sun, tanning beds) is absolutely contraindicated as melanin would be redistributed and migrate toward upper epidermis building a "light-blocker" to any treatment.
- Also exclude self-tanning lotions, which give the skin a competing artificial coloration through a chemical reaction with the amino acids of the stratum corneum.
- Tanned skin CANNOT be "defied" by selecting a darker skin type. In other words, don't try to trick the system by choosing a darker skin type.
- On areas with slower "de-tanning" past the minimum solar exposure of three to four weeks, recommend gentle exfoliation of the area one week prior to treatment.
- Always err on the side of caution in treatment settings. More aggressive settings can be added but can never be taken away.

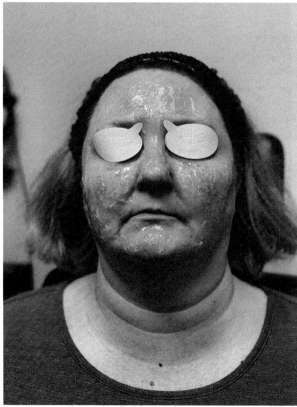

FIGURE 22-10 Patient at end of first treatment with proper erythematous flush.

Treatment order matters. Treat deeper and larger targets first and then work more superficially. If performing skin treatments, utilize those settings first and then move on to the MGD settings for the face and V2 distribution. Next, if choosing to treat lids perform those and then finally spot treat and perform any "aesthetic" clean up.

DISCUSSION OF DEVICE SETTINGS

The authors' experiences are primarily with the M22 (Lumenis, Inc., Santa Clara, CA.) The Lumenis system has a sophisticated graphical user interface that includes presets for a wide array of dermatologic conditions. Settings are based on the work of Mitchel Goldman, MD, who used cut-off filters appropriate for vascular lesions and pigmentary targets while avoiding light of wavelengths harmful to the epidermis.[24,25] The MGD-specific settings are based on the work of Rolando Toyos, MD.[15] The MGD-specific settings treating the eyelids are based on the work of Laura Periman, MD.[23] *Settings will vary by IPL device, and an operator's manual specific to a given device should be consulted.*

Cut-off filters, pulse duration, fluence, and number of pulses (single, double, triple) per treatment session are chosen to assure safety and selective photothermolysis.

Number of pulses are single, double, or triple. The energy is spread over 1 pulse or 3. One pulse with equal energy is a more aggressive setting than a triple pulse with equal energy because the energy is spread out over the 3 pulses.

Pulse durations are selected to slowly heat vessels to coagulation while avoiding purpura. This allows patients to return to normal activities quickly rather than suffering from purpura for one or two weeks. Longer pulse durations are less aggressive.

Energy levels (fluence in J/cm^2) are governed by clinical response. If tissue reactions do not occur, fluence levels may be increased by 1 J/cm^2 (Lumenis M22) or 2 J/cm^2. A good rule of thumb is to use mild to moderate erythema as the clinical treatment end point. The higher the fluence level the more aggressive the treatment.

Cut-off filters are selected to optimize targeting of the chromophore while filtering out wavelengths damaging to the epidermis. These vary by skin type and target chromophore. The filters available are 515, 560, 590, 615, 640, 695, and 755 nm. For example, with the 515 nm filter, all wavelengths below 515 nm are cut and all wavelengths above 515 nm are kept until 1,200 nm. The smaller the number, the more superficial in the tissue and the more aggressive the treatment becomes.

For stubborn telangiectasias, the 530- to 650- and 900- to 1,200-nm vascular filter is a good option for earlier vessel clearance. This filter targets the chromophore oxyhemaglobin (HbO_2) primarily and deoxyhemaglobin (Hb) secondarily. When exposed at 530 to 650 nm, HbO_2 and Hb absorptions are optimal and melanin competition weaker than at shallower wavelengths. When exposed at 900 to 1,200 nm, HbO_2 absorption band starts again at 900 nm when the coefficient is high enough for effective light conversion. As absorption remains less than in the first 530 to 650 nm band, it allows deeper penetration. The rejected 650 to 900 nm band allows "concentration" of the light intensity in the more effective absorption bands.

MEIBOMIAN GLAND DYSFUNCTION

Meibomian gland dysfunction can be effectively treated with IPL. See Table 22.2 for specific settings.

HORDEOLUM/CHALAZIA

Use the exact settings utilized for lids with a double pass. Then stack 2 to 3 pulses on the affected area. As these occur on the eyelid, utilization of laser grade corneal shields is mandatory and pulses need to be delivered 2 mm away from the lash line.[23] See Table 22.3 for specific settings on the Lumenis M22.

PIGMENTARY LESIONS

Sample device settings for pigmentary abnormalities such as the photofacial and lentigines are shown in Tables 22.4 and 22.5. As hyperpigmentation improves, lower filters and higher energy levels may be used. Darkening of the target usually represents the end point of treatment. Skin types I to III typically need a 590-nm cut-off filter for severe hyperpigmentation or a 560 nm filter for mild to moderate hyperpigmentation would be appropriate because epidermal cells of lighter skin absorb only small amounts of light (compared to epidermal cells of skin types IV and V). This allows more light to be absorbed by the target pigment.

See Table 22.4 for treatment settings for pigment and aging sun damage.

VASCULAR LESIONS

Superficial vascular abnormalities require 515- to 590-nm cut-off filters, which provide wavelengths in the absorption spectrum of hemoglobin and are safe to use in fair-skinned patients. In skin types I and II, 515- and 560-nm filters, single or double pulses, and 2.0- to 4.0-ms pulse durations work well. For smaller telangiectasias, shorter pulse durations suffice to heat correspondingly small targets. Conversely, larger target vessels require longer pulse durations for heating. Finally, deeper vessels require (1) longer wavelengths that penetrate more deeply into the skin and (2) longer pulse durations to heat these deeper targets. For skin types III and IV, longer wavelengths, longer multiple pulse durations (3.0–4.0 ms), and longer delay times are considered safer.[21] An example with Lumenis M22 for vascular settings is shown in Tables 22.6 and, 22.7A, B, and C. *Settings will vary by IPL device, and an operator's manual specific to a given device should be consulted.*

When utilizing IPL you can target multiple layers of the skin in one treatment session. The deeper tissue must be targeted initially working more superficially with the settings. If the initial pass is too superficial then erythema occurs and blocks the deeper targeted tissue on the second pass. So, treat deeper and larger areas to smaller and more superficial areas. An example of a patient who has significant flushing of the skin along with erythematous and ocular rosacea and Fitzpatrick skin type II is seen in Figure 22.10 and treated as seen in Video 22.1. The author treated this patient effectively over a period of four treatments.

POSTTREATMENT INSTRUCTIONS

To date, there is no universal agreement about the therapy that patients should receive after IPL treatment such as meibomian gland expression immediately post procedure.

For two days after treatment, patients may experience redness, slight swelling, and a "sunburned" feeling. These are normal reactions. Pigmented areas may also appear darker. Superficial pigment darkens, dries, and sloughs off in seven to ten days resembling coffee grounds. Deeper pigment darkens, and then slowly fades as the body absorbs the remnants of the damaged pigment. In addition to discussing expected posttreatment sequelae, patients are given the following instructions:

- Apply sunscreen every day (30 Sun Protection Factor or greater).
- If the treated area is red and irritated after treatment, apply an ice pack or cold compresses.
- In caring for the treated area, use only gentle cleansers and lotions until healing is complete. Avoid perfumes and products with alcohol or acid.
- If a blister develops, apply an antibiotic ointment until the blister dries. When a scab forms, apply Aquaphor healing ointment. Do not pick the blister or scab because a scar may form.
- Call the clinician's office if any problems, questions, or concerns arise.

RECOMMENDATIONS FOR FOLLOW-UP

Most patients require three to five treatment sessions to achieve satisfactory results. Patients may return for additional treatments no sooner than two to four weeks after the most recent treatment. Patients should be instructed to call or return sooner if adverse effects occur.

POTENTIAL COMPLICATIONS AND THEIR TREATMENT

Modern IPL systems cause minimal and transient adverse effects such as crusting (2%), purpura (4%), a burning sensation during treatment (45%), hyperpigmentation and hypopigmentation (8%–15%), erythema, and mild swelling or edema (25%).[26] Crusted areas heal within seven days, and purpura resolves within two to five days. Hyperpigmentation is treated daily with topical hydroquinone (4%–6%) and sunscreen.[26] Swelling and edema are treated with cold ice packs before the patient leaves the office and with cold compresses for an additional 24 hours. If blisters develop, patients should apply ice during the first 24 hours and antibacterial ointment when the blisters rupture. If a hypertrophic scar develops (rare), intralesional steroids may be used to diminish the scar.[26]

VIDEOS OF PROCEDURE

Video 22.1—This is an IPL procedure being performed with the Lumenis M22 on a patient with keratoconjunctivitis sicca and MGD secondary to ocular and facial rosacea and skin type II. Patient is being prepped in this video.

First Pass: medium to deep depth 590 nm, triple pulse, 3.5 to 30 ms, 20 J/cm^2.

Second Pass: shallow depth 560 nm, triple pulse, 3.0 to 25 ms, 18 J/cm^2. Toyos settings over V2 with double pass: 590 nm filter, triple pulse 6.0 ms pulse, 50 ms rest, 12 J/cm^2.

Eyelids: Periman Protocol with LASER Grade Corneal Shields: small rectangle light guide 3 pulses per lid with double pass, staying 2 mm away from the lash line (Total 24 pulses) with 590 nm filter, triple pulse 5.0 ms pulse, 50 ms rest, 12 J/cm^2.

Video courtesy of Selina R. McGee.

Video 22.2—This is the continuation of the IPL procedure being performed with the Lumenis M22 on a patient with keratoconjunctivitis sicca and MGD secondary to ocular and facial rosacea and skin type II. Patient is being actively treated in this video.

First Pass: medium to deep depth 590 nm, triple pulse, 3.5 to 30 ms, 20 J/cm^2.

Second Pass: shallow depth 560 nm, triple pulse, 3.0 to 25 ms, 18 J/cm^2. Toyos settings over V2 with double pass: 590 nm filter, triple pulse 6.0 ms pulse, 50 ms rest, 12 J/cm^2.

Eyelids: Periman Protocol with LASER Grade Corneal Shields: Small rectangle light guide 3 pulses per lid with double pass, staying 2 mm away from the lash line (Total 24 pulses) with 590 nm filter, triple pulse 5.0 ms pulse, 50 ms rest, 12 J/cm^2.

Video courtesy of Selina R. McGee.

Video 22.3—This is an IPL procedure being performed with the Lumenis M22 on a patient for photodamage and skin type III. First and only pass: 560 nm, double pulse, 4.0 ms pulse, 20 ms rest, 17 J/cm^2 with the 15 × 35 mm crystal.

Video courtesy of Selina R. McGee.

Video 22.4—This video reviews the use of corneal metal shields to treat eyelids.

Video by Selina R. McGee.

Video 22.5—This video reviews Dr. McGee's postoperative procedure and care for the IPL patient.

Video courtesy of Selina R. McGee.

EFFICACY

DED is a multifactorial disease.[27] Potential mechanisms whereby IPL could achieve clinical improvement include selective photothermolysis of abnormal blood vessels below the skin surrounding the eyes, activation of fibroblasts and enhancing the synthesis of new collagen fibers,[28] decreasing *Demodex* and the bacterial load on the eyelids, interference with the inflammatory cycle by regulation of antiinflammatory agents and matrix metalloproteinases,[28,29] reducing the turnover of skin epithelial cells and decreasing the risk of physical obstruction of the meibomian glands, and heating the meibomian glands and liquefying the meibum.[30] Due to its multifactorial nature, it is possible that multiple treatment mechanisms of action are helping to reduce patient signs and symptoms of MGD and DED. As IPL expands and is utilized more to treat MGD and DED, the eye care community will learn and be able to expand on this thought process.

REFERENCES

1. Bitter PH. Noninvasive rejuvenation of photodamaged skin using serial, full-face intense pulsed light treatments. *Dermatol Surg*. 2000;26:835–842.
2. Nelson JD, Craig JP, Akpek EK, et al. TFOS DEWS II introduction. *Ocul Surf*. 2017;15(3):269–275.
3. Nichols KK, Foulks GN, Bron AJ, et al. The international workshop on meibomian gland dysfunction: Executive summary. *Invest. Ophthalmol Vis Sci*. 2011;52(4):1922–1929. doi:10.1167/iovs.10-6997a
4. Chhadva P, Goldhardt R Galor A. Meibomian gland disease: the role of gland dysfunction in dry eye disease. *Ophthalmology*. 2017;124(11S):S20–S26. doi:10.1016/j.ophtha.2017.05.031
5. Schaller M, et al. Rosacea treatment update: recommendations from the global ROSacea COnsensus (ROSCO) panel. *BJD*. 2016 Nov 12. 465–471. doi:10.1111/bjd.15173
6. Papageorgiou P, Clayton W, Norwood S, Chopra S, Rustin M. Treatment of rosacea with intense pulsed light: significant improvement and long-lasting results. *Br J Dermatol*. 2008;159(3):628–632.
7. Geerling G, Baudouin C, Aragona P, et al. Emerging strategies for the diagnosis and treatment of meibomian gland dysfunction: Proceedings of the OCEAN group meeting. *Ocul Surf*. 2017;15(2):179–192. doi:10.1016/j.jtos.2017.01.006
8. Dell SJ. Intense pulsed light for evaporative dry eye disease. *Clin Ophthalmol*. 2017;11:1167–1173. doi:10.2147/OPTH.S139894
9. Jiang X, Lv H, Song H, et al. Evaluation of the safety and effectiveness of intense pulsed light in the treatment of meibomian gland dysfunction. *J Ophthalmol*. 2016;2016:1910694.
10. Toyos R, McGill W, Briscoe D. Intense pulsed light treatment for dry eye disease due to meibomian gland dysfunction; a 3-year retrospective study. *Photomed Laser Surg*. 2015;33(1):41–46. doi:10.1089/pho.2014.3819
11. Rong B, Tang Y, Liu R, et al. Long-Term effects of intense pulsed light combined with meibomian gland expression in the treatment of meibomian gland dysfunction. *Photomed Laser Surg*. 2018;36(10):562–567. doi:10.1089/pho.2018.4499
12. Craig JP, Chen Y-H and Turnbull PRK. Prospective trial of intense pulsed light for the treatment of meibomian gland dysfunction. *Invest. Ophthalmol. Vis. Sci*. 2015;56(3):1965–1970. doi:10.1167/iovs.14-15764.
13. Vora GK, Gupta PK. Intense pulsed light therapy for the treatment of evaporative dry eye disease. *Curr Opin Ophthalmol*. 2015;26(4):314–318.
14. Gupta PK, Vora GK, Matossian C, Kim M, Stinnett S. Outcomes of intense pulsed light therapy for treatment of evaporative dry eye disease. *Can J Ophthalmol*. 2016;51(4):249–253.

15. Toyos R, Buffa C, Youngerman S. Case report: dry–eye symptoms improve with intense pulsed light treatment. *EyeWorld (ASCRS)*. 2005 Jan 1;33(1):41–46.

16. Vegunta S, Patel D, Shen JF. Combination therapy of Intense Pulsed Light Therapy and Meibomian Gland Expression (IPL/MGX) can improve dry eye symptoms and meibomian gland function in patients with refractory dry eye: A retrospective analysis. *Cornea*. 2016;35(3):318–322.

17. Giannaccare G, Taroni L, Senni C, Scorcia V. Intense pulsed light therapy in the treatment of meibomian gland dysfunction: Current perspectives. *Clin Optom (Auckl)*. 2019;11:113–126. doi:10.2147/OPTO.S217639

18. Dell S, Gaster R, Barbarino S, Cunningham D. Prospective evaluation of intense pulsed light and meibomian gland expression efficacy on relieving signs and symptoms of dry eye disease due to meibomian gland dysfunction. *Clin Ophthalmol*. 2017;11:817–827.

19. Kirn T. Intense pulsed light eradicates *Demodex* mites. *Skin Allergy News*. 2002;33(1):37.

20. Gilbert D, Gilbert G. Intense pulsed light. *J Cosmet Dermatol*. 2007;(23):1–7.

21. Lumenis (2015). M22 Intense Pulsed Light (IPL) CD-20003888 Rev. A

22. Sharma AN and Patel BC. Laser fitzpatrick skin type recommendations. [Updated 2020 May 4]. In: StatPearls [Internet]. Treasure Island (FL): StatPearls Publishing; 2020 Jan.

23. The Dry Eye Master YouTube website. Accessed 2020.

24. Goldman MP, Weiss RA, Weiss MA. Intense pulsed light as a nonablative approach to photoaging. *Dermatol Surg*. 2005;31(9 Pt 2):1179–1187.

25. Goldman MP. Treatment of benign vascular lesions with the Photoderm VL high-intensity pulsed light source. *Adv Dermatol*. 1997;13:503–521.

26. Prieto VG, Sadick NS, Lloreta J, Nicholson J, Shea CR. Effects of intense pulsed light on sun-damaged human skin, routine, and ultrastructural analysis. *Lasers Surg Med*. 2002;30(2):82–85. doi:10.1002/lsm.10042

27. DEWS The definition and classification of dry eye disease: report of the definition and classification subcommittee of the international dry eye workshop. *Ocul Surf*. 2007;5(2):75–92.

28. Huang J, Luo X, Lu J, et al. IPL irradiation rejuvenates skin collagen via the bidirectional regulation of MMP-1 and TGF-β1 mediated by MAPKs in fibroblasts. *Lasers Med Sci*. 2011;26(3):381–387.

29. Cuerda-Galindo E, Díaz-Gil G, Palomar-Gallego M, Linares-García, Valdecasas R. Increased fibroblast proliferation and activity after applying intense pulsed light 800–1,200 nm. *Ann Anat*. 2015;198:66–72.

30. Liu R, Rong B, Tu P, et al. Analysis of cytokine levels in tears and clinical correlations after intense pulsed light treating meibomian gland dysfunction. *Am J Ophthalmol*. 2017;183:81–90. doi:10.1016/j.ajo.2017.08.021

23

Non-ablative Lasers in Aesthetics

Selina R. McGee

Skin aging is a complex and dynamic process. Bone loss, muscle atrophy, loss of collagen and elastin, as well as skin thinning all contribute and will manifest in various ways, such as wrinkles and decreased volume. Due to the anatomy and structures of the periorbital region this is the first area to be affected and noticed by the observer and patients alike.[1] The unique properties of reduced epidermis and dermis thickness as well as the functional sensitivity of its components require specialized periorbital skin rejuvenating treatments. See Figure 23.1 showing how the face ages..

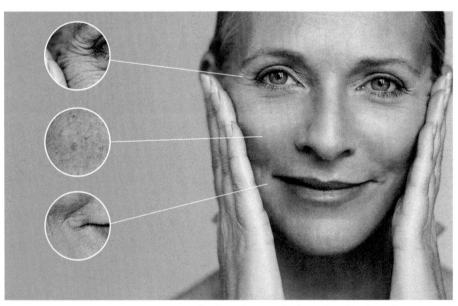

FIGURE 23-1 Photo demonstrating how the face ages resulting in rhytids, photodamage, and volume loss. (Photo courtesy of Selina R. McGee, OD, FAAO)

Since about 1997, aesthetic treatments have moved to become less invasive and more preventative in nature.

Achieving maximum aesthetic results typically requires a multipronged approach. The goal of skin rejuvenation is overall improvement in the many aspects of cutaneous changes secondary to ultraviolet light exposure and intrinsic aging. Patients who are interested in skin rejuvenation but are unable or unwilling to have significant downtime typically are good candidates for non-ablative procedures. Proper patient selection is critical to ensuring desired outcomes. Patients with realistic expectations between the ages of 35 and 65 and only mild to moderate rhytids are ideal.[1]

Different types of devices can be used to achieve cosmetically pleasing results. These devices can be used in conjunction with each other, sometimes even during the same treatment session and include: radiofrequency (RF), intense pulsed light (IPL), and lasers, which can be either ablative or non-ablative in nature.[2] Neurotoxin, dermal fillers, platelet rich plasma, skin peels, and a medical grade skin care regimen round out the complete approach for the aesthetic patient. This chapter will serve to educate about non-ablative technology. It is up to the practitioner to determine what treatments need to be customized to the patient.

MECHANISM OF ACTION, LASER PHYSICS, AND TARGET TISSUE

Aesthetic lasers target chromophores: water, melanin, oxyhemaglobin, and exongenous chromophores such as carbon-based ink found in tattoos.[1] Lasers produce monochromatic light and are named by the specific wavelength they produce. Due to this nature no laser can supply all the wavelengths needed for different targets.

Understanding light interactions with skin is essential to appropriately treating and achieving results as well as knowing laser and light-based wavelengths, fluences, and pulse durations. There are numerous energy-delivering devices, light-based devices and lasers on the market currently. Fully understanding how they work and what target they work best on is essential to incorporating them into patient care.

IPL therapy can be used to effectively treat vascular and pigmented lesions that may be seen in photodamaged skin and is also used to reduce unwanted hair. IPL is discussed extensively in Chapter 22. The reader is invited to review the relevant sections.

Non-ablative laser therapies treat the target chromophores of water, melanin, and oxyhemaglobin and leave the surrounding skin intact. As the stratum corneum remains intact, the skin maintains its defense function to microbial infection and highly minimizes the risk of potential side effects as compared to ablative techniques. Due to the nature of treatment there is less downtime and less risk of infection versus ablative laser therapies. Lasers falling below the infrared range of 2,000 nm are non-ablative.[3]

Ablative lasers such as the CO_2 10,600 nm or the Erbium:YAG 2,940 nm ablate the target chromophore as well as vaporize surrounding tissue and have significant downtime typically ranging from three to ten days if fractionated and 7 to 14 days if unfractionated. Due to corneum stratum breakdown there is a higher risk of infection as the skin's defense system is open.[4] High risk yields high reward though as these treatments can produce significant results. More discussion on ablative technology will be made in Chapter 24.

Fractional laser treatments introduced by Anderson and Parrish utilize fractional photothermolysis to generate microthermal zones.[5] This means that the energy is delivered in columns rather than complete ablation. When this technology is utilized it creates micro-wounds in the skin surrounded by intact tissue. This heating, up to mid-reticular dermis, serves as the stimulus for inflammatory mediator release, fibroblast activation, neocollagenesis, and dermal remodeling. Furthermore, the impacted coagulation columns act like elimination channels, which expel pigment and explain the clinical lightening of lentigines and melasma.[5]

When delivered this way it allows deeper penetration into the tissue without compromising more superficial tissues. Typically, multiple treatments are required to achieve best results, but there is less downtime, an average of three days, associated with each treatment (Fig. 23.2). Fractional technology can be found in both ablative and non-ablative lasers.[2]

Q-switched means that instead of the laser operating in a continuous wave (CW) it stores energy and is able to produce an increased pulse or higher pulse energy and longer pulse duration. This also allows the laser to shatter pigment including those

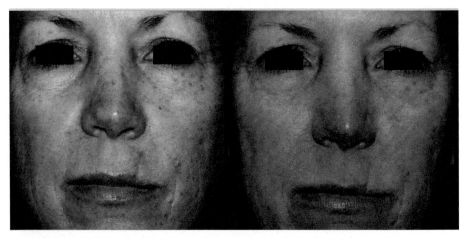

FIGURE 23-2 A patient who had ResurFx, a non-ablative laser at 1,565 nm. (Photo courtesy of R. Saluja, MD)

in tattoos and pigmented lesions that can then be absorbed by phagocytosis and expelled through the lymphatic system (Fig. 23.3).[2]

Picosecond lasers entered the market specifically for tattoo removal as they pulse at a picosecond versus a nanosecond (Fig. 23.4).[6] They have expanded capabilities, but since tattoo removal doesn't typically take place in the periorbital area the discussion about picosecond lasers will be limited here.

RF technology is used for bulk heating of tissue and is primarily used for skin tightening and collagen remodeling (Figs. 23.5–23.7). Water is the only chromophore it targets making the device "colorblind," therefore it can be used on any skin type. Elevation of dermal layer temperature leads to a transient denaturation of structural collagen fibrils, which is followed by contraction and tightening of the skin. Heat is applied to the epidermis creating an inflammatory phase that last one to three days. Early contraction of blood vessels during the initial heat of 39°C to 42°C is followed by vasodilation in order to increase blood supply, which can last multiple hours to one to three days. Macrophages, neutrophils, and other cells infiltrate the damaged area to remove dead/damaged tissue and destroy bacteria. The proliferative phase will last up to three weeks in which there is an ongoing process to repair tissue. During days two to three there is fibroblast activity that is induced in damaged tissue. Fibroblasts multiply, sending mediators to stimulate repair, combining with damaged tissue. Fibroblasts will begin collagen synthesis usually around day 7 up to day 21. Old collagen is removed by collagenase during this time as well. The maturation phase starts at week three

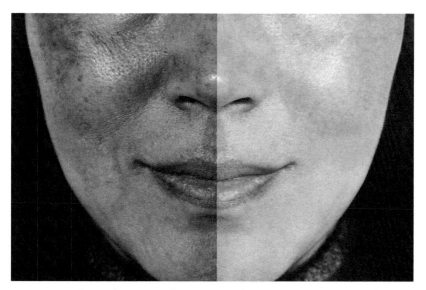

FIGURE 23-3 Photo of a patient demonstrating less pigment due to photodamage. (Photo courtesy of Selina R. McGee, OD, FAAO)

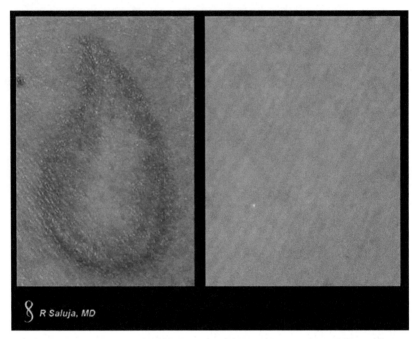

FIGURE 23-4 Tattoo removal with Picosure. (Photo courtesy of R. Saluja, MD)

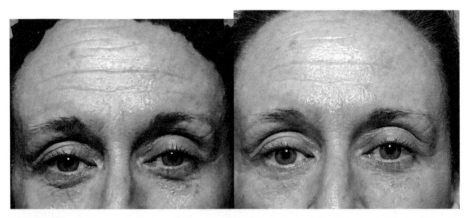

FIGURE 23-5 Before and after patient with the TempSure Envi by Cynosure. (Photo courtesy of Selina R. McGee, OD, FAAO)

and will continue for six months and sometimes beyond where new collagen is generated and elastin becomes more uniform and its quality is improved.[7] Typically 2 to 4 treatments performed four weeks apart are generally needed to see a clinically measurable response.[7] There are multiple studies in the literature on the effectiveness of RF technology in the periorbital region.[7] The author introduces the technology here as it

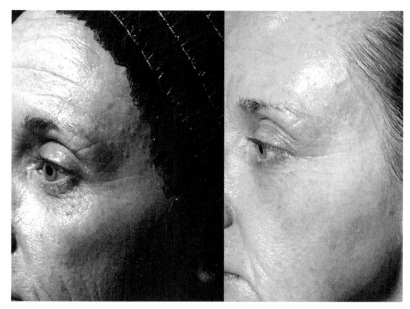

FIGURE 23-6 Before and after with TempSure Envi RF technology. (Photo courtesy of Selina R. McGee, OD, FAAO)

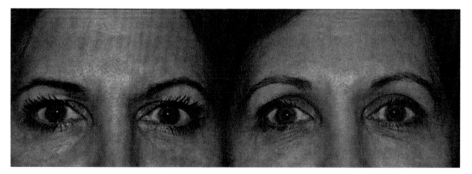

FIGURE 23-7 Patient with less dermatochalasis, increased MRD-1, and improved rhytids treated with RF technology by Cynosure. (Photo courtesy of R. Saluja, MD)

is a noninvasive option with no downtime to rejuvenate skin and can be used in conjunction with other treatment modalities being discussed to attain a synergistic effect.

Selective photothermolysis is the mechanism of action of laser therapy as it targets chromophores melanin, oxyhemaglobin, and water. Photons of light produced by the laser are absorbed by the specific chromophore within a specific target, producing heat. The heat dissipates and when sufficient energy is delivered faster than the rate of cooling, heat accumulates within the target and selectively destroys it. Tissue absorption and scattering determine penetration of laser light into the skin. Longer wavelengths can penetrate deeper into the skin, but as the wavelength is increased into the far-infrared region, light is heavily absorbed by water, which limits its penetration.[5] Since soft tissue is an organic composite mainly composed of water and structural proteins, it is very helpful to know laser absorption and tissue penetration by wavelength. Wavelengths or "color" of light in the infrared range (2,000 nm and above) are ablative in nature due to the absorption of water and limited penetration.[5] It is also imperative to understand that thermal relaxation time (TRT), which largely determines the ideal pulse duration for selective thermolysis, in seconds is directly proportional to the square of the target size in millimeters. For example, a 0.2-mm telangiectasia, typical for rosacea, cools in about 0.04 seconds (40 ms). The optimal laser or IPL pulse duration is typically approximately equal to the TRT, so in this example a pulsed dye (595 nm) laser operated at ~20 to 40 ms would be appropriate.[1]

The following list of lasers may not be all-inclusive as the market is increasing at a fairly rapid rate and is meant to serve as a guide and introduce familiarity to wavelengths and target chromophores (Fig. 23.8).

CO_2 lasers 10,600 nm: This is a gas laser in the mid infra-red spectrum that is highly absorbed in water. It is hypothesized that CO_2 lasers cause immediate contraction of the ablated areas by denaturing existing old collagen.[1,6] This laser is ablative and will be discussed in more detail in Chapter 24.

Erbium 2,940 nm: This is a solid-state laser that is highly absorbed in water and is used for laser resurfacing and skin rejuvenation. This frequency is much closer to the peak absorption range of water and thus has an absorption coefficient 16 times greater than the CO_2 laser. This greater absorption decreases the penetration depth into the epidermis by a factor of 10. This is an advantage, as more precise ablation of skin is possible with even less damage to surrounding tissue.[1,6] This laser is ablative and will be discussed in more depth in Chapter 24.

1,540 to 1,565 nm: These lasers are considerably less absorbed by intracellular water than the ablative 10,600 nm CO_2 and the 2,940 nm Erbium:YAG lasers, making them non-ablative. They are typically used for skin resurfacing procedures including periorbital wrinkles.[8]

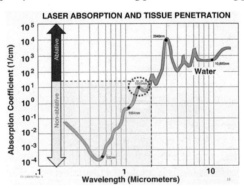

FIGURE 23-8 Absorption peaks as they relate to wavelength. (Reprinted with permission from Ross EV, McKinlay JR, Anderson RR. Why does carbon dioxide resurfacing work? A review. *Arch Dermatol.* 1999;135(4):444–454.)

Nd:YAG 1,064 nm: This is absorbed by many chromophores. It is highly absorbed in hemoglobin so it works well for the treatment of vascular conditions. Melanin absorbs this wavelength and it is useful for hair removal and tattoo pigment.[1,6]

Alexandrite 755 nm: This laser is highly absorbed by melanin, and it is considered by some to be the gold standard for hair reduction with those that have light skin and dark hair.[1,6]

Pulsed dye 577 to 585 nm: These lasers are absorbed by hemoglobin so they are used in vascular treatments and vascular staining such as port wine stains.[1,6]

INDICATIONS

Common indications for aesthetic lasers are dyschromia, skin laxity and irregular texture, soft tissue coagulation, vascular lesions, and hair removal.

VASCULAR LESIONS AND PIGMENTED LESIONS

Oxyhemaglobin and deoxyhemaglobin are the main chromophores for vascular lasers. Fitzpatrick skin typing must be taken into consideration as melanin can compete for absorption resulting in unfavorable results like hyperpigmentation or hypopigmentation and scarring can occur. Selective photothermolysis for blood vessels needs to reach approximately 70°C to damage the blood vessel wall resulting in its destruction. The composition, structure, and history of the vascular lesion need to be determined prior to treatment. Once ascertained, then appropriate treatment can be decided. IPL, as discussed in Chapter 22, is well suited to treat telangiectasias and pigment in the periocular/midface region, as well as the pulsed dye lasers, and the Nd:YAG 1064 (Figs. 23.9 and 23.10).[3,9,10]

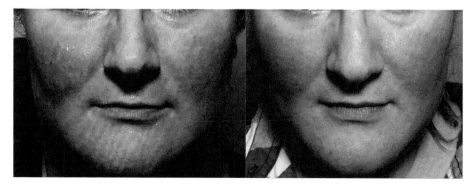

FIGURE 23-9 A patient with improvement of telangiectasic vessels, pustules, and erythema related to rosacea. This patient was treated with IPL. (Photo courtesy of Selina R. McGee, OD, FAAO)

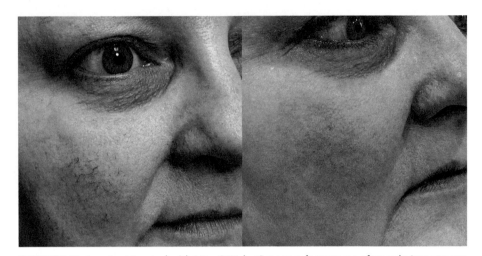

FIGURE 23-10 A patient treated with Max G IPL by Cynosure for rosacea after only 1 treatment. (Photo courtesy of Selina R. McGee, OD, FAAO)
Settings will vary by device, and an operator's manual specific to a given device should be consulted.

DISCUSSION OF DEVICE SETTINGS

Wavelength: the "color" of light.

Pulse durations: can be single or repeated and the time of the pulse and between pulses may vary.

Energy levels: also known as fluence in J/cm^2, are governed by clinical response and are the "dose" of light. The higher the fluence level the more aggressive the treatment.

Exposure spot size: scan patterns and sizes can be customized to the patient and the area of treatment for more or less coverage. The pattern and size should allow the beams to be placed in an even perpendicular fashion to the skin.

Density: within a particular scan size, density can also be increased or decreased. Avoid high energy and high density since this is not general practice and can lead to an increased risk of adverse events.[5]

PATIENT SELECTION

The easiest patients to treat have fair skin (Fitzpatrick skin types I–III). Darker skin types can also be treated (Fitzpatrick skin type IV–VI)—with caution—by using lower energies, longer pulse durations, longer delay times, and aggressive skin cooling techniques. Patients must be willing to undergo multiple treatments at varying intervals. Most patients need a series of 3 to 5 treatments and then will continue to need a maintenance treatment every four to six months.[1] These treatments are currently not covered by private insurance; therefore, patients must be willing to assume responsibility for the cost of treatments. Patients' medical history, medications, and previous cosmetic treatments must also be discussed.

FITZPATRICK SKIN TYPING SCALE

The Fitzpatrick skin phototypes (types) were constructed based on an individual's skin color and their tendency to burn or tan when exposed to sunlight. There are six skin types characterized by Tables 23.1 and 23.2.[11]

CONTRAINDICATIONS

Contraindications for laser treatment include the following[1]:

- Active herpes simplex virus (HSV) infection
- Exposure to sun, remaining suntan, or artificial tanning in the three to four weeks preoperative

TABLE 23.1 FITZPATRICK SKIN TYPE

FITZPATRICK SKIN TYPE	SKIN COLOR BEFORE SUN EXPOSURE	EYE COLOR	HAIR COLOR	SUN REACTION
Skin type I	Ivory	Light blue, light gray, or light green	Red or light blonde	Skin always freckles, always burns and peels, and never tans
Skin type II	Fair or pale	Blue, gray, or green	Blonde	Skin usually freckles, burns and peels often, and rarely tans
Skin type III	Fair to beige, with golden undertones	Hazel or light brown	Dark blonde or light brown	Skin usually freckles, burns and peels often, and rarely tans
Skin type IV	Olive or light brown	Dark brown	Dark brown	Doesn't really freckle, burns rarely, and tans often
Skin type V	Dark brown	Dark brown to black	Dark brown to black	Rarely freckles, almost never burns, and always tans
Skin type VI	Deeply pigmented dark brown to darkest brown	Brownish black	Black	Never freckles, never burns, and always tans darkly

TABLE 23.2 FITZPATRICK TYPES I, II, AND III WRINKLE AND ELASTOSIS

CLASS	WRINKLING	SCORE
I	Fine wrinkles (rhytids)	1–3
II	Fine to moderate depth wrinkles, moderate number of lines	4–6
III	Fine to deep wrinkles, numerous lines with or without redundant skin folds	7–9

- Active lupus erythematous
- Dysplastic nevi
- Significant concurrent skin conditions or any inflammatory skin conditions
- Open lacerations or abrasions
- Chronic or cutaneous viral, fungal, or bacterial diseases
- Unreasonable expectations
- Tattoos (unless that is the desired target)
- Skin types V and VI
- Unmanaged cardiovascular disease or diabetes
- Medical history of keloids
- Pregnancy or lactation

PRETREATMENT PATIENT EDUCATION

The following should be discussed with patients prior to performing laser treatment:

- Results are not guaranteed.
- Not all red and brown areas, or rhytids will disappear. Red and brown spots removed by treatment may recur, especially with excessive sun exposure. Rhytids may return or deepen.
- Deep wrinkle lines will not be removed by the treatment.
- Adverse effects include redness, swelling, burning, pain, crust formation, bruising, hyperpigmentation and hypopigmentation, and scar formation.
- Multiple treatment sessions (typically three to five) are required for optimal results.
- Maintenance treatments are often recommended four to six months after the initial series. In addition, patients should be quoted a price for the treatment course.[1]

PRETREATMENT PATIENT INSTRUCTIONS

A review of the national database of drugs and the wavelengths causing photo-sensitive reactions of each drug with each laser wavelength is recommended prior to treatment.

Patients are given the following instructions prior to treatment:

- Isotretinoin (Accutane) should not be taken for six months prior to treatment.
- Apply sunscreen four to six weeks preoperatively: Sun Protection Factor (SPF) 30 to 50 utilized every day.
- Sun exposure and tan skin will result in a need to reschedule your appointment.
- Do not apply makeup or lotions on your day of treatment, or be prepared to remove them at our office.
- If you have a history of cold sores, take your prescribed medication (e.g., valacyclovir [Valtrex], famciclovir [Famvir], acyclovir [Zovirax]) on the day before, day of, and five days posttreatment.

PHOTOGRAPHY INFORMED CONSENT

Since these treatments are being performed on the face, photography informed consent is necessary. An example may read like this:

> I hereby authorize (**physician name**), of (**name of practice**), and/or his/her associates or licensees to take pre-procedural and post-procedural photographs, slides.
>
> I consent to the use of these images for the purposes of pre-procedural planning and post-procedural evaluation by (**physician name**) and/or the staff of (**name of practice**), and I understand that they shall be made a part of my medical record.

INFORMED CONSENT

Informed consent should contain the following information as well as the alternative treatments available, followed by written consent. The following suggested template should serve as a guide.

> This is an informed consent document. It has been prepared to help inform you about laser treatment procedures of skin, risks, and alternative treatments.
>
> It is important that you read this information carefully and completely.
>
> Conditions such as wrinkles, sun damaged skin, unsightly veins, and some types of skin lesions/disorders may be treated with the laser. Certain surgical procedures may use the laser as a cutting instrument. In some situations, laser treatments may be performed at the time of other surgical procedures.
>
> Alternative forms of treatment include not undergoing the proposed laser skin treatment procedure. Other forms of skin treatment (chemical peel) or surgical procedures may be substituted. In certain situations, the laser may offer a specific therapeutic advantage over other forms of treatment.

Alternatively, laser treatment procedures in some situations may not represent a better alternative to other forms of surgery or skin treatment when indicated. Risks and potential complications are associated with alternative forms of treatment that involve skin treatments or surgical procedures.

There are both risks and complications associated with all laser treatment procedures of the skin. Risks involve both items that specifically relate to the use of laser energy as a form of surgical therapy and to the specific procedure performed. An individual's choice to undergo a procedure is based on the comparison of risk to potential benefits. Although the majority of patients do not experience these complications, you should discuss each of them with your physician to make sure you understand the risks, potential complications, and consequences of laser skin treatment.

Infection

HSV infections around the mouth or other areas of the face can occur following a laser treatment. This applies to both individuals with a past history of HSV infections and individuals with no known history of HSV infections in the mouth area. Specific medications may be prescribed and taken both prior to and following the laser treatment procedure in order to suppress an infection from this virus. Should any type of skin infection occur, additional treatments including antibiotics may be necessary.

Scarring

Although normal healing after the procedure is expected, abnormal scars may occur both in the skin and deeper tissues. In rare cases, keloid scars may result. Scars may be unattractive and of different color than the surrounding skin. Additional treatments may be needed to treat scarring.

Burns

Laser energy can produce burns. Adjacent structures including the eyes may be injured or permanently damaged by the laser beam. Burns are rare yet represent the effect of heat produced within the tissues by laser energy. Additional treatment may be necessary to treat laser burns.

Color Change

Laser treatments may potentially change the natural color of your skin. Skin redness usually lasts two weeks to three months and occasionally six months following laser skin treatment. There is the possibility of irregular color variations within the skin including areas that are both lighter and darker.

Visible Skin Patterns

Laser treatment procedures may produce visible patterns within the skin. The occurrence of this is not predictable.

Patient Failure to Follow Through

Patient follow through following a laser skin treatment procedure is important. Post-operative instructions concerning appropriate restriction of activity and use of sun protection need to be followed in order to avoid potential complications, increased pain, and unsatisfactory result. Your physician may recommend that you utilize a long-term skin care program to enhance healing following a laser skin treatment.

Damaged Skin

Skin that has been previously treated with chemical peels or dermabrasion, or damaged by burns, or radiation therapy may heal abnormally or slowly following treatment by lasers or other surgical techniques. The occurrence of this is not predictable. Additional treatment may be necessary.

Unsatisfactory Result

There is the possibility of an unsatisfactory result from these procedures. Laser procedures may result in unacceptable visible deformities, skin slough, loss of function, and permanent color changes in the skin. You may be disappointed with the final result from laser treatments.

Allergic Reactions

In rare cases, local allergies to tape, preservatives used in cosmetics, or topical preparations have been reported. Systemic reactions that are more serious may result from drugs used during medical procedures and prescription medicines. Allergic reactions may require additional treatment.

Lack of Permanent Results

Laser or other treatments may not completely improve or prevent future skin disorders, lesions, or wrinkles. Additional procedures or surgery may be necessary to further tighten loose skin.

Delayed Healing

It may take longer than anticipated for healing to occur after laser treatments. Skin healing may result in thin, easily injured skin. This is different from the normal redness in skin after a laser treatment.

Unknown Risks

There is the possibility that additional risk factors of laser skin treatments may be discovered.

Additional Treatment or Surgery Necessary

There are many variable conditions that influence the long-term result of laser skin treatments. Even though risks and complications occur infrequently, the risks cited are the ones that are particularly associated with these procedures. Other complications and risks can occur but are even more uncommon. Should complications occur, procedures, surgery, or other treatments may be necessary. The practice of medicine and surgery is not an exact science. Although good results are expected, there is no guarantee or warranty expressed or implied on the results that may be obtained.

It is important that you read the aforementioned information carefully and have all of your questions answered before signing the consent on the next page.

Informed Consent for Laser-Based Treatments

I hereby authorize certified personnel to perform the following laser light energy procedure and skin tightening treatments.

I recognize that during the course of the procedure and medical treatment, unforeseen conditions may necessitate different procedures than those above. I therefore authorize the above physician to perform such other procedures that are in the exercise of his or her professional judgment necessary and desirable. The authority granted under this paragraph shall include all conditions that require treatment and are not known to my physician at the time the procedure is begun.

I consent to the administration of such anesthetics considered necessary or advisable. I understand that all forms of anesthesia involve risk and the possibility of complications, injury, and sometimes death.

I acknowledge that no guarantee has been given by anyone as to the results that may be obtained.

I Consent to the Treatment or Procedure and the Above Listed Items
[Signed by the patient, physician, witness and date] at (physician's practice name)

PROCEDURE PROTOCOL

- *Tray setup:* The setup tray may include laser grade eye shields, cooling devices, smoke evacuator, chlorhexidine wipes, washcloth, hair band, and nonsterile gloves. In addition, cleanser and sunscreen lotion may be available for use by the patient.
- *Patient prep:* Immediately before applying topical anesthesia (if utilizing) cleanse the area to be treated with warm soapy water; rinse and dry well.
- *Topical anesthetic:* Follow the guidelines of the manufacturing health care professional for application dosage, occlusion, and timing. Topical anesthetic must be

applied at the medical facility under the supervision of a licensed practitioner and should not be applied to large areas because of the potential risk of systemic absorption. Potential complications include death.[12,13] Do not apply cream to patients with a history of allergic reactions to benzacaine, tetracaine, or lidocaine. Do not apply cream to patients taking Class I antiarrhythmic drugs. Apply a thin film of cream to the area that will be treated, using a tongue depressor. Wait for 30 to 60 minutes for the cream to work. Remove the excess cream prior to treatment.

- Wipe with alcohol-free antisepsis (e.g., water-based chlorhexidine)
- Dry skin thoroughly
- Immediately before session
  - Put eyewear on the patient as per treatment area. There are many case reports in the literature of corneal abrasions post-laser therapy.[14,15] This can be due to chemical, mechanical, or thermal damage. To best prevent this, use laser grade corneal shields of the largest size available. Currently, at the time of publication it is 26 mm. Be extremely careful to not get anything under the shield upon insertion, such as coupling gel or anesthetic cream, as this may cause a severe chemical burn. The patient will not know until later because of the instillation of topical anesthetic eye drops prior to inserting the shields.

Safety Concerns

- Post the laser warning sign on the entrance door.
- Do not leave laser unattended when in operation.
- Never look directly in the aperture of the treatment head even when wearing adequate safety goggles.
- Avoid directing the laser beam anywhere other than the intended treatment area.
- The aiming beam is ON by default when turning the system ON.
- Do not allow reflective or flammable items within the operating field.
- Always enter STANDBY mode when the laser is not being operated and accommodate connected treatment head in the cradle.

Safety Goggles

- Must be worn in the operating room by **all personnel** every time the system is ON
- Must be identified and marked by the specific wavelength filter optical density >6
- Must be without scratches, cracks, or optical coating peel

Adequate Epidermal Cooling

Cooling devices are utilized to protect the epidermis and, reduce pain and erythema as well as improve the absorption of the energy into the target chromophore.[16] Typically, each laser system will have a specific recommendation for the device. This coupled with clinician choice and ease of use will drive the decision of what method and device to utilize.

PROCEDURE TECHNIQUE GENERAL

- Prior to laser resurfacing, test patch (3–5 spots) shall be conducted with treatment settings in a small inconspicuous area, but still in the requested anatomical treatment zone.
- Use same technique and parameters as for overall treatments.
- Selection of treatment parameters should be considered carefully and care should be employed to evaluate patch testing following an appropriate period of time.
- At least 15 to 30 minutes for skin types I to IV.
- At least 48 to 72 hours for skin types V and VI after patch testing, to observe tissue reaction. Patients, in particular with darker skin types (Fitzpatrick IV to VI), with sensitive skin, or without pretreatment regimen, may develop delayed healing, hyperpigmentation, or hypopigmentation.[1]
- Depending upon the actual treatment, various protocols exist that are machine-dependent such as the optical energies, fluency, number of passes, and other considerations for treatment.
- Apply handpiece perpendicular to the skin.
- Take precaution to not bulk heat the tissue.
- Please refer to manufacturer's white papers, peer-to-peer cite review, or other protocols that may be obtained concerning the actual condition and treatment parameters for your device.

CLINICAL END POINTS

- Visual skin response is gentle edema that appears with a delay of around 2 to 5 minutes[17] as seen in Figure 23.11.
- Uniform and acceptable erythema at 5 to 10 minutes.[18]

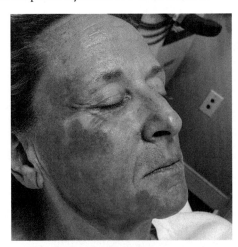

FIGURE 23-11 A typical clinical endpoint with edema and erythema with a 1540 nm. Note the areas where overlap needs to be placed. (Photo courtesy of Selina R. McGee, OD, FAAO)

- Excessive vasoconstriction is not desired as it may indicate selection of too high energies and densities.[19]
- Patients may experience a mild sting feel replaced by dissipating warmth and short-term itchiness.[1]

PROCEDURE CHECKLIST

- Patient education form read and understood
- Pretreatment instructions reviewed and understood
- Informed consent signed
- Skin type identified
- Pretreatment test site confirmed with no adverse reaction
- Confirm that patient has taken prophylactic antiviral medication (if positive history of HSV) and has no contraindications for treatment
- Pretreatment photograph taken
- Set up procedure tray including eye shields
- Select treatment parameters
- Perform laser treatment
- Provide verbal and written posttreatment instructions to patient
- Complete procedure note including device settings
- Subsequent treatment scheduled

HOW TO CHOOSE THE CORRECT LIGHT SOURCE FOR SELECTIVE PHOTOTHERMOLYSIS?

- Define clinical indication—what is the end goal?
- Choose correct light wavelength (nm) based on target chromophore.
- Is CW or pulsed source needed based on skin type and target?
- Choose correct pulse duration.
- Choose pulse frequency.
- Choose exposure spot size.
- Choose appropriate light dose (fluency).
- Set cooling parameters.
- Test target area and observe clinical end point.
- Proceed or adjust if needed.

PROCEDURE FOR PERIORBITAL WRINKLES

Periorbital wrinkles can be either dynamic or static. Dynamic wrinkles are caused by repeated muscular contractions or facial expressions like the lateral canthal rhytids (Fig. 23.12). Static wrinkles are caused by a loss of elasticity in the skin due to aging

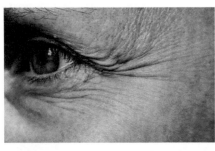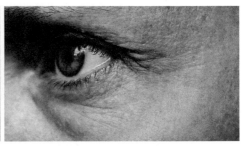

FIGURE 23-12 Improvement in lateral canthul rhytids. (Photo courtesy of Selina R. McGee, OD, FAAO)

and environmental factors such as sun exposure or smoking, like the skin beneath the lower eyelid.[8] Optimal patient selection would be a patient who has a wrinkling class I–II and elastosis score 1 to 6.[11] Results on rhytids may improve with the adjunctive use of botulinum toxin. Wait after post-procedure edema has subsided before injecting to avoid any risk of diffusion. Botulinum toxin does not absorb laser light, but the associated swelling makes it difficult to evaluate the action of the muscle for proper titration of injections. If done before laser skin treatment, allow a minimum of 1.5 months between the two treatments.

KEY PROCEDURAL POINTS

- Utilize a white makeup pencil to cover pigment that patients want to keep.
- Tanning of all forms (sun, tanning beds) is absolutely contraindicated as melanin would be redistributed and migrate toward upper epidermis building a "light-blocker" to any treatment.
- Also exclude self-tanning lotions that give the skin a competing artificial coloration through a chemical reaction with the amino acids of the stratum corneum.
- Tanned skin CANNOT be "defied" by selecting a darker skin type. In other words don't try to trick the system by choosing a darker skin type.
- On areas with slower "de-tanning" passed the minimum solar exposure of three to four weeks, recommend gentle exfoliation of the area one week prior to treatment.

POSTTREATMENT INSTRUCTIONS

After treatment, patients may experience redness, swelling, and a "sunburned" feeling. These are normal reactions.

- Immediately apply a cool (not iced) compresses and/or cool thermal water spray or utilize a dynamic cooling device.
- Apply sunscreen every day (30 SPF or greater).
- In caring for the treated area, use only gentle cleansers and lotions until healing is complete. Avoid perfumes and products with alcohol or acid. Care should be taken to prevent trauma to the treated site. Avoid hot baths, massage, and exercise until healed.
- If a blister develops, apply an antibiotic ointment until the blister dries. When a scab forms, apply Aquaphor healing ointment. Do not pick the blister or scab because a scar may form.
- Fillers or other injectables should not be done within two weeks before/after treatment.
- Call the physician's office if any problems, questions, or concerns arise.

RECOMMENDATIONS FOR FOLLOW-UP

Most patients require three to five treatment sessions to achieve satisfactory results. Patients may return for additional treatments no sooner than three to four weeks after the most recent treatment. Patients should be instructed to call or return sooner if adverse effects occur.

POSTOPERATIVE EXPECTATIONS

Erythema

Posttreatment erythema is commonly observed, is transient, and may typically last from one to five days. A higher level of erythema might be observed on sensitive light skin.

Edema

Edema is usually transient and may typically last from one to two days. A higher level of swelling might be observed on sensitive anatomical areas and thin skin.

"Bronzed" Appearance

Some patients may develop a "bronzed" appearance, within the first few days after treatment, due to the presence of melanin being sloughed off and to the coagulated zones in phagocytosis process. Discrete dry flaking of the stippled light-colored microdots typically is seen at three to ten days that feels like fine sandpaper.[1]

ADVERSE EVENTS

Occasionally

Xerosis and pruritus likelihood in the event of no/poor postoperative soothing care; it will typically will resolve by day five or six, is minimally bothersome, and responds well to moisturization.

Very Rarely

Burns: likelihood of burns is extremely rare and highly reduced by following all treatment instructions.

Might turn into post-inflammatory hyperpigmentation (PIH) or hypopigmentation (Fig. 23.13A & B). Likelihood of transient PIH or hypopigmentation is highly reduced by following all treatment instructions. Should it occur, it may mostly affect skin types IV to VI. PIH may become apparent between two weeks and two months after treatment.[1]

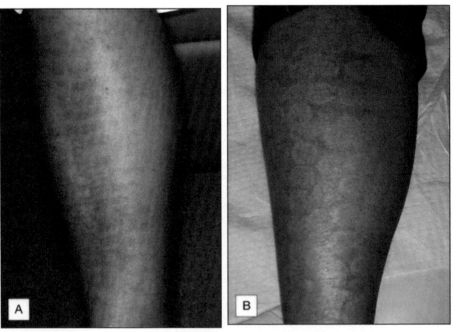

FIGURE 23-13 Permanent (A) hyperpigmentation and (B) hypopigmentation. (Reprinted with permission from HurzaGJ, *Lasers and Lights*, 4th Edition, Elsevier, 2018.)

PIH is usually reversible over time. It can take between three and 6 months and can be easily concealed in the meantime with makeup.

Hypopigmentation may be clinically apparent one to six months after treatment and is more commonly observed on darker skin types. It is most often related to the usage of inappropriate laser parameters.

Sun exposure must imperatively be avoided; it may actually worsen the change of pigmentation and its duration.

Scarring

In very rare cases, raised keloid scars may appear. To reduce the chance of scarring, it is important to carefully follow all posttreatment instructions and exclude patients who have a genetic tendency for scarring.[20]

- Scarring may last 6 to 24 months but could also remain permanent.
- Scarring may be treated with injections of intralesional corticosteroids.

EFFICACY

Skin rejuvenation devices, whether intended to target water, melanin, or oxyhemaglobin, have entered the market at a rapid rate over the past decade. Patients desire these treatments because of the little to no downtime associated with the procedures. There are evidence-based medicine and studies documenting mild to moderate improvement in the lax and droopy skin of the forehead and eyebrows, eyelids, and periorbital wrinkles with non-ablative skin resurfacing, IPL, and RF technologies.[7] These procedures provide a safe and effective means of improving many aspects of photoaged skin. It is up to the practitioner to investigate the claims and it is critical to research the therapeutic principles and modality of particular devices. Each device will have best practices as well as specific settings unique to that instrument that will make the procedures safe and effective. As discussed in Chapters 22, 23, and 24 of this book, there is more than one way to address specific issues. It is up to the clinician to understand and be able to incorporate each modality in a synergistic way that achieves the end goals for the patients safely and efficiently.

REFERENCES

1. Hurza GJ. *Lasers and Lights*, 4th Edition. Amsterdam: Elsevier; 2018.
2. Goldman MP. One laser for a cosmetic/dermatologic practice. *J Clin Aesthet Dermatol.* 2011;4(5): 18–21.
3. Goldberg DJ. *Laser Dermatology*, 2nd Edition. Blackwell Publishing; 2008.
4. Campbell T, Goldman MP. Complications of fractional CO_2 laser, a review of 373 treatments. *Dermatol Surg.* 2010;36:1645–1650.

5. Anderson RR, Parrish JA. Selective photothermolysis: Precise microsurgery by selective absorption of pulsed radiation. *Science*. 1983;220(4596):524–527.doi:10.1126/science.6836297

6. Patil UA, Dhami LD. Overview of lasers. *Indian J Plast Surg*. 2008;41(Suppl):S101–S113.

7. Narins DJ, Narins RS. Non-surgical radiofrequency facelift. *J Drugs Dermatol*. 2003;2:495–500.

8. Tierney EP, Hanke CW, Watkins L. Treatment of lower eyelid rhytids and laxity with ablative fractionated carbon-dioxide laser resurfacing: case series and review of the literature. *J Am Acad Dermatol*. 2011;64(4):730-740. doi:10.1016/j.jaad.2010.04.023

9. Bitter PH. Noninvasive rejuvenation of photodamaged skin using serial, full-face intense pulsed light treatments. *Dermatol Surg*. 2000;26:835–842.

10. Goldman MP, Weiss RA,Weiss MA. Intense pulsed light as a nonablative approach to photoaging. *Dermatol Surg*. 2005;31(9 Pt 2):1179–1187.

11. Sharma AN, Patel BC. Laser Fitzpatrick Skin Type Recommendations. [Updated 2020 May 4]. In: *StatPearls* [Internet]. Treasure Island, FL: StatPearls Publishing; January 2020.

12. Sobanko JF, Miller CJ, Alster TS. Topical anesthetics for dermatologic procedures: a review. *Dermatol Surg*. 2012;38(5):709–721. doi:10.1111/j.1524-4725.2011.02271.x

13. Railan D, Alster TS. Use of topical lidocaine for cosmetic dermatologic procedures. *J Drugs Dermatol*. 2007;6(11):1104–1108.

14. Boonsiri M, Marks KC, Ditre CM. Benzocaine/lidocaine/tetracaine cream: report of corneal damage and review. *J Clin Aesthet Dermatol*. 2016;9(3):48–50.

15. Huang A, Phillips A, Adar T, Hui A. Ocular injury in cosmetic laser treatments of the face. *J Clin Aesthet Dermatol*. 2018;11(2):15–18.

16. Das A, Sarda A, De A. Cooling devices in laser therapy. *J Cutan Aesthet Surg*. 2016;9(4):215–219. doi:10.4103/0974-2077.197028

17. Goldman MP. Laser resurfacing. In: Draelos Z, ed. *Cosmetic Dermatology: A Comprehensive Medical and Surgical Text*. New Jersey: Wiley–Blackwell; 2010. pp. 393–408.

18. Preissig J, Hamilton K, Markus R. Current laser resurfacing technologies: a review that delves beneath the surface. *Semin Plast Surg*. 2012;26(3):109–116. doi:10.1055/s-0032-1329413

19. Shah S, Alam M. Laser resurfacing pearls. *Semin Plast Surg*. 2012;26(3):131–136. doi:10.1055/s-0032-1329417

20. Bowman PH, Fosko SW, Hartstein ME. Periocular reconstruction. *Semin Cutan Med Surg*. 2003;22(4):263–272.

24 Ablative Lasers in Aesthetics

Selina R. McGee

The carbon dioxide (CO_2) laser with a wavelength of 10,600 nm has long been the gold standard in dermatology for skin resurfacing since its introduction in the mid-90s. At this wavelength, the laser has an absorbing chromophore of water and is utilized to vaporize tissue. The effects of wrinkle eradication and tightening lax tissue are excellent but with a significant downtime of two weeks, erythema for months, and postoperative complications such as hypopigmentation and infections, there are some authors that believe it is just on the edge of being the gold standard.[1] Significant strides have been made to reduce downtime and adverse events in the past two decades to this class of lasers. The introduction of the Erbium:YAG lasers, fractional photothermolysis as introduced by Manstein et al., and non-ablative fractional devices are some examples.[2] These concepts are discussed in detail in Chapter 23.

MECHANISM OF ACTION

Ablative lasers such as the CO_2 10,600 nm, the Erbium:YAG 2940 nm, and the Yttrium-Scandium-Gallium-Garnet (YSGG 2780 nm) ablate the target chromophore water as well as vaporize surrounding tissue. When done in a continuous wave (CW) it is called full-field resurfacing.[3] The original lasers removed the entire top layer of the skin to the depth specified. CO_2 lasers are thought to have the efficacious component of not only tissue ablation but also coagulation.[3] The Erbium:YAG 2940 nm is a solid-state laser that is highly absorbed in water and is used for laser resurfacing and skin rejuvenation. This frequency is much closer to the peak absorption range of water and thus has an absorption coefficient 16 times greater than the CO_2 laser (Fig. 24.1).

This greater absorption decreases the penetration depth into the epidermis by a factor of 10. This is an advantage, as more precise ablation of skin is possible with even less damage to surrounding tissue, resulting in less downtime and less complications like hypopigmentation.[3] Anderson and Manstein introduced fractional photothermolysis to generate microthermal zones.[4] This means that the energy is

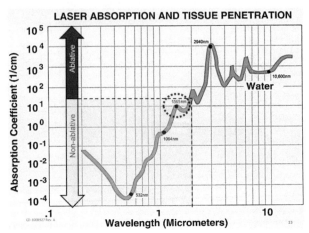

FIGURE 24-1 Laser absorption and tissue penetration as it relates to wavelength and absorption coefficient.[3] (Reprinted with permission from Ross EV, McKinlay JR, Anderson RR. Why does carbon dioxide resurfacing work? A review. Arch Dermatol. 1999;135(4):444–454.)

delivered in columns rather than complete ablation. When this technology is utilized it creates micro-wounds in the skin surrounded by intact tissue. This heating, up to mid-reticular dermis, serves as the stimulus for inflammatory mediator release, fibroblast activation, neocollagenesis, and dermal remodeling. Furthermore, the impacted coagulation columns act like elimination channels, which expel pigment and explain the clinical lightening of lentigines and melasma. When delivered this way it allows deeper penetration into the tissue without compromising more superficial tissues.[5] Typically, multiple treatments are required to achieve best results, but there is less downtime, an average of three days, associated with each treatment. Combinations to mimic CO_2 results for periorbital rhytids with non-ablative or ablative fractional technology are indeed efficacious.[6–9] Figure 24.2 shows a patient treated very effectively for lateral canthus rhytids with the Icon platform by Cynosure. However, it takes more lasers, or a multi-platform laser, and certainly can be time consuming.[10]

INDICATIONS

The most common indications for both full-field and fractional laser resurfacing are superficial dyschromias, textural anomalies, superficial to deep rhytids, scarring from acne, and surgical incisions. Xanthelasma has also been successfully treated.[1]

Settings will vary by device, and an operator's manual specific to a given device should be consulted.

Discussion of Device Settings—see Chapter 23 for more extensive discussion.

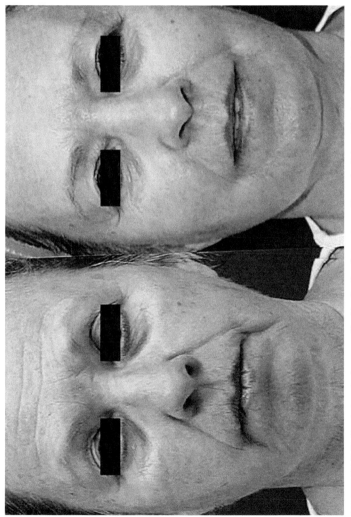

FIGURE 24-2 Patient treated very effectively for lateral canthus rhytids with the Icon platform by Cynosure. (Photo courtesy of R. Saluja, MD)

PATIENT SELECTION

The easiest patients to treat have fair skin (Fitzpatrick skin types I–III). Darker skin types can also be treated (Fitzpatrick skin type IV–VI)—with caution—by using lower energies, longer pulse durations, longer delay times, and aggressive skin cooling techniques.[11]

The Fitzpatrick skin phototypes (types) were constructed based on an individual's skin color and their tendency to burn or tan when exposed to sunlight. There are six skin types characterized by the Fitzpatrick Skin Typing Scale (Tables 24.1 and 24.2).[9]

TABLE 24-1 FITZPATRICK SKIN TYPING SCALE

FITZPATRICK SKIN TYPE	SKIN COLOR BEFORE SUN EXPOSURE	EYE COLOR	HAIR COLOR	SUN REACTION
Skin type I	Ivory	Light blue, light gray, or light green	Red or light blonde	Skin always freckles, always burns and peels, and never tans
Skin type II	Fair or pale	Blue, gray, or green	Blonde	Skin usually freckles, burns and peels often, and rarely tans
Skin type III	Fair to beige, with golden undertones	Hazel or light brown	Dark blonde or light brown	Skin usually freckles, burns and peels often, and rarely tans
Skin type IV	Olive or light brown	Dark brown	Dark brown	Doesn't really freckle, burns rarely, and tans often
Skin type V	Dark brown	Dark brown to black	Dark brown to black	Rarely freckles, almost never burns, and always tans
Skin type VI	Deeply pigmented dark brown to darkest brown	Brownish black	Black	Never freckles, never burns, and always tans darkly

TABLE 24-2 FITZPATRICK TYPES I, II, AND III WRINKLE AND ELASTOSIS

CLASS	WRINKLING	SCORE
I	Fine wrinkles (rhytids)	1–3
II	Fine to moderate depth wrinkles, moderate number of lines	4–6
III	Fine to deep wrinkles, numerous lines with or without redundant skin folds	7–9

These treatments are currently not covered by private insurance; therefore, patients must be willing to assume responsibility for the cost of treatments. Since more aggressive treatments sometimes need to be performed under general anesthesia these conversations come about while a patient has already scheduled another cosmetic surgery and built time-off into their recovery. These in-depth conversations are important to have during consultation. Fully evaluate patient needs, end result, efficacy, risks, cost, and downtime when choosing what is best for the patient.

EXPECTED BENEFITS

The potential improvement is dependent on the device used and depth and degree of injury produced. There are many options and combination of options to achieve results. Practitioners use combination therapy with superficial full-field treatment combined with fractional treatment while others use fractional ablative and non-ablative therapy (Fig. 24.3).[1]

Still others, and the author, use intense pulsed light (IPL) with fractional non-ablative resurfacing and radiofrequency.[12–15] IPL addresses the superficial dyschromias and vasculature; the laser addresses texture and rhytids and radiofrequency tightens skin by building collagen through dermal heating and tissue damage.

CONTRAINDICATIONS

Absolute Contraindications for Laser Treatment Include the Following:

- Active bacterial, fungal, or viral infection
- Appendageal abnormality
- Skin grafts
- X-ray irradiated skin
- Extensive electrolysis
- Isotretinoin (Accutane) should not be taken for six months to two years prior to treatment

Relative Contraindications Include the Following:

- Unrealistic expectations
- Keloid formation
- Previous deep chemical peel, deep dermabrasion, or deep laser resurfacing
- Prophylactically treat herpes simplex virus (HSV), three days prior to surgery and continue through epithelialization

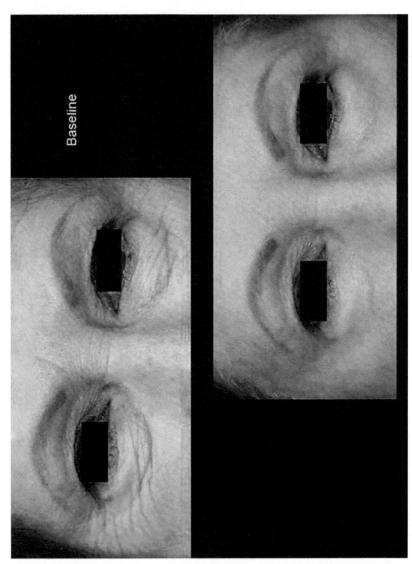

FIGURE 24-3 Before and after of patient treated with combination therapy. (Photo courtesy of R. Saluja, MD)

PRETREATMENT PATIENT EDUCATION

The following should be discussed with patients prior to performing laser treatment:

- Results are not guaranteed.
- Postoperative care is critical.
- Set realistic expectations.
- Adverse effects include redness, swelling, burning, pain, crust formation, bruising, hyperpigmentation and hypopigmentation, and scar formation.
- Multiple treatment sessions (typically three to five) are required for optimal results when utilizing fractional technology.

PRETREATMENT PATIENT INSTRUCTIONS

Review possible photosensitizing medications.
Patients are given the following instructions prior to treatment:

- Apply sunscreen four to six weeks preoperatively: Sun Protection Factor (SPF) 30 to 50 utilized every day.
- If there is a history of cold sores, take your prescribed medication (e.g., valacyclovir [Valtrex], famciclovir [Famvir], acyclovir [Zovirax]) on the day before, day of, and until skin re-epithelizes.

PHOTOGRAPHY INFORMED CONSENT AND INFORMED CONSENT

Since these treatments are being performed on the face, photography informed consent is necessary. An example may read like this:

> I hereby authorize (**physician name**), of (**name of practice**), and/or his/her associates or licensees to take pre-procedural and post-procedural photographs, slides.
>
> I consent to the use of these images for the purposes of pre-procedural planning and post-procedural evaluation by (**physician name**) and/or the staff of (**name of practice**), and I understand that they shall be made a part of my medical record.

Informed consent should contain the following information as well as the alternative treatments available, followed by written consent. The following suggested template should serve as a guide.

> This is an informed consent document. It has been prepared to help inform you about laser treatment procedures of skin, risks, and alternative treatments.

It is important that you read this information carefully and completely.

Conditions such as wrinkles, sun damaged skin, unsightly veins, and some types of skin lesions/disorders may be treated with the laser. Certain surgical procedures may use the laser as a cutting instrument. In some situations, laser treatments may be performed at the time of other surgical procedures.

Alternative forms of treatment include not undergoing the proposed laser skin treatment procedure. Other forms of skin treatment (chemical peel) or surgical procedures may be substituted. In certain situations, the laser may offer a specific therapeutic advantage over other forms of treatment. Alternatively, laser treatment procedures in some situations may not represent a better alternative to other forms of surgery or skin treatment when indicated. Risks and potential complications are associated with alternative forms of treatment that involve skin treatments or surgical procedures.

There are both risks and complications associated with all laser treatment procedures of the skin. Risks involve both items that specifically relate to the use of laser energy as a form of surgical therapy and to the specific procedure performed. An individual's choice to undergo a procedure is based on the comparison of risk to potential benefits. Although the majority of patients do not experience these complications, you should discuss each of them with your physician to make sure you understand the risks, potential complications, and consequences of laser skin treatment.

Infection

HSV infections around the mouth or other areas of the face can occur following a laser treatment. This applies to both individuals with a past history of HSV infections and individuals with no known history of HSV infections in the mouth area. Specific medications may be prescribed and taken both prior to and following the laser treatment procedure in order to suppress an infection from this virus. Should any type of skin infection occur, additional treatments including antibiotics may be necessary.

Scarring

Although normal healing after the procedure is expected, abnormal scars may occur both in the skin and deeper tissues. In rare cases, keloid scars may result. Scars may be unattractive and of different color than the surrounding skin. Additional treatments may be needed to treat scarring.

Burns

Laser energy can produce burns. Adjacent structures including the eyes may be injured or permanently damaged by the laser beam. Burns are rare yet represent the effect of heat produced within the tissues by laser energy. Additional treatment may be necessary to treat laser bums.

Color Change

Laser treatments may potentially change the natural color of your skin. Skin redness usually lasts two weeks to three months and occasionally six months following laser skin treatment. There is the possibility of irregular color variations within the skin including areas that are both lighter and darker.

Visible Skin Patterns

Laser treatment procedures may produce visible patterns within the skin. The occurrence of this is not predictable.

Patient Failure to Follow Through

Patient follow through following a laser skin treatment procedure is important. Post-operative instructions concerning appropriate restriction of activity and use of sun protection need to be followed in order to avoid potential complications, increased pain, and unsatisfactory result. Your physician may recommend that you utilize a long-term skin care program to enhance healing following a laser skin treatment.

Damaged Skin

Skin that has been previously treated with chemical peels or dermabrasion, or damaged by burns, or radiation therapy may heal abnormally or slowly following treatment by lasers or other surgical techniques. The occurrence of this is not predictable. Additional treatment may be necessary.

Unsatisfactory Result

There is the possibility of an unsatisfactory result from these procedures. Laser procedures may result in unacceptable visible deformities, skin slough, loss of function, and permanent color changes in the skin. You may be disappointed with the final result from laser treatments.

Allergic Reactions

In rare cases, local allergies to tape, preservatives used in cosmetics, or topical preparations have been reported. Systemic reactions that are more serious may result from drugs used during medical procedures and prescription medicines. Allergic reactions may require additional treatment.

Lack of Permanent Results

Laser or other treatments may not completely improve or prevent future skin disorders, lesions, or wrinkles. Additional procedures or surgery may be necessary to further tighten loose skin.

Delayed Healing

It may take longer than anticipated for healing to occur after laser treatments. Skin healing may result in thin, easily injured skin. This is different from the normal redness in skin after a laser treatment.

Unknown Risks

There is the possibility that additional risk factors of laser skin treatments may be discovered.

Additional Treatment or Surgery Necessary

There are many variable conditions that influence the long-term result of laser skin treatments. Even though risks and complications occur infrequently, the risks cited are the ones that are particularly associated with these procedures. Other complications and risks can occur but are even more uncommon. Should complications occur, procedures, surgery, or other treatments may be necessary. The practice of medicine and surgery is not an exact science. Although good results are expected, there is no guarantee or warranty expressed or implied on the results that may be obtained.

It is important that you read the aforementioned information carefully and have all of your questions answered before signing the consent on the next page.

Informed Consent for Laser-Based Treatments

I hereby authorize certified personnel to perform the following laser light energy procedure and skin tightening treatments.

I recognize that during the course of the procedure and medical treatment, unforeseen conditions may necessitate different procedures than those above. I therefore authorize the above physician to perform such other procedures that are in the exercise of his or her professional judgment necessary and desirable. The authority granted under this paragraph shall include all conditions that require treatment and are not known to my physician at the time the procedure is begun.

I consent to the administration of such anesthetics considered necessary or advisable. I understand that all forms of anesthesia involve risk and the possibility of complications, injury, and sometimes death.

I acknowledge that no guarantee has been given by anyone as to the results that may be obtained.

I Consent to the Treatment or Procedure and the Above Listed Items

[Signed by the patient, physician, witness and date] at (physician's practice name)

PROCEDURE PROTOCOL

Patient Prep

Immediately before applying topical anesthesia, if utilizing when patient isn't sedated, cleanse the area to be treated with warm soapy water, rinse, and dry well.

Topical Anesthetic

Follow the guidelines of the manufacturing health care professional for application dosage, occlusion, and timing. Topical anesthetic must be applied at the medical facility under the supervision of a licensed practitioner and should not be applied to large areas because of the potential risk of systemic absorption. Potential complications include death.[16,17] Do not apply cream to patients with a history of allergic reactions to benzacaine, tetracaine, or lidocaine. Do not apply cream to patients taking class I antiarrhythmic drugs. Apply a thin film of cream to the area that will be treated, using a tongue depressor. Wait for 30 to 60 minutes for the cream to work. Remove the excess cream prior to treatment.

- Wipe with alcohol-free antisepsis (e.g., water-based chlorhexidine)
- Dry skin thoroughly
- Immediately before session
    - Put eyewear on the patient per treatment area. There are many case reports in the literature of corneal abrasions post-laser therapy. This can be due to chemical, mechanical, or thermal damage.[5,18–20] To best prevent this, use laser grade corneal shields of the largest size available. Currently, at the time of publication it is 26 mm. Be extremely careful to not get anything under the shield upon insertion, like coupling gel or anesthetic cream. This may cause a severe chemical burn. The patient will not know until later because of the instillation of topical anesthetic eye drops prior to inserting the shields.

Safety Concerns

- Post the laser warning sign on the entrance door.
- Do not leave laser unattended when in operation.
- Fire is a rare occurrence but the laser should never be fired on paper products or gauze; avoid alcohol-based cleansers.
- Never look directly in the aperture of the treatment head even when wearing adequate safety goggles.
- Avoid directing the laser beam anywhere other than the intended treatment area.
- The aiming beam is ON by default when turning the system ON.
- Do not allow reflective or flammable items within the operating field.
- Always enter STANDBY mode when the laser is not being operated and accommodate connected treatment head in the cradle.

Safety Goggles

- Must be worn in the operating room by **all personnel** every time the system is ON
- Must be identified and marked by the specific wavelength filter Optical density >6
- Must be without scratches, cracks, or optical coating peel

Adequate Epidermal Cooling

Cooling devices are utilized to protect the epidermis, reduce pain and erythema, and improve the absorption of the energy into the target chromophore.[20] Typically, each laser system will have a specific recommendation for the device. This coupled with clinician choice and ease of use will drive the decision of what method and device to utilize.

PROCEDURE TECHNIQUE: GENERAL

- Prior to laser resurfacing, test patch (3–5 scans) shall be conducted with treatment settings in a small inconspicuous area, but still in the requested anatomical treatment zone
- Use same technique and parameters as for overall treatments
- Selection of treatment parameters should be considered carefully and care should be employed to evaluate test patching following an appropriate period of time
- A common mistake made by beginning laser users is to "turn down" the power of a surgical CO_2 laser in a misguided attempt to exercise caution. Unfortunately, turning down the power can cause burns because the process turns from rapid, precise vaporization with minimal thermal damage to bulk heating of the skin from unwanted residual heat.[1] For example, immediate contraction of the skin is always a sign that substantial thermal injury of the dermis has occurred.
- At least 15 to 30 minutes for skin types I to IV after test patches.
- At least 48 to 72 hours for skin types V and VI after test patches, to observe tissue reaction. Patients, in particular those with darker skin types (Fitzpatrick IV to VI), with sensitive skin or without pretreatment regimen, may develop delayed healing, hyperpigmentation or hypopigmentation
- Depending upon the actual treatment, various protocols exist that are machine dependent, such as the optical energies, fluency, number of passes, and other considerations for treatment.
- Apply hand piece perpendicular to the skin.
- Take precaution to not bulk heat the tissue; tissue contraction is an immediate sign of this.
- Expected clinical end point after laser treatment of pigmented lesions, using a Q-switched 755 nm alexandrite laser for solar lentigines. Immediate response observed with epidermal whitening due to steam bubbles (Fig. 24.4).[1]
- Please refer to manufacturer's white papers, peer-to-peer cite review, or other protocols that may be obtained concerning the actual condition and treatment parameters for your device.

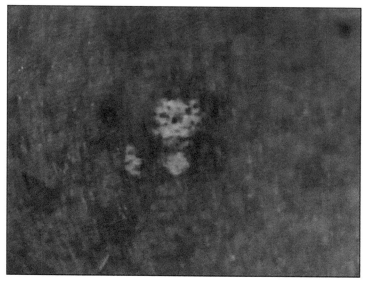

FIGURE 24-4 Immediate response observed with epidermal whitening due to steam bubbles. (Reprinted with permission from Hurza GJ. *Lasers and Lights*, 4th ed. Elsevier; 2018.)

PROCEDURE CHECKLIST

- Patient education form read and understood.
- Pretreatment instructions reviewed and understood.
- Informed consent signed.
- Skin type identified.
- Pretreatment test site confirmed with no adverse reaction.
- Confirm that patient has taken prophylactic antiviral medication (if positive history of HSV) and has no contraindications for treatment.
- Pretreatment photograph taken.
- Set up procedure tray including eye shields.
- Select treatment parameters.
- Perform laser treatment.
- Provide verbal and written posttreatment instructions to patient.
- Complete procedure note including device settings.
- Subsequent treatment scheduled.

HOW TO CHOOSE THE CORRECT LIGHT SOURCE FOR SELECTIVE PHOTOTHERMOLYSIS?

- Define clinical indication: What is the end goal? Example: A patient who desires maximum effects with least downtime may choose a combination of techniques.
- Choose correct light wavelength (nm) based on target chromophore.

- Is CW or pulsed source needed based on skin type and target?
- Choose right pulse duration.
- Choose pulse frequency.
- Choose exposure spot size.
- Choose appropriate light dose (fluency).
- Set cooling parameters.
- Test target area and observe clinical end point.
- Proceed or adjust if needed.

POSTTREATMENT INSTRUCTIONS

For full-field procedures, most recommend an occlusive ointment or dressing. One author suggests using Flexzan Foam Adhesive Dressing for CO_2 patients and Aquaphor for Erbium:YAG until after epithelialization is complete and then a nonocclusive moisturizer thereafter.[1,21] Sunscreen every day (30 SPF or greater) is mandatory. A skin care regimen is appropriate and although there is controversy over what is in these regimens, a combination of 4% hydroquinone and low-strength Retin-A (tretinoin) is still used.[1]

RECOMMENDATIONS FOR FOLLOW-UP

Most patients require three to five treatment sessions to achieve satisfactory results if utilizing fractional technology (Fig. 24.5). Patients may return for additional treatments no sooner than three to four weeks after the most recent treatment. Patients should be instructed to call or return sooner if adverse effects occur.

POSTOPERATIVE EXPECTATIONS AND COMPLICATIONS

- Erythema is normal after laser resurfacing. It is directly related to the depth of ablation and the amount of surrounding thermal damage. Eventually, this will improve but can take months. If the patient desires resolution faster, topical corticosteroids may be utilized as well as IPL or a vascular laser treatment. A higher level of erythema might be observed on sensitive light skin. Telangiectasias can also occur commonly as they are now more visible with less photodamage overlying it. These can also be treated with a vascular laser.[22]
- Acne or milia are also common postoperatively. An over-occlusion with topical products can occur and can be discontinued to treat the acne. Oral antibiotics and or acne laser treatments may also be used for stubborn cases.

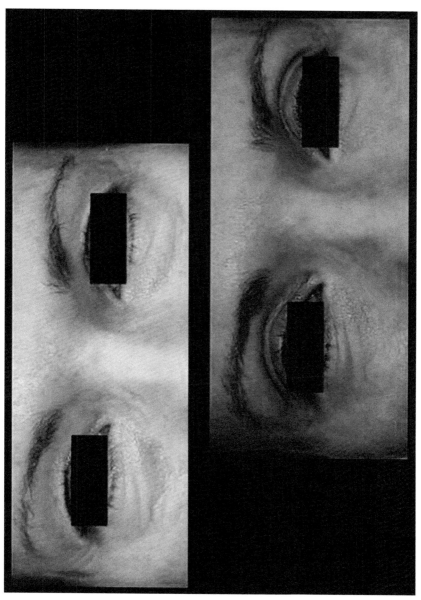

FIGURE 24-5 Result in the periorbital area. (Photo courtesy of R. Saluja, MD)

- Hypopigmentation is the complication that is most disconcerting. It's more commonly seen in CO_2 full-field treatments. It is much more rare with Erbium:YAG and rarer still with all fractional treatments. There are not many effective treatments for hypopigmentation to date. Hypopigmentation may be clinically apparent one to six months after treatment and is more commonly observed on darker skin types and often related to the usage of inappropriate laser parameters.

- Postinflammatory hyperpigmentation (PIH) is very common. Topical bleaching creams with retinoids are the usual treatment. For stubborn cases IPL can be performed. Should it occur, it may mostly affect skin types IV to VI. PIH may become apparent between two weeks and two months after treatment. PIH is usually reversible over time. It can take between three and six months and can be easily concealed in the meantime with makeup. Sun exposure must imperatively be avoided since it may actually worsen the change of pigmentation and its duration.

- Full-field laser treatments are controlled first- or second-degree burns. Too aggressive a treatment can turn a mild burn to a deeper burn unintentionally. Infections can also convert first- or second-degree burns to third-degree burns. Infection can be viral, bacterial, or fungal. The most common is due to HSV. Ensure patients are prophylactically treated and understand the importance of taking the prescribed medication appropriately. Topical soaks with dilute vinegar solution help to create a local environment undesirable to fungus.[19]

- Scarring can occur with these lasers. Potent topical corticosteroids, as well as intralesional corticosteroids, and vascular laser or IPL treatments as well as fractional lasers have all been utilized to improve hypertrophic scars after laser resurfacing. When patients are very slow to reepithelialize, this can also lead to scarring. These patients need a culture or biopsy to determine the underlying mechanism causing the issue.

- Ectropion can be caused by tightening the lower skin without properly assessing the eyelid structures and support system. Carefully examine lid structure and function with the lid snap test. Synechia can also occur when epidermal surfaces heal together, like those of the lower eyelid. Manual manipulation of the tissue until the line opens can prevent cyst formation.[19]

EFFICACY

Laser surgeon's should continue to customize treatments to individual patients for best possible outcomes. Systematic and meticulous preoperative and postoperative care as well as a comprehensive consultation is critical to achieve excellent patient results with the least risk for permanent long-term complications.[22]

REFERENCES

1. Hurza GJ. *Lasers and Lights*. 4th Edition. Elsevier; 2018.
2. Goldberg DJ. *Laser Dermatology*. 2nd Edition. Blackwell Publishing; 2008.
3. Ross EV, McKinlay JR, Anderson RR. Why does carbon dioxide resurfacing work? A review. *Arch Dermatol*. 1999;135(4):444–454.

4. Manstein D, Herron SG, Sink RK, et al Fractional photothermolysis: a new concept for cutaneous remodeling using microscopic patterns of thermal injury. *Lasers Surg Med.* 2004;34(5):426–438. https://doi.org/10.1002/lsm.20048

5. Huang A, Phillips A, Adar T, Hui A. Ocular injury in cosmetic laser treatments of the face. *J Clin Aesthet Dermatol.* 2018;11(2):15–18.

6. Bowman PH, Fosko S, Hartstein M, et al. *Semin Cutan Med Surg.* 2003;22(4):263–272.

7. Balzani A, Chilgar RM, Nicoli M, et al. Novel approach with fractional ultrapulse CO_2 laser for the treatment of upper eyelid dermatochalasis and periorbital rejuvenation. *Lasers Med Sci.* 2013;28:1483–1487. https://doi.org/10.1007/s10103-012-1255-4

8. Tierney EP, Hanke CW, Watkins L. Treatment of lower eyelid rhytides and laxity with ablative fractionated carbon-dioxide laser resurfacing: case series and review of the literature. *J Am Acad Dermatol.* 2011;64(4):730–740. doi:10.1016/j.jaad.2010.04.023

9. Toyos MM. Continuous wave fractional CO_2 laser for the treatment of upper eyelid dermatochalasis and periorbital rejuvenation. *Photomed Laser Surg.* 2017;35(5):278–281. doi:10.1089/pho.2016.4225

10. Goldman MP. One laser for a cosmetic/dermatologic practice. *J Clin Aesthet Dermatol.* 2011;4(5):18–21.

11. Sharma AN, Patel BC. Laser Fitzpatrick Skin Type Recommendations. [Updated 2020 May 4]. In: StatPearls [Internet]. Treasure Island (FL): StatPearls Publishing; 2020 Jan.

12. Bitter PH. Noninvasive rejuvenation of photodamaged skin using serial, full-face intense pulsed light treatments. *Dermatol Surg.* 2000;26:835–842.

13. Goldman MP, Weiss RA, Weiss MA. Intense pulsed light as a nonablative approach to photoaging. *Dermatol Surg.* 2005;31(9 Pt 2):1179–1187.

14. Goldman MP. Laser resurfacing. In: Draelos Z, ed. *Cosmetic Dermatology: A Comprehensive Medical and Surgical Text.* Wiley–Blackwell; 2010. pp. 393–408.

15. Preissig J, Hamilton K, Markus R. Current laser resurfacing technologies: a review that delves beneath the surface. *Semin Plast Surg.* 2012;26(3):109–116. doi:10.1055/s-0032-1329413

16. Railan D, Alster TS. Use of topical lidocaine for cosmetic dermatologic procedures. *J Drugs Dermatol.* 2007;6(11):1104–1108.

17. Sobanko JF, Miller CJ, Alster TS. Topical anesthetics for dermatologic procedures: a review. *Dermatol Surg.* 2012;38(5):709–721. doi:10.1111/j.1524-4725.2011.02271.x

18. Boonsiri M, Marks KC, Ditre CM. Benzocaine/lidocaine/tetracaine cream: report of corneal damage and review. *J Clin Aesthet Dermatol.* 2016;9(3):48–50.

19. Blanco G, Clavero A, Soparkar CN, Patrinely JR. Periocular laser complications. *Semin Plast Surg.* 2007;21(1):74–79. doi:10.1055/s-2007-967752.

20. Das A, Sarda A, De A. Cooling devices in laser therapy. *J Cutan Aesthet Surg.* 2016;9(4):215–219. doi:10.4103/0974-2077.197028.

21. Shah S, Alam M. Laser resurfacing pearls. *Semin Plast Surg.* 2012;26(3):131–136. doi:10.1055/s-0032-1329417

22. Avram MR. *Laser and Light Source Treatments for the Skin.* JP Medical LTD; March 20, 2014.

INDEX

Note: Page numbers in italic and bold refer to figures and tables, respectively.